GENDER-AFFIRMING
PSYCHIATRIC CARE

GENDER-AFFIRMING
PSYCHIATRIC CARE

Edited by

Teddy G. Goetz, M.D., M.S.
Alex S. Keuroghlian, M.D., M.P.H.

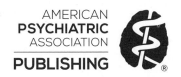

AMERICAN
PSYCHIATRIC
ASSOCIATION
PUBLISHING

If you wish to buy 50 or more copies of the same title, please go to www. appi.org/specialdiscounts for more information.

Copyright © 2023 American Psychiatric Association Publishing

ALL RIGHTS RESERVED

First Edition

Manufactured in the United States of America on acid-free paper
27 26 25 24 23   5 4 3 2 1

American Psychiatric Association Publishing
800 Maine Avenue SW, Suite 900
Washington, DC 20024-2812
www.appi.org

Library of Congress Cataloging-in-Publication Data
Names: Goetz, Teddy G., editor. | Keuroghlian, Alex S., editor. | American
   Psychiatric Association Publishing, issuing body.
Title: Gender-affirming psychiatric care / edited by Teddy G. Goetz, Alex
   S. Keuroghlian.
Description: First edition. | Washington, DC : American Psychiatric
   Association Publishing, [2023] | Includes bibliographical references and
   index.
Identifiers: LCCN 2023016038 (print) | LCCN 2023016039 (ebook) | ISBN
   9781615374724 (paperback ; alk. paper) | ISBN 9781615374731 (ebook)
Subjects: MESH: Health Services for Transgender Persons | Mental Health
   Services | Transgender Persons--psychology | Healthcare Disparities |
   Social Determinants of Health | United States
Classification: LCC RC451.4.G39 (print) | LCC RC451.4.G39 (ebook) | NLM
   WA 305 AA1 | DDC 362.2086/7--dc23/eng/20230727
LC record available at https://lccn.loc.gov/2023016038
LC ebook record available at https://lccn.loc.gov/2023016039

British Library Cataloguing in Publication Data
A CIP record is available from the British Library.

Contents

Contributors

Noah Adams, M.S.W., Ph.D.   he/him
Ph.D. Student, Ontario Institute for Studies in Education, University of Toronto, Toronto, Ontario, Canada; Junior Fellow, Center for Applied Transgender Studies, Chicago, Illinois; Transgender Professional Association for Transgender Health, Toronto, Ontario, Canada

Rodrigo Aguayo-Romero, Ph.D.   they/them
Research Scientist, Whitman-Walker Institute, Washington, DC

Valeria Karina Anaya, M.D.   she/her
Child, Adolescent, and General Psychiatrist; Adjunct Voluntary Professor, Keck School of Medicine, Los Angeles, California; Psychiatrist, Reswell-Pasadena, Pasadena, California; Co-Director, Refugee Health Alliance, Tijuana, Mexico

Sebastian M. Barr, Ph.D.   he/him
Independent Practice, Connecticut River Valley, Massachusetts

Stephanie Bi, M.D.   she/her
Resident Physician, Hospital of the University of Pennsylvania, Philadelphia, Pennsylvania

Jack Bruno, M.S.W.   he/him
Operations Coordinator, The Fenway Institute, Boston, Massachusetts

Evelyn Callahan, Ph.D., M.Sc.   they/them
Research Fellow, The Bartlett School of Sustainable Construction, University College London, London, United Kingdom

Juwan Campbell, M.A.   they/them
Programmer/Analyst, The Fenway Institute, Boston, Massachusetts

Alexander Chen, J.D.   he/him
Founding Director, LGBTQ+ Advocacy Clinic, Harvard Law School, Cambridge, Massachusetts

Jaimie Cory, M.Ed. she/her
Doctoral Student, Department of Counseling and Educational Development, The University of North Carolina at Greensboro, Greensboro, North Carolina; Licensed Clinical Mental Health Counselor Associate, Banyan Tree Counseling and Wellness, Winston-Salem, North Carolina

Steph deNormand, M.A. they/them
Trans Health Program Manager, Fenway Health, Boston, Massachusetts

Zackary Derrick, B.A., M.P.H. they/them
Master's Student, School of Public Health and Social Policy, University of Victoria, Victoria, British Columbia, Canada

Gene Dockery, Ph.D. they/them
Assistant Clinical Professor of Counseling, Seattle University, Seattle, Washington

Brett Dolotina, B.S. they/them
Project Coordinator, Spatial Epidemiology Lab, Columbia University Mailman School of Public Health, New York, New York

Dallas M. Ducar, M.S.N., A.P.R.N. she/her
Chief Executive Officer, Transhealth; Assistant Professor, University of Virginia School of Medicine and Nursing, Charlottesville, Virginia; Assistant Professor, Columbia University, New York, New York

Mason Dunn, J.D. he/him
Deputy Director of Education and Training Programs, The Fenway Institute, Boston, Massachusetts

Emerson J. Dusic, M.P.H. they/them
Ph.D. Candidate, Institute of Public Health Genetics, University of Washington, Seattle, Washington

Kristen Eckstrand, M.D., Ph.D. she/they
Clinical Assistant Professor, Department of Psychiatry, University of Pittsburgh; Medical Director, UPMCLGBTQ+ Health, University of Pittsburgh Medical Center, Pittsburgh, Pennsylvania

Laura Erickson-Schroth, M.D. she/they
Chief Medical Officer, The Jed Foundation; Assistant Professor of Psychiatry, Columbia University Medical Center, New York, New York

Morgan Faeder, M.D., Ph.D. he/him
Assistant Professor of Psychiatry and Neurology, University of Pittsburgh
School of Medicine, Pittsburgh, Pennsylvania

Dan E. Ferrari Funk, M.A. they/them
Director of Data Analytics, The Fenway Institute, Boston, Massachusetts

Fiona (Fi) Fonseca, M.D., Ph.D. they/them
Consultation-Liaison Psychiatry Fellow, Mayo Clinic, Rochester, Minnesota

Henri M. Garrison-Desany, Ph.D., M.S.P.H. any pronouns
Yerby Post-Doctoral Fellow, Department of Social and Behavioral Sciences,
Harvard T. H. Chan School of Public Health, Boston, Massachusetts

Seran Gee, J.D. they/them
Equal Justice Works Fellow, Transgender Legal Defense and Education
Fund, Somerville, Massachusetts

Teddy G. Goetz, M.D., M.S. they/them
Resident Physician, Department of Psychiatry, University of Pennsylvania,
Philadelphia, Pennsylvania

Chris Grasso, M.P.H. she/her
Associate Vice President for Informatics and Data Services, The Fenway Institute, Boston, Massachusetts

Victoria Grieve, Pharm.D. she/her
Assistant Professor, Department of Pharmacy and Therapeutics, University
of Pittsburgh School of Pharmacy, Pittsburgh, Pennsylvania

Vern Harner, Ph.D., M.S.W. they/them
Assistant Professor, School of Social Work and Criminal Justice, University
of Washington at Tacoma, Tacoma, Washington

Aude Henin, Ph.D. she/her
Co-Director, Child Cognitive-Behavioral Therapy Program, Department of
Psychiatry, Massachusetts General Hospital and Harvard Medical School,
Boston, Massachusetts

Brendon Holloway, M.S.W. he/him
Doctoral Student, Graduate School of Social Work, University of Denver,
Denver, Colorado

Robert P. Holloway, M.D. he/him
Clinical Associate Professor of Psychiatry and the Behavioral Sciences, Pediatrics, and Anesthesiology, Keck School of Medicine, University of Southern California, Los Angeles, California

Hannah Janeway, M.D. they/them
Assistant Clinical Professor of Emergency Medicine, David Geffen School of Medicine at UCLA, Los Angeles, California; Co-Founder/Co-Director, Refugee Health Alliance, Tijuana, Mexico

Kevin Johnson, M.D. he/him
Psychiatrist, Crouse Addiction Treatment Services, Crouse, New York

Michelle Joy, M.D. she/her
Clinical Associate Professor of Psychiatry, University of Pennsylvania; Director of Behavioral Health Emergency Services, Corporal Michael J. Crescenz VA Medical Center, Philadelphia, Pennsylvania

Shanna K. Kattari, Ph.D., M.Ed., C.S.E., A.C.S. they/them
Associate Professor, School of Social Work and Department of Women's and Gender Studies, University of Michigan, Ann Arbor, Michigan

Alex S. Keuroghlian, M.D., M.P.H. any pronouns
Associate Chief, Public and Community Psychiatry, Department of Psychiatry, Massachusetts General Hospital; Michele and Howard J. Kessler Chair and Director, Division of Public and Community Psychiatry, Massachusetts General Hospital; Associate Professor of Psychiatry, Harvard Medical School; Director, Division of Education and Training, The Fenway Institute, Boston, Massachusetts

Hyun-Hee "Heather" Kim, M.D. she/they
Psychiatrist/Clinical Instructor, Department of Psychiatry, Massachusetts General Hospital, Boston, Massachusetts

Lisa Krinsky, M.S.W., L.I.C.S.W. she/her
Director, LGBTQIA+ Aging Project; The Fenway Institute, Boston, Massachusetts

Clair Kronk, Ph.D. she/her
Postdoctoral Fellow, Yale Center for Medical Informatics, New Haven, Connecticut; Senior Fellow, Center for Applied Transgender Studies (CATS), Chicago, Illinois

Madeleine Lipshie-Williams, M.D. they/them
Psychiatry Specialist, Sylmar, California

Em Matsuno, Ph.D. they/them
Assistant Professor, Counseling and Counseling Psychology, Arizona State University, Phoenix, Arizona

Gabrielle Morgan, B.S. she/her
Transgender Outreach and Engagement Specialist, LGBTQIA+ Aging Project; Store Manager, The Fenway Institute, Boston, Massachusetts

Sarah Noble, D.O. she/they
Medical Director, Outpatient Behavioral Health, Einstein Medical Center; Clinical Assistant Professor of Psychiatry and Human Behavior, Thomas Jefferson University, Philadelphia, Pennsylvania

Néstor Noyola, Ph.D. he/him
Postdoctoral Fellow in Psychology, Department of Psychiatry, Massachusetts General Hospital and Harvard Medical School, Boston, Massachusetts

Jae A. Puckett, Ph.D. they/them
Assistant Professor, Department of Psychology, Michigan State University, East Lansing, Michigan

Roz Queen, B.S. she/they
Research Assistant, School of Health Information Science, University of Victoria, British Columbia, Canada

Sari L. Reisner, Sc.D. he/him
Director, Transgender Research, Division of Endocrinology, Diabetes and Hypertension, Brigham and Women's Hospital; Harvard Medical School; The Fenway Institute; Department of Epidemiology, Harvard T.H. Chan School of Public Health

Arjee Javellana Restar, Ph.D., M.P.H. she/her
Assistant Professor, Department of Epidemiology, University of Washington School of Public Health, Seattle, Washington; Researcher, Department of Social and Behavioral Sciences, Yale University School of Public Health, New Haven, Connecticut

Jae Sevelius, Ph.D. they/them
Professor, Department of Psychiatry, Columbia University, New York, New York

Scout Silverstein, M.P.H.   they/them
Senior Program Development Lead, Equip Health, Carlsbad, California

Melissa Simone, Ph.D.   they/them
Postdoctoral Scholar, Division of Epidemiology and Community Health, University of Minnesota School of Public Health, Minneapolis, Minnesota

Simón(e) Sun, Ph.D.   she/they
Postdoctoral Fellow, Cold Spring Harbor Laboratory Postdoctoral Fellow, Cold Spring Harbor, New York

Reubs J. Walsh, B.A., M.Sc., Ph.D.   they/them
Postdoctoral Fellow, Einstein Lab of Cognitive Neurosciences, Gender and Health, Department of Psychology, University of Toronto, Toronto, Ontario, Canada; Junior Fellow, Center for Applied Transgender Studies, Chicago, Illinois

Alann Weissman-Ward, M.D.   he/him
Family Medicine Specialist, Syracuse, New York

Tobias Wiggins, Ph.D.   he/him
Assistant Professor, Women's and Gender Studies, Athabasca University, Athabasca, Alberta, Canada

Talen Wright, M.Sc., B.Sc.   she/her
Ph.D. Student, Division of Psychiatry, Institute of Mental Health, Faculty of Brain Sciences, University College London, London, United Kingdom

Disclosures

The following contributors have indicated a financial interest in or other affiliation with a commercial supporter, manufacturer of a commercial product, and/or provider of a commercial service as listed below:

Morgan Faeder, M.D., Ph.D.: *Salary:* Oakstone CME.

Dan E. Ferrari Funk, M.A.: *Salary, Grant/Research Support:* Fenway Health.

Aude Henin, Ph.D.: *Royalties:* Oxford University Press.

Alex S. Keuroghlian, M.D., M.P.H.: *Royalties:* McGraw Hill.

Sari L. Reisner, Sc.D.: *Royalties:* McGraw Hill.

The following contributors stated that they had no competing interests during the year preceding manuscript submission:

Noah Adams, M.S.W., Ph.D.; Rodrigo Aguayo-Romero, Ph.D.; Valeria Karina Anaya, M.D.; Sebastian M. Barr, Ph.D.; Stephanie Bi, M.D.; Jack Bruno, M.S.W.; Evelyn Callahan, Ph.D., M.Sc.; Juwan Campbell, M.A.; Alexander Chen, J.D.; Jaimie Cory, M.Ed.; Steph deNormand, M.A.; Zackary Derrick, B.A., M.P.H.; Gene Dockery, Ph.D.; Brett Dolotina, B.S.; Dallas M. Ducar, M.S.N., A.P.R.N.; Mason Dunn, J.D.; Emerson J. Dusic, M.P.H.; Kristen Eckstrand, M.D., Ph.D.; Laura Erickson-Schroth, M.D.; Morgan Faeder, M.D., Ph.D.; Dan E. Ferrari Funk, M.A.; Fiona Fonseca, M.D., Ph.D.; Henri M. Garrison-Desany, Ph.D., M.S.P.H.; Seran Gee, J.D.; Teddy G. Goetz, M.D., M.S.; Chris Grasso, M.P.H.; Victoria Grieve, Pharm.D.; Vern Harner, Ph.D., M.S.W.; Aude Henin, Ph.D.; Brendon Holloway, M.S.W.; Robert P. Holloway, M.D.; Hannah Janeway, M.D.; Kevin Johnson, M.D.; Michelle Joy, M.D.; Shanna K. Kattari, Ph.D., M.Ed., C.S.E., A.C.S.; Alex S. Keuroghlian, M.D., M.P.H.; Hyun-Hee "Heather" Kim, M.D.; Lisa Krinsky, M.S.W., L.I.C.S.W.; Clair Kronk, Ph.D.; Madeleine Lipshie-Williams, M.D.; Em Matsuno, Ph.D.; Gabrielle Morgan, B.S.; Sarah Noble, D.O.; Néstor Noyola, Ph.D.; Jae A. Puckett, Ph.D.; Roz Queen, B.S.; Sari L. Reisner, Sc.D.; Arjee Javellana Restar, Ph.D., M.P.H.; Jae Sevelius, Ph.D.; Scout Silverstein, M.P.H.; Melissa Simone, Ph.D.; Simón(e) Sun, Ph.D.; Reubs J. Walsh, B.A., M.Sc., Ph.D.; Alann Weissman-Ward, M.D.; Tobias Wiggins, Ph.D.; Talen Wright, M.Sc., B.Sc.

Foreword

WELCOME to *Gender-Affirming Psychiatric Care*! This volume represents the first textbook dedicated to providing affirming, intersectional, and evidence-informed psychiatric care for transgender, non-binary, and/or gender-expansive (TNG) people.

For millennia, outside of European colonial influences, gender diversity has flourished to varying degrees among hundreds of Indigenous communities around the world. In comparison, the field of psychiatry is but a hundred-year blip. Your reading these words was far from inevitable. We launch this handbook into a specific, complicated cultural moment. Just 50 years ago, the American Psychiatric Association stopped classifying homosexuality as a psychiatric diagnosis. In 2013, DSM-5 (American Psychiatric Association 2013) replaced *gender identity disorder* (pathologizing gender) with *gender dysphoria* (pathologizing distress from gender-body incongruence). The decade since has brought unprecedented visibility and recognition of gender diversity, chased by ongoing political backlash against people's autonomy over identification, embodiment, expression, reproduction, and family making. That backlash targets those who have been systematically marginalized and erased on the basis of race, class, ability, religion, immigration status, body size, and more.

Where will this collision leave us? As medical and mental health professionals? As TNG people? These identity categories are far from mutually exclusive: this textbook is a proud, intentional product of voices from this nexus. In her seminal article "Situated Knowledges," science, technology, and society studies scholar Donna Haraway argued that scientific neutrality is a fallacy, as training and personal perspective influence the questions we think to ask and accordingly shape the answers that we find (Haraway 1988). Who conducts work matters; voices shape the stories that get told. As editors, we approached every stage of this project with expertise gleaned from both professional and lived experiences. We are both TNG psychiatrists, and carry many other identities (individually or together) that directly informed this work, such as queer, chronically ill, neurodivergent, Jewish, Middle Eastern, immigrant, child of civil war refugees, and descendent of

xix

genocide survivors. We are also both obscenely privileged in many respects, for example as English-speaking American physicians who had access to rarefied medical education and training at some of the world's best-resourced academic institutions.

We did our best to choose authors while prioritizing lived experience, diversity of perspectives, and community impact of prior work over academic titles. The following 26 chapters were written by a total of 56 authors, 50 of whom are TNG (89%). Each chapter has at least one TNG author, and the authorship of chapters focusing on specific intersectional identities is composed of community voices. Contributors collaborated to offer interdisciplinary perspectives from the fields of psychiatry, psychology, social work, nursing, pharmacy, epidemiology, public health, law, sociology, gender studies, business, community activism, and more. To our knowledge, this is the first book on TNG health produced by field experts who bring lived experience to their clinical and scholarly work. We explicitly name this process to demonstrate that such a representation is more than possible: it fuels the authenticity, relevance, and quality of our work. We hope that future efforts similarly lead with community member expertise to drive conversations about health equity.

During the editing process, we have struggled with terminology, which is as dynamic as gender itself. Our field's lexicon is constantly evolving and will continue to do so after the publication of this textbook. We made decisions here to the best of our ability, acknowledging the inherent imperfection of our linguistic framework. The following list represents choices made at the time of sending to press, with input from many fellow interdisciplinary TNG scholars and community members. We sought to use consistent definitions where possible, with some exceptions when intentional conceptual distinctions were necessary. Below, we briefly explain some such choices:

- *Inclusion without bias:* How to refer to the communities in question throughout this handbook? Although they are often shorthanded *trans* or *trans+*, we wanted to explicitly include gender-expansive people who do not specifically identify as trans. Similarly, we chose not to limit the acronym to *transgender and non-binary* (TGNB), to avoid excluding people who do not identify in those ways yet are not cisgender. We avoided *transgender and gender nonconforming* (TGNC) because gender nonconformity typically connotes gender expression, not gender identity (e.g., a cisgender girl with a buzzcut who plays hockey and a cisgender boy with painted nails who does ballet would both be cisgender and gender nonconforming). We were down to two options: *transgender and gender diverse* (TGD) and *transgender, non-binary, and/or gender expansive* (TNG; this can be interchanged with *transgender, non-binary, and/*

or gender diverse with the same acronym, although it seemed more accurate to refer to one person as *gender expansive* rather than *gender diverse*). The former offers a more concise phrase; the latter explicitly names non-binary identities and the individual, overlapping, and fluid nature of gender categories. We decided to use TNG throughout the text. Although this solution is imperfect, we hope it is sufficient, and we watch with fascination as language continues to evolve.

- *The "big acronym":* Similarly, there are many different acronyms for broader not-straight, not-cisgender, not-endosex communities, including *lesbian, gay, bisexual, transgender, queer, intersex, asexual, and more* (LGBTQIA+) or the more truncated LGBTQ+. Some include Two-Spirit (2S) in this acronym (2SLGBTQIA+), to explicitly name and acknowledge Indigenous identities and knowledges. We want to be specific in our terminology and to be inclusive in content rather than with lip-service alone; accordingly, we sought to include the *IA* when the work includes and pertains to intersex and asexual people and the *2S* when the work includes and pertains to Two-Spirit people. That being said, we ultimately deferred to the judgment of each chapter's authors.

- *To hyphenate or not to hyphenate:* The word "non(-)binary" can be written with or without the hyphen (non-binary vs. nonbinary). Some prefer non-binary, as the hyphen is grammatically customary for prefixes modifying an existing word in this way (e.g., "non-toxic"). Others prefer nonbinary because as words become more broadly accepted, the hyphens are often dropped (e.g., "nondescript"). Alternatively, the two forms may function as distinct words: nonbinary as a specific identity versus non-binary as an umbrella term referring to *not binary* genders (e.g., nonbinary, agender, genderqueer, genderfluid). We invited authors to use their preference, with intrachapter consistency.

- *Does a space change the meaning?* Per community consensus, *trans man* and *trans woman* are written as two words, with *trans* serving as any other descriptive adjective modifying a noun. Yet opinions diverge when it comes to the adjacent terms *transmasculine/trans masculine* and *transfeminine/trans feminine*. Some dislike the appearance of the compound adjective (without a space) because it is similar to the unacceptable and alienating *transman/transwoman*. Others prefer the single-word versions for accuracy: gender is not equal to expression. Transmasculine people may be feminine, androgynous, or otherwise not identify with "masculinity"; vice versa for transfeminine people. We asked each team of authors to consistently use one spacing and look forward to the ongoing evolution of community conversations.

- *Prejudice, bias, or fear?* Multiple, distinct terms for a negative stance against TNG people include the following:

- *Transphobia* (corollary *homophobia*), literally "fear of" TNG people; defined in psychology as "an emotional disgust toward individuals who do not conform to society's gender expectations" (Hill and Willoughby 2005, p. 533). Such sentiment can prompt implicit and explicit anti-TNG hostility, stereotypes, tropes, and discrimination; the term focuses on an individual's internal reactions. Further, the misnomer insidiously removes accountability for external actions; for instance, the ongoing (successful) use of the *gay/trans panic defense* to shift blame from a defendant to the LGBTQIA+ person they attacked, claiming the victim's existence sparked fear (National LGBTQ+ Bar Association and Foundation 2022).
- *Cisgenderism* (alternate *cissexism*; corollary *heterosexism*) is a more recent term that crucially challenges the normativity of cisgender experience and the separation of TNG people as a distinct class of humans, to the end of recognizing how individual acts fit within the broad systemic marginalization of TNG people (Ansara and Hegarty 2012). Cisgenderism is defined as a "cultural and systemic ideology that denies, denigrates, or pathologizes self-identified gender identities that do not align with assigned gender at birth as well as resulting behavior, expression, and community" and privileges cisgender experiences as having greater inherent worth (Lennon and Mistler 2014, p. 63). Although *cisgenderism* is sometimes conflated with *cisnormativity* (see next item), here *cisgenderism* will be used as defined above.
- *Cisnormativity* (corollary *heteronormativity*) is one aspect of cisgenderism: the indirect discrimination that occurs when cisgender experiences are assumed to be the neutral, default state; for example, naming an obstetrics and gynecology practice a *women's health center* is cisnormative, because it assumes the practice will only serve patients with one gender.

• *Who is providing care?* Acknowledging this handbook (and gender-affirming care, broadly) as a rich, interdisciplinary collaboration, we refer to practitioners delivering mental health care as *clinicians* (not *physicians* or *providers*) to explicitly include counselors, nurses, psychologists, social workers, and all mental health professionals.
• *Who is receiving care?* We supported author preference in choosing to refer to people receiving care as either *patients* or *clients*, with intrachapter consistency.

In this undertaking, it was imperative to consider our positionality as psychiatrists, trained and working within a field built on the work (and assumptions) of European, white, cisgender men, including their colonial, Anglocentric, cisheteropatriarchal worldview and pathologization of experiences that did not fit their own "norm." We acknowledge that such biases remain explicitly and implicitly within psychiatric training and practice and, despite our best efforts, undoubtedly have influenced this handbook. We have attempted to shift the norm/reference value away from the mythical man-woman binary and instead center the widespread historical legacy of gender diversity, with particular attention to (and authorship from) Two-Spirit and other Indigenous identities and roles that colonizers attempted to destroy. Our effort was constrained by space and remains just a start; we encourage you to continue reading work from Two-Spirit and all TNG Indigenous scholars, activists, and community members, to continue learning from the ancestral heritage of gender diversity.

The textbook begins with a discussion of epidemiology, minority stress and resilience, the neuroscience of gender, and psychopharmacological considerations for prescribing with TNG people. Chapters 5–10 are dedicated to providing intersectional gender-affirming care for and meeting the access needs of a series of specific, multiply marginalized communities: those who are Two-Spirit, Black, Asian American, and Pacific Islander; those who are neurodivergent and disabled; and migrants, refugees, and unhoused people. Chapters 11 and 12 help readers develop clinical tools to provide trauma-informed care and mitigate their own transphobic countertransference across settings. Chapters 13 and 14 focus on working with TNG people, and their families, in a developmentally appropriate manner across the life span, from children and adolescents to older adults. The chapters that follow are organized by psychiatric clinical specialty area and pertain to affirming gender identity in the context of eating disorders, substance use disorders, pregnancy, and serious mental illness. We then consider the specific care needs of populations who carry the compounding traumas of incarceration and gender identity conversion efforts, followed by guidance for providing an assessment in support of gender-affirming surgery. The final chapters explore systems-level change, including collecting gender identity information in electronic health records, building gender-affirming clinical environments, mental health law and policy considerations, and a case study of how TNG leaders can reimagine and transform delivery of gender-affirming mental health care. These chapters are not mutually exclusive in their content and considerations. We have done our best to remove redundancy and cross-reference pertinent chapters where beneficial.

We hope that this handbook, although necessarily not comprehensive, can serve as a guide for broadening readers' understanding of the richness and complexity of gender-affirming mental health care. We were limited by spatial constraints: there could have been dozens more chapters, and our exclusion of any topic is not a statement about its lack of importance. We hope this is just a starting point for more continued discourse, and in future handbooks we look forward to reading and learning about all of the compelling topics not highlighted here. We hope these chapters leave you with as many questions as answers. We hope they inspire you to create space for, listen to, and actionably affirm TNG people with lived experience in your own spheres. There is so much work to be done. Thank you for joining us.

Teddy G. Goetz, M.D., M.S.
Alex S. Keuroghlian, M.D., M.P.H.

REFERENCES

American Psychiatric Association: Diagnostic and Statistical Manual of Mental Disorders, 5th Edition. Arlington, VA, American Psychiatric Association, 2013

Ansara YG, Hegarty P: Cisgenderism in psychology: pathologising and misgendering children from 1999 to 2008. Psychol Sex 3(2):137–160, 2012

Haraway D: Situated knowledges: the science question in feminism and the privilege of partial perspective. Fem Stud 14(3):575–599, 1988

Hill DB, Willoughby BL: The development and validation of the genderism and transphobia scale. Sex Roles 53(7):531–544, 2005

Lennon E, Mistler BJ: Cisgenderism. Transgend Stud Q 1(1–2):63–64, 2014

National LGBTQ+ Bar Association and Foundation: LGBTQ+ "Panic" Defense. March 11, 2022. Available at: https://lgbtqbar.org/programs/advocacy/gay-trans-panic-defense/. Accessed August 28, 2022.

Content Warning: This book contains discussions of trauma; gender identity conversion efforts; prejudice toward TNG people (ageism, cisgenderism, misogyny, misogynoir, racism, sexism, transphobia, xenophobia) and those with autism, disabilities, eating disorders, mental illness, neurodivergence, and substance use disorders; historical negation and abuse; and pathologization of gender expression.

CHAPTER 1

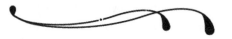

Epidemiological Overview of Mental Health Outcomes Among Transgender, Nonbinary, and/or Gender-Expansive (TNG) People

Arjee Javellana Restar, Ph.D., M.P.H.
E.J. Dusic, M.P.H.
Rodrigo Aguayo-Romero, Ph.D.
Sari L. Reisner, Sc.D.

TNG people experience a disproportionately high burden of mental health conditions, and TNG mental health is a public health priority that clinicians, researchers, program designers, and policymakers must address. U.S. federal and state programs that combat negative mental health outcomes in general continue to largely ignore TNG populations, despite evidence that timely intervention is needed.

In this chapter, we review recent epidemiological evidence regarding mental health outcomes among TNG people. Based on our teams' knowledge and expertise in the field, and as members of TNG communities ourselves, we focus on the mental health outcomes that we observe to be most prevalent and influential among TNG communities in the United States. We highlight epidemiological findings on anxiety, depression, suicide, and substance use disorders, while acknowledging the vast array of other mental health outcomes that disproportionately affect TNG populations (see Chapter 8, "DoubleQueer," regarding autism and ADHD and Chapter 18, Affirming Gender Identity in the Setting of Serious Mental Illness," regarding severe mental illness). We also note positive mental health outcomes, such as quality of life and resilience, that can be leveraged and strengthened to address these mental health inequities.

ANXIETY AND PTSD

Anxiety disorders are characterized by excessive or persistent fear and anxiety, typically lasting ≥6 months, and related behaviors such as avoidance (American Psychiatric Association 2013, 2015). Anxiety disorders are distinguished by the specific feared or avoided situations and the content of related cognitions or beliefs (American Psychiatric Association 2013).

Studies consistently demonstrate a high prevalence of anxiety disorders and symptoms in TNG populations (Bockting et al. 2013; Budge et al. 2013; Puckett et al. 2019), with a three- to fivefold greater burden of anxiety than cisgender populations (Brown and Jones 2016; Dragon et al. 2017; Hanna et al. 2019; Lipson et al. 2019; Reisner et al. 2015; Wanta et al. 2019). The 2007–2014 National Inpatient Sample, the largest publicly available all-payer inpatient hospitalization database in the United States, comprises 25,233 TNG and >254 million cisgender inpatient hospital encounters (age at hospitalization 57.2 ± 20.8 years; 68.7% white). Discharge records demonstrated threefold higher prevalence of anxiety disorder diagnostic codes for TNG (23.9%) versus cis (7.3%) encounters (OR=3.44; 95% CI 3.32–3.56; $P<0.001$), after adjusting for demographics, hospital characteristics, and comorbidities (Hanna et al. 2019). All-payer claims data from 1999–2018 electronic health records (EHRs) in 26 U.S. health care systems show an overall prevalence of DSM-5 (American Psychiatric Association 2013) anxiety disorders of 31.0% among TNG patients (those with the diagnostic code for *gender dysphoria* or equivalent; $n=10{,}270$) and only 6.0% among patients without such a diagnosis (presumed to be cisgender; >53 million; no further demographic data available) (Wanta et al. 2019).

Similar patterns have been observed for anxious symptomatology. Lipson et al. (2019) reported on 2015–2017 data from the Healthy Minds Study, a representative sample of 1,237 TNG (2.1% of the overall sample) and 63,994 cis undergraduate and graduate students from 71 U.S. college campuses (66.5% ages 18–22 years; 65.0% white). Nearly half (49.8%) of TNG versus 23.8% of cisgender students met criteria for probable anxiety disorder based on the self-reported Generalized Anxiety Disorder 7-item scale (GAD-7) with standard cutoff ≥ 10, representing threefold increased odds (OR=3.18; 95% CI 2.70–3.73; $P<0.001$) (Lipson et al. 2019).

Anxiety-related morbidity appears early in the life course for TNG populations (Bauer et al. 2021; Becerra-Culqui et al. 2018; Reisner et al. 2015; Tordoff et al. 2022). For example, Becerra-Culqui et al. (2018) evaluated mental health diagnoses in 1,333 TNG youth matched (by year of birth, race/ethnicity, site, and membership year) to 10 cisgender male and 10 cisgender female youth in the STRONG cohort, an EHR cohort of Kaiser Permanente sites (Georgia, Northern California, and Southern California) from 2006 to 2014. TNG youth had a significantly higher rate of anxiety disorder diagnostic codes than cisgender youth. In TNG children ages 3–9 years, anxiety diagnoses ranged from 11.8% to 15.6%, a four- to sixfold elevated prevalence relative to cisgender male and female children; in TNG adolescents ages 10–17, the prevalence of anxiety diagnoses was 37.2%–38.9%, four- to fivefold higher than in cisgender adolescent comparators (Becerra-Culqui et al. 2018). Regarding anxiety symptomatology, an observational study of 104 youths (ages 13–20, 15.8±1.6 years; 64.4% white) seeking gender-affirming care from 2017 to 2018 at an urban multidisciplinary gender clinic in Seattle found that 50.0% had a probable anxiety disorder (GAD-7 score ≥10) at baseline (Tordoff et al. 2022).

There are multiple types of anxiety disorders, including generalized anxiety disorder, panic disorder, social anxiety disorder, and phobic disorders. Wanta et al. (2019) found a higher prevalence of each anxiety disorder type in EHRs for TNG compared with cisgender patients: 12.0% versus 2.0% generalized anxiety disorder, 4.4% versus 0.74% panic disorder, 2.1% versus 0.06% social phobia, and 0.87% versus 0.08% agoraphobia. Symptoms of social anxiety are high in TNG individuals, are associated with gender minority stress (Kaplan et al. 2019; Testa et al. 2015), and show improvement with gender-affirming medical interventions (Butler et al. 2019). There is an absence of representative population data assessing distinct types of anxiety disorders among TNG populations, highlighting the importance of including measures of gender identity and gender modality status in national survey, EHR, and cohort studies. Research is needed that distinguishes between types of anxiety disorders in prevalence estimation and disorder characterization to inform treatment approaches in TNG populations, particularly because treatments may differ depending on anxiety type (Millet et al. 2017).

The epidemiological research on anxiety in TNG populations is plagued by multiple measurement-related issues: lack of differentiation in types of anxiety disorders, heterogeneity of measures (e.g., diagnostic instrument; screener for elevated symptomatology), unstandardized methods of outcome ascertainment (e.g., provider-administered clinical interview; self-report screener; EHR diagnosis codes), inconsistency in time frame of assessment (e.g., past 7 days; lifetime), and varying categorization of frequency and severity (e.g., binary cutoff of frequency corresponding to probable diagnosis; mild/moderate/severe categorization of symptom severity). Regardless, anxiety is clearly extremely prevalent in TNG populations. Evidence-informed interventions for anxiety are urgently needed, particularly those considering TNG-specific risk factors, such as stigma, that may uniquely contribute to the high prevalence and burden of anxiety disorders and symptoms in this population (Valentine and Shipherd 2018).

PTSD warrants specific attention in TNG mental health, particularly in the context of widespread traumatic experiences of gender minority stress, stigma, and violence (James et al. 2016) and the fear and anxiety elicited by actual or anticipated exposures to these stressors (see Chapter 11, "Trauma-Informed Mental Health Care"). TNG populations have a high burden of PTSD diagnosis and symptomatology (Barr et al. 2022; Dragon et al. 2017; McDowell et al. 2019; Poteat et al. 2020; Reisner et al. 2016), including in subpopulations such as veterans (Blosnich et al. 2017; Brown and Jones 2016; Livingston et al. 2022). Dragon et al. (2017) examined diagnostic codes from 2010–2015 Medicare claim records for >39 million patients (TNG age 53.1 ± 16.6 years; 76.8% white; cisgender age 70.9 ± 12.4; 78.1% white); they found PTSD prevalence of 22.7% in TNG patients versus 1.6% in cisgender peers. Brown and Jones (2016) assessed 5,135 TNG veterans matched 1:3 to 15,405 cisgender veterans seeking Veteran's Health Administration care from 1996 to 2013 (age 55.8 ± 13.5 years; 80% non-Hispanic white) and found significantly higher prevalence of both PTSD (38.7% TNG vs. 3.1% cisgender; OR = 2.82; 95% CI 2.60–3.06; $P < 0.0001$) and panic disorder (9.3% TNG vs. 2.5% cisgender; OR = 2.06; 95% CI 1.80–2.36; $P < 0.0001$) diagnoses among TNG veterans. Estimates of PTSD diagnosis in TNG community samples, based on self-reported symptoms, range from 42% to 44% depending on the subpopulation (McDowell et al. 2019; Reisner et al. 2016). Self-reported PTSD symptom severity is positively correlated with exposure to gender minority stress, stigma, and discrimination, with adjustment for other traumatic stressors (e.g., childhood abuse) (Barr et al. 2022; Reisner et al. 2016). Additional research is needed on PTSD in TNG populations, including representative studies, comparisons by gender identity and race/ ethnicity, and characterization of PTSD from repeated or prolonged trauma, acute stress disorder, and secondhand ("vicarious") trauma resulting from exposure to trauma of others in TNG communities.

DEPRESSION

Research has consistently shown a high prevalence of depression diagnosis among TNG populations in the United States. Although measures of depression outcomes in these studies vary—by diagnostic instrument, clinical cutoff points, duration (e.g., lifetime vs. past week), severity (e.g., mild, moderate, major), and methods (e.g., structured clinical interview, inventories of depressive symptoms, diagnosis in medical records, or self-report)—depressive symptoms are consistently elevated. For example, in a 2016 analysis using data from the Growing Up Today Study, which is a national cohort of 7,831 young adults, more TNG young adults clinically met elevations in depressive symptoms than their cisgender counterparts (52% of TNG people vs. 27% of cisgender women and 25% of cisgender men) using the Center for Epidemiologic Studies Depression Scale (CESD, cutoff point ≥10) (Reisner et al. 2016a). The high rates of depression were also similar when disaggregating TNG adult populations by gender. For example, studies report depression prevalence estimates as high as 64.2% in trans women (CESD ≥16), 63.0% in trans men (CESD ≥20), and 46.0% in nonbinary adults (CESD ≥10) (Nemoto et al. 2014; Nuttbrock et al. 2013; Reisner and Hughto 2019). Moreover, within-group disparities have been observed in large probability studies that examined depression by race/ethnicity, with TNG Hispanic adults having higher odds of depression compared with white TNG adults and Black TNG adults having higher odds of depression compared with Black cisgender adults, highlighting the need for intersectional research and intervention approaches to address depression within diverse TNG communities (Nemoto et al. 2014; Nuttbrock et al. 2013; Reisner and Hughto 2019). Together, these findings indicate that reducing depression in TNG populations is a critical public health priority.

The body of research on social and structural determinants of depression among TNG populations is still emerging (Reisner et al. 2016a), but a quantitative systematic review by Rowniak et al. (2019) identified a range of studies (both cross-sectional and prospective observational) in which gender-affirming care, particularly access to hormone use for those who desired it, resulted in significant improvements in depression.

SUICIDE

Rates of suicidality among TNG people are alarmingly high, and suicide has been identified as a public health crisis for TNG populations (dickey and Budge 2020). A systematic review of mainstream and gray North American literature from 1997 to 2017 reported an average lifetime prevalence of 46.6% for suicidal ideation and 27.2% for suicidal attempts among TNG people; the highest rates of lifetime suicide attempts reported were among First Nations (55.3%) and biracial/multiracial (50.9%) people (Adams and Vincent 2019). A meta-synthesis by Adams et al. (2017a) of mainstream and gray North American literature from 1997 to 2016 reported that lifetime suicidal ideation was highest among trans women (51.7%), followed by trans men (45.4%) and gender-nonconforming people (30.0%). The number of lifetime suicide attempts was highest among trans men (32.3%), followed by trans women (31.0%) and gender-nonconforming people (25.6%) (Adams et al. 2017a). The review also found that external minority stressors (gender-based violence, discrimination, stigma, rejection, lack of social support, nonaffirmation), internal minority stressors (internalized stigma, expectations of rejection, identity concealment), and depressive and PTSD symptoms were associated with suicidal ideation. Meanwhile, physical, sexual, and verbal aggression, victimization, non-suicide self-injury, and substance misuse were associated with lifetime suicide attempts (Adams and Vincent 2019).

A secondary analysis of the 2015 U.S. Transgender Survey, one of the largest national studies to date, indicated that about half of the study participants (48.5%) reported suicidal ideation in the past year (Yockey et al. 2022), particularly in certain subpopulations (e.g., transgender veterans) (Barboza et al. 2016; Tucker et al. 2019). For example, older TNG people reported lower odds of past-year suicidal ideation than younger ones (18–25 years old). Asian and Pacific Islander TNG people had decreased odds of suicidal ideation compared with white TNG people. TNG people with incomes lower than $49,999 (or no income) had significantly higher odds of suicidal ideation than those with incomes $100,000 or higher. Trans women, nonbinary/genderqueer individuals, and individuals who lived part time as one gender and part time as another had significantly higher odds of suicidal ideation than trans men (Yockey et al. 2022).

A secondary analysis of the population-based 2017 Youth Risk Behavior Survey found that, compared with cisgender boy peers, TNG students were approximately four times more likely to report suicidal ideation (43.9% TNG vs. 11.0% cisgender boys), four times more likely to report suicide planning (39.3% vs. 10.4%), and six times more likely to have attempted suicide (34.6% vs. 5.5%) (Johns et al. 2019).

Data on associations between gender-affirming procedures and suicidality remain inconclusive (Wolford-Clevenger et al. 2018). However, two large-scale studies that included TNG youth found that use of gender-affirming hormone therapy (GAHT) among those who desired it was associated with lower odds of suicidal ideation than among those who desired but did not receive GAHT (Green et al. 2022; Turban et al. 2020). A systematic review from Baker et al. (2021) about the effect of GAHT on psychological outcomes noted that more research is needed to further examine the relationship between GAHT and death by suicide. Protective factors against suicidal ideation and behaviors include social support, which is consistently reported in the literature as reducing risk for suicidal ideation (Wolford-Clevenger et al. 2018). Improved access to gender-affirming care and structural policy changes that reduce minority stress are needed to reduce the risk of suicidality among TNG people (Perez-Brumer et al. 2015; Wolford-Clevenger et al. 2018).

SUBSTANCE USE DISORDER

Rates of substance use and substance use disorder (SUD) are consistently higher in TNG people than cis peers (Connolly and Gilchrist 2020; Hughto et al. 2021; Ruppert et al. 2021), with differences emerging in adolescence (Day et al. 2017; De Pedro et al. 2017). A large body of literature details the prevalence of substance use in TNG populations; it is largely focused on transgender women (Connolly and Gilchrist 2020; Ruppert et al. 2021), however, and it often fails to include comparative data with reference groups (Ruppert et al. 2021), which can provide more context about the magnitude of SUD disparities. Additionally, when comparisons are made between TNG and cisgender individuals, TNG subpopulations are often aggregated in analyses (Ruppert et al. 2021). Across the existing body of work, measurement of SUD is inconsistent: some studies use measures such as the Cannabis Use Disorder Identification Test for problematic cannabis use or Alcohol Use Disorders Identification Test for hazardous drinking, whereas others use DSM-5 criteria or ask more generally about substance use behaviors (Adamson and Sellman 2003; American Psychiatric Association 2022; de Meneses-Gaya et al. 2009; Ruppert et al. 2021).

TNG people are at increased vulnerability to heavy episodic drinking, binge drinking, and alcohol use disorders, compared with cis peers (Connolly and Gilchrist 2020; Ruppert et al. 2021). In a sample of Canadian TNG adults, 33.2% reported monthly episodic drinking in the last year, a figure 1.5 times greater than general population estimates (Scheim et al. 2016). Of TNG cohorts, transgender men and trans masculine individuals report the highest rates of alcohol use (Ruppert et al. 2021; Scheim et al. 2016). Cannabis use is extremely prevalent: >40% of TNG participants endorsed regular cannabis use in one sample (Walsh et al. 2020), and lifetime cannabis use in TNG youth has been estimated to be ≤2 times greater than that of cisgender youth (Benotsch et al. 2013). As with alcohol, relatively few studies compare cannabis use between TNG subpopulations, but existing data identify transgender men and nonbinary individuals as having the highest levels of cannabis use (Connolly et al. 2020; Gonzalez et al. 2017; Ruppert et al. 2021). Nicotine use also warrants attention. TNG individuals, particularly trans men, report significantly higher rates of cigarette, e-cigarette, and smokeless tobacco use than cisgender individuals (Ruppert et al. 2021).

Many studies and reviews group drug use into one category broadly titled "illicit substances" (Christian et al. 2018; Gonzalez et al. 2017; Keuroghlian et al. 2015; Ruppert et al. 2021). TNG people are more likely than cis peers to report methamphetamine, cocaine, and injection drug use (Connolly and Gilchrist 2020). Most research in this area focuses on trans women, who have the greatest prevalence of illicit drug use (Connolly and Gilchrist 2020; Ruppert et al. 2021) and need for help to stop using these substances (Connolly et al. 2020). Opportunities for future work include exploring how substances are used in combination and further characterizing SUD in TNG subpopulations—for instance, there is a lack of research on illicit substance use in transgender men and trans masculine and nonbinary individuals.

Little work to date discusses prescription drug misuse in TNG populations. TNG individuals may be more frequently exposed to prescription pain medications, as they disproportionately experience chronic and acute pain related to gender-affirming surgeries (Girouard et al. 2019; Scheim et al. 2017). Although access to gender-affirming care may improve mental health and reduce susceptibility to SUD, it is important to consider the potential risk that comes with increased exposure to pain from gender-affirming surgeries. Future work is necessary to clarify the relationship between access to gender-affirming care and drug use, as well as to inform gender-affirming adaptation of prevention and treatment interventions, for trans people with SUD (Glynn and van den Berg 2017). This should include expanding targeted national initiatives—strategic plans combating SUDs, including nonmedical use of prescription opioids in the context of national trends in the opioid epidemic, are desperately needed.

POSITIVE MENTAL HEALTH OUTCOMES

In line with the general positive mental health literature, epidemiological studies on positive mental health outcomes such as quality of life and resilience among TNG people remain understudied. One systematic review found three studies linking improvement in general quality of life with having access to gender-affirming care among TNG adults who desire it (Rowniak et al. 2019). Another systematic review that included seven studies (one randomized clinical trial, two pre-post designs, two prospective cohorts, and two cross-sectional studies) found no evidence that GAHT decreased the quality of life among trans women and trans men (White Hughto and Reisner 2016); as of 2021, no additional publications addressed quality of life (Baker et al. 2021). More research is needed to understand the impact of GAHT on nonbinary people's quality of life.

Similarly, although epidemiological studies on resilience among TNG populations also remain underexplored, scholars have recognized the importance of resilience in promoting mental health, including the role of social networks and peer, romantic, sexual, and community relationships in buffering the negative mental health sequelae of social, environmental, and structural stressors (McCann and Brown 2017; Stone et al. 2020). A narrative review of 19 quantitative studies (McCann and Brown 2017) found that developing resilience via individual coping skills and bolstering social connectedness can positively influence quality of life and lessen psychological distress in TNG populations, particularly in the face of discrimination and other significant challenges. Moreover, although the emerging field of resilience studies has focused on the wider needs of populations placed marginally, there is a need to ensure that TNG people are fully integrated, included, and represented in this work. Treatment approaches that leverage and build on resilience promise to improve mental health outcomes in TNG populations (Budge et al. 2021; Matsuno and Israel 2018).

CONCLUSION, FUTURE DIRECTIONS, AND IMPLICATIONS FOR TNG POPULATIONS

In this chapter, we discuss the existing literature on certain mental health outcomes among TNG populations, highlighting select areas for future work. As psychiatric epidemiological research among TNG populations continues to emerge, it needs to include the spectrum of TNG communities, particularly trans men and nonbinary people, who remain underrepresented in TNG research and are likely vulnerable to negative mental health outcomes. Applying gender-inclusive and gender-specific approaches to study designs (Restar et al. 2021a, 2021b) can help align sampling methods with research objectives, analyses, and recommendations—particularly in psychiatric research, which has a legacy of pathologizing TNG people. For instance, in light of the known high prevalence of anxiety, depression, and suicidality in TNG populations, creating or adapting existing evidence-informed interventions that are effective requires understanding intervention components that are applicable across all TNG groups or specific and tailored to one or more groups.

Moreover, research on positive mental health outcomes (such as quality of life and resilience) is warranted among TNG populations. Ways to improve quality of life and factors important to enhance and sustain resilience at individual, community, and structural levels continue to be an underexplored area of research.

Interventions must attend to those shared resiliencies and vulnerabilities that affect the mental health status of all populations (e.g., social support; childhood abuse), alongside TNG-specific resiliencies and vulnerabilities (e.g., TNG activism; cisgenderist bullying). Life course considerations, including data about the onset and emergence of mental health conditions in TNG youth, particularly during important milestones such as internal and external disclosure of TNG identity (Restar et al. 2019), necessitate further attention and investigation. Ways to improve quality of life and resilience during these developmental periods could counter the negative impacts of stigma and discrimination that tend to be associated with these milestones. Such components are integral to developmentally situated mental health interventions among TNG populations, including early-in-life interventions to prevent the negative mental health sequelae of traumatic social stressors such as stigma and discrimination.

Our review also has implications for the broader field of public health, particularly mental health. Public, local, state, and federal public health initiatives and programs that address adverse mental health outcomes at a population level, particularly those already operating with strong structural and investment support, must begin adopting gender-transformative changes that abolish barriers to accessing mental health services (Restar et al. 2021a, 2021b). The future of TNG health, including the autonomy to receive life-saving gender-affirming therapy, counseling, and care services, remains socially and politically precarious. Researchers working in psychiatry must work in an interdisciplinary (and ethical) way (Adams et al. 2017b), side by side with TNG researchers and community stakeholders, to focus on strengthening and building multilevel interventions. New mental health interventions are needed that focus on addressing mental health at the individual level, but as this handbook explores, they should also address the social, environmental, and structural stressors that negatively contribute to the mental health and well-being of TNG populations. Lastly, identifying and strengthening factors that are linked to positive mental health outcomes, including evidence-based policies that target gender-based discrimination, could yield supportive and sustainable strategies for clinicians, researchers, program designers, and policymakers to counteract adverse mental health outcomes for TNG populations.

REFERENCES

Adams N, Hitomi M, Moody C: Varied reports of adult transgender suicidality: synthesizing and describing the peer-reviewed and gray literature. Transgend Health 2(1):60–75, 2017a 28861548

Adams N, Pearce R, Veale J, et al: Guidance and ethical considerations for undertaking transgender health research and Institutional Review Boards adjudicating this research. Transgend Health 2(1):165–175, 2017b 29098202

Adams NJ, Vincent B: Suicidal thoughts and behaviors among transgender adults in relation to education, ethnicity, and income: a systematic review. Transgend Health 4(1):226–246, 2019 31637302

Adamson SJ, Sellman JD: A prototype screening instrument for cannabis use disorder: the Cannabis Use Disorders Identification Test (CUDIT) in an alcohol-dependent clinical sample. Drug Alcohol Rev 22(3):309–315, 2003 15385225

American Psychiatric Association: Diagnostic and Statistical Manual of Mental Disorders, 5th Edition. Arlington, VA, American Psychiatric Association, 2013

American Psychiatric Association: Anxiety Disorders: DSM-5® Selections. Arlington, VA, American Psychiatric Association Publishing, 2015

American Psychiatric Association: Diagnostic and Statistical Manual of Mental Disorders, 5th Edition, Text Revision. Washington, DC, American Psychiatric Association, 2022

Baker KE, Wilson LM, Sharma R, et al: Hormone therapy, mental health, and quality of life among transgender people: a systematic review. J Endocr Soc 5(4):bvab011, 2021

Barboza GE, Dominguez S, Chance E: Physical victimization, gender identity and suicide risk among transgender men and women. Prev Med Rep 4:385–390, 2016 27547721

Barr SM, Snyder KE, Adelson JL, Budge SL: Posttraumatic stress in the trans community: the roles of anti-transgender bias, non-affirmation, and internalized transphobia. Psychol Sex Orientat Gend Divers 9(4):410–421, 2022

Bauer GR, Pacaud D, Couch R, et al; Trans Youth CAN! Research Team: Transgender youth referred to clinics for gender-affirming medical care in Canada. Pediatrics 148(5):e2020047266, 2021 34620727

Becerra-Culqui TA, Liu Y, Nash R, et al: Mental health of transgender and gender nonconforming youth compared with their peers. Pediatrics 141(5):e20173845, 2018 29661941

Benotsch EG, Zimmerman R, Cathers L, et al: Non-medical use of prescription drugs, polysubstance use, and mental health in transgender adults. Drug Alcohol Depend 132(1-2):391–394, 2013 23510637

Blosnich JR, Marsiglio MC, Dichter ME, et al: Impact of social determinants of health on medical conditions among transgender veterans. Am J Prev Med 52(4):491–498, 2017 28161034

Bockting WO, Miner MH, Swinburne Romine RE, et al: Stigma, mental health, and resilience in an online sample of the US transgender population. Am J Public Health 103(5):943–951, 2013 23488522

Brown GR, Jones KT: Mental health and medical health disparities in 5135 transgender veterans receiving healthcare in the Veterans Health Administration: a case-control study. LGBT Health 3(2):122–131, 2016 26674598

Budge SL, Adelson JL, Howard KAS: Anxiety and depression in transgender individuals: the roles of transition status, loss, social support, and coping. J Consult Clin Psychol 81(3):545–557, 2013 23398495

Budge SL, Sinnard MT, Hoyt WT: Longitudinal effects of psychotherapy with transgender and nonbinary clients: a randomized controlled pilot trial. Psychotherapy (Chic) 58(1):1–11, 2021 32567869

Butler RM, Horenstein A, Gitlin M, et al: Social anxiety among transgender and gender nonconforming individuals: the role of gender-affirming medical interventions. J Abnorm Psychol 128(1):25–31, 2019 30489112

Christian R, Mellies AA, Bui AG, et al: Measuring the health of an invisible population: lessons from the Colorado Transgender Health Survey. J Gen Intern Med 33(10):1654–1660, 2018 29761263

Connolly D, Gilchrist G: Prevalence and correlates of substance use among transgender adults: a systematic review. Addict Behav 111:106544, 2020 32717497

Connolly D, Davies E, Lynskey M, et al: Comparing intentions to reduce substance use and willingness to seek help among transgender and cisgender participants from the Global Drug Survey. J Subst Abuse Treat 112:86–91, 2020 32199550

Day JK, Fish JN, Perez-Brumer A, et al: Transgender youth substance use disparities: results from a population-based sample. J Adolesc Health 61(6):729–735, 2017 28942238

de Meneses-Gaya C, Zuardi AW, Loureiro SR, et al: Alcohol Use Disorders Identification Test (AUDIT): an updated systematic review of psychometric properties. Psychol Neurosci 2(1):83–97, 2009

De Pedro KT, Gilreath TD, Jackson C, Esqueda MC: Substance use among transgender students in California public middle and high schools. J Sch Health 87(5):303–309, 2017 28382667

dickey lm, Budge SL: Suicide and the transgender experience: a public health crisis. Am Psychol 75(3):380–390, 2020 32250142

Dragon CN, Guerino P, Ewald E, Laffan AM: Transgender Medicare beneficiaries and chronic conditions: exploring fee-for-service claims data. LGBT Health 4(6):404–411, 2017 29125908

Girouard MP, Goldhammer H, Keuroghlian AS: Understanding and treating opioid use disorders in lesbian, gay, bisexual, transgender, and queer populations. Subst Abus 40(3):335–339, 2019 30759045

Glynn TR, van den Berg JJ: A systematic review of interventions to reduce problematic substance use among transgender individuals: a call to action. Transgend Health 2(1):45–59, 2017 28861547

Gonzalez CA, Gallego JD, Bockting WO: Demographic characteristics, components of sexuality and gender, and minority stress and their associations to excessive alcohol, cannabis, and illicit (noncannabis) drug use among a large sample of transgender people in the United States. J Prim Prev 38(4):419–445, 2017 28405831

Green AE, DeChants JP, Price MN, Davis CK: Association of gender-affirming hormone therapy with depression, thoughts of suicide, and attempted suicide among transgender and nonbinary youth. J Adolesc Health 70(4):643–649, 2022 34920935

Hanna B, Desai R, Parekh T, et al: Psychiatric disorders in the U.S. transgender population. Ann Epidemiol 39:1–7.e1, 2019 31679894

Hughto JMW, Quinn EK, Dunbar MS, et al: Prevalence and co-occurrence of alcohol, nicotine, and other substance use disorder diagnoses among US transgender and cisgender adults. JAMA Netw Open 4(2):e2036512, 2021 33538824

James SE, Herman JL, Rankin S, et al: The Report of the 2015 U.S. Transgender Survey. Washington, DC: National Center for Transgender Equality, 2016. Available at https://transequality.org/sites/default/files/docs/usts/USTS-Full-Report-Dec17.pdf. Accessed July 17, 2023.

Johns MM, Lowry R, Andrzejewski J, et al: Transgender identity and experiences of violence victimization, substance use, suicide risk, and sexual risk behaviors among high school students—19 states and large urban school districts, 2017. MMWR Morb Mortal Wkly Rep 68(3):67–71, 2019 30677012

Kaplan SC, Butler RM, Devlin EA, et al: Rural living environment predicts social anxiety in transgender and gender nonconforming individuals across Canada and the United States. J Anxiety Disord 66:102116, 2019 31357038

Keuroghlian AS, Reisner SL, White JM, Weiss RD: Substance use and treatment of substance use disorders in a community sample of transgender adults. Drug Alcohol Depend 152:139–146, 2015 25953644

Lipson SK, Raifman J, Abelson S, Reisner SL: Gender minority mental health in the U.S.: results of a national survey on college campuses. Am J Prev Med 57(3):293–301, 2019 31427032

Livingston NA, Lynch KE, Hinds Z, et al: Identifying posttraumatic stress disorder and disparity among transgender veterans using nationwide Veterans Health Administration electronic health record data. LGBT Health 9(2):94–102, 2022 34981963

Matsuno E, Israel T: Psychological interventions promoting resilience among transgender individuals: transgender resilience intervention model (TRIM). Couns Psychol 46(5):632–655, 2018

McCann E, Brown M: Discrimination and resilience and the needs of people who identify as Transgender: a narrative review of quantitative research studies. J Clin Nurs 26(23-24):4080–4093, 2017 28597989

McDowell MJ, Hughto JMW, Reisner SL: Risk and protective factors for mental health morbidity in a community sample of female-to-male trans-masculine adults. BMC Psychiatry 19(1):16, 2019 30626372

Millet N, Longworth J, Arcelus J: Prevalence of anxiety symptoms and disorders in the transgender population: a systematic review of the literature. Int J Transgend 18(1):27–38, 2017

Nemoto T, Bödeker B, Iwamoto M, Sakata M: Practices of receptive and insertive anal sex among transgender women in relation to partner types, sociocultural factors, and background variables. AIDS Care 26(4):434–440, 2014 24160715

Nuttbrock L, Bockting W, Rosenblum A, et al: Gender abuse, depressive symptoms, and HIV and other sexually transmitted infections among male-to-female transgender persons: a three-year prospective study. Am J Public Health 103(2):300–307, 2013 22698023

Perez-Brumer A, Hatzenbuehler ML, Oldenburg CE, Bockting W: Individual- and structural-level risk factors for suicide attempts among transgender adults. Behav Med 41(3):164–171, 2015 26287284

Poteat TC, Reisner SL, Miller M, Wirtz AL; American Cohort to Study HIV Acquisition Among Transgender Women (LITE): Vulnerability to COVID-19-related harms among transgender women with and without HIV infection in the eastern and southern U.S. J Acquir Immune Defic Syndr 85(4):e67–e69, 2020 33136755

Puckett JA, Matsuno E, Dyar C, et al: Mental health and resilience in transgender individuals: what type of support makes a difference? J Fam Psychol 33(8):954–964, 2019 31318262

Reisner SL, Hughto JMW: Comparing the health of non-binary and binary transgender adults in a statewide non-probability sample. PLoS One 14(8):e0221583, 2019 31454395

Reisner SL, Vetters R, Leclerc M, et al: Mental health of transgender youth in care at an adolescent urban community health center: a matched retrospective cohort study. J Adolesc Health 56(3):274–279, 2015 25577670

Reisner SL, White Hughto JM, Gamarel KE, et al: Discriminatory experiences associated with posttraumatic stress disorder symptoms among transgender adults. J Couns Psychol 63(5):509–519, 2016 26866637

Restar A, Jin H, Breslow AS, et al: Developmental milestones in young transgender women in two American cities: results from a racially and ethnically diverse sample. Transgend Health 4(1):162–167, 2019 31482132

Restar A, Jin H, Operario D: Gender-inclusive and gender-specific approaches in trans health research. Transgend Health 6(5):235–239, 2021a 34993295

Restar AJ, Sherwood J, Edeza A, et al: Expanding gender-based health equity framework for transgender populations. Transgend Health 6(1):1–4, 2021b 33644317

Rowniak S, Bolt L, Sharifi C: Effect of cross-sex hormones on the quality of life, depression and anxiety of transgender individuals: a quantitative systematic review. JBI Database Syst Rev Implement Reports 17(9):1826–1854, 2019 31021971

Ruppert R, Kattari SK, Sussman S: Review: Prevalence of addictions among transgender and gender diverse subgroups. Int J Environ Res Public Health 18(16):8843, 2021 34444595

Scheim AI, Bauer GR, Shokoohi M: Heavy episodic drinking among transgender persons: disparities and predictors. Drug Alcohol Depend 167:156–162, 2016 27542688

Scheim AI, Bauer GR, Shokoohi M: Drug use among transgender people in Ontario, Canada: disparities and associations with social exclusion. Addict Behav 72:151–158, 2017 28411424

Stone AL, Nimmons EA, Salcido R Jr, Schnarrs PW: Multiplicity, race, and resilience: transgender and non-binary people building community. Sociol Inq 90(2):226–248, 2020

Testa RJ, Habarth J, Peta J, et al: Development of the Gender Minority Stress and Resilience Measure. Psychol Sex Orientat Gend Divers 2(1):65–77, 2015

Tordoff DM, Wanta JW, Collin A, et al: Mental health outcomes in transgender and nonbinary youths receiving gender-affirming care. JAMA Netw Open 5(2):e220978, 2022 35212746

Tucker RP, Testa RJ, Reger MA, et al: Current and military-specific gender minority stress factors and their relationship with suicide ideation in transgender veterans. Suicide Life Threat Behav 49(1):155–166, 2019 29327446

Turban JL, King D, Carswell JM, Keuroghlian AS: Pubertal suppression for transgender youth and risk of suicidal ideation. Pediatrics 145(2):e20191725, 2020 31974216

Valentine SE, Shipherd JC: A systematic review of social stress and mental health among transgender and gender non-conforming people in the United States. Clin Psychol Rev 66:24–38, 2018 29627104

Walsh CF, O'Connell RP, Kvach E: Patterns of healthcare access and utilization among nonurban transgender and nonbinary patients at a large safety net health system in Colorado. Ann LGBTQ Public Popul Health 1(3):186–199, 2020

Wanta JW, Niforatos JD, Durbak E, et al: Mental health diagnoses among transgender patients in the clinical setting: an all-payer electronic health record study. Transgend Health 4(1):313–315, 2019 31701012

White Hughto JM, Reisner SL: A systematic review of the effects of hormone therapy on psychological functioning and quality of life in transgender individuals. Transgend Health 1(1):21–31, 2016 27595141

Wolford-Clevenger C, Frantell K, Smith PN, et al: Correlates of suicide ideation and behaviors among transgender people: a systematic review guided by ideation-to-action theory. Clin Psychol Rev 63:93–105, 2018 29960203

Yockey A, King K, Vidourek R: Past-year suicidal ideation among transgender individuals in the United States. Arch Suicide Res 26(1):70–80, 2022 32780685

CHAPTER 2

Stigma and Mental Health Inequities

The Gender Minority Stress and Resilience Framework

Em Matsuno, Ph.D.
Jae A. Puckett, Ph.D.
Sebastian M. Barr, Ph.D.

TRANSGENDER, nonbinary, and/or gender-expansive (TNG) people often experience structural and enacted stigma, such as a hostile sociocultural climate, discrimination, rejection, victimization, and nonaffirmation related to their gender identity or expression. This stigma can lead to the development of proximal stressors, such as expecting others to reject them, internalizing negative beliefs about TNG identities, concealing their identity, and experiencing worsened gender dysphoria. Stressors also stem from the general pervasive stigma against TNG people and oppressive systems and cultural norms that seek to invalidate or eliminate them (Price et al. 2021; Puckett et al. 2021), despite long-standing community resistance to such oppressive systems. These added layers of stressors explain the heightened mental health risks documented among TNG people (Lefevor et al. 2019; Testa et al. 2017). In this chapter, we discuss mental health disparities experienced by TNG people, summarize minority stress theory (MST), describe the unique minority stress experiences of TNG people, provide an updated model (Figure 2–1), describe the factors that lead to resilience among TNG people, and briefly provide clinical recommendations based on MST.

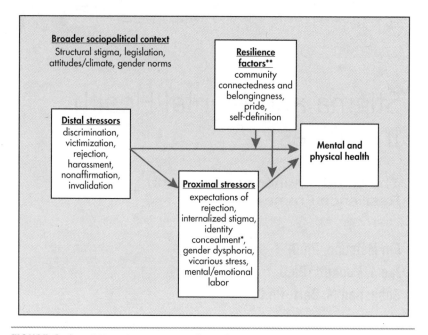

FIGURE 2–1.   **Minority stress and resilience factors affecting the health of TNG people.**

*Identity concealment can be an act of affirmation for some TNG people.
**Other experiences may promote resilience, such as social advocacy, role models, critical consciousness, etc. For an expanded resilience model, see the Transgender Resilience Intervention Model (TRIM) (Matsuno and Israel 2018).

MENTAL HEALTH DISPARITIES

Research has consistently documented that TNG communities experience mental health disparities compared with the general population. TNG people are more likely than cisgender peers to carry a broad range of mental health diagnoses, including anxiety disorders, trauma-related disorders, mood disorders, and schizophrenia spectrum disorders (Barr et al. 2021; Bockting et al. 2013; Valentine and Shipherd 2018). Many studies have also documented higher levels of experienced distress, symptoms, and manifestations of psychological distress, such as self-injury and suicidal behavior, among TNG participants (e.g., Downing and Przedworski 2018; Thoma et al. 2019). This mental health risk has been weaponized against TNG communities to pathologize gender diversity and to suggest that there is fundamental psychological instability within TNG communities (Davy 2015; Puckett 2019). This conclusion is at odds with a large evidence base (including multiple systematic reviews; e.g., McNeil et al. 2017; Valentine and Shipherd

2018) confirming what TNG communities have long expressed (Serano 2009): mental health risk is linked to the unique factors of oppression (i.e., gender minority stress) that TNG people face in cisnormative and transnegative societies and is not inherent to or generative of TNG identities.

MINORITY STRESS THEORY

Virginia Brooks (1981) was the first author to use the term *minority stress* to describe the added social stressors experienced by lesbian women. Meyer (2003) extended this work to include lesbian, gay, and bisexual (LGB) people and created the minority stress model, a conceptual model that posits that a stressful social environment causes mental health problems among LGB people. The minority stress model separates *distal stressors*—external and "objective" stressful events and conditions—from *proximal stressors*—the internal experiences of social stressors. The model identifies experiences of prejudice (such as discrimination and violence) as distal stressors, and expectations of rejection, concealment, and internalized homophobia as proximal stressors. Meyer (2003) also hypothesized that coping and social support could buffer the negative impact of minority stressors. This model was extended to TNG people (Hendricks and Testa 2012) and then expanded to recognize the unique stressors that TNG people experience, such as nonaffirmation of their gender (Testa et al. 2015). In the following section, we describe the major minority stressors identified in the literature, while attending to how these stressors may vary or look different among subgroups of TNG populations.

TNG-Specific Minority Stressors

Distal Stressors

Discrimination, victimization, rejection, and structural stigma. It is well documented that TNG people experience discrimination in several areas of life. *Discrimination* refers to instances when TNG people are denied equal treatment, services, or opportunities. TNG people experience high levels of discrimination in work, housing, and health care. The U.S. Transgender Survey found that 16% of TNG people who have been employed have lost a job due to biases associated with their gender identity or expression (James et al. 2016). TNG people are commonly discriminated against in the hiring process or are denied promotions (Bardales 2013), which contributes to high rates of unemployment, housing insecurity, and economic disparities (James et al. 2016; Kattari and Begun 2017). TNG people are three times more likely to be unemployed and live in poverty than the general population, and these disparities are worse among TNG Black, Indigenous, and people of color

(BIPOC) and trans women (James et al. 2016). One in three TNG people has experienced houselessness in their lifetime, through employment discrimination or being evicted or denied housing owing to their TNG identity (James et al. 2016).

Health care is rife with anti-TNG discrimination. TNG individuals report being denied care outright because clinicians refuse to work with people who are TNG, as well as experiencing incompetent care, mistreatment, harassment, and violence from health care clinicians (James et al. 2016; Puckett et al. 2018). Many TNG people, out of fear of being mistreated, avoid going to see a doctor, which has harmful health implications.

Since the inception of gender-affirming medical interventions, such as hormone therapy and gender-affirming surgeries, TNG people have experienced significant discrimination and barriers to receiving care. Insurance companies often refuse to cover gender-affirming medical care, despite scientific evidence showing that these procedures improve quality of life and mental health (Murad et al. 2010; White Hughto and Reisner 2016). Unfortunately, gatekeeping practices among mental health clinicians are prevalent, especially toward nonbinary people or those whose experience does not match the binary medicalized narrative of the transgender experience (e.g., extreme dysphoria, binary experience of gender, "consistent and persistent" transgender identification since early childhood) (Johnson 2016; Puckett et al. 2018). Since 2021, anti-TNG political groups have been heavily promoting laws to ban gender-affirming health care for TNG minors, thereby delaying the possibility of gender-affirming medical interventions until age 18. Given the well-documented mental health risks of gatekeeping practices (Schulz 2018), discrimination in this area has devastating mental health consequences.

TNG people with intersecting marginalized identities (e.g., TNG BIPOC, trans women, and transfeminine people) are more likely to experience gender minority stressors than TNG people with more privileged intersecting identities (James et al. 2016). Multiple marginalized identities may also have a compounding impact in terms of the effects of discrimination on mental health. Research has found that individuals with more identities toward which discrimination may be directed are more affected by it (Smith and Pössel 2022).

Unfortunately, many TNG people, particularly transfeminine BIPOC, also experience *victimization* (i.e., violence, harassment, intimate partner violence, and other forms of intimidation), leading to increased experiences of PTSD and other negative mental health outcomes (Barr et al. 2022; Wirtz et al. 2020). In 2021, the deadliest year for TNG people in recent U.S. history, at least 59 TNG people were murdered in the United States, the vast majority of whom were Black and Latinx trans women (Human Rights Campaign

2021). Nevertheless, anti-TNG violence continues to be largely ignored by the mainstream media. Harassment and violence appear to be highest among those who are perceived by others as transgender or gender nonconforming, those who work in the underground economy (e.g., sex work), and BIPOC (James et al. 2016). TNG people have a low prevalence of reporting violent crimes to police, as police are often perpetrators of harassment and violence toward TNG people or may blame TNG people for experiencing violence (Yerke and DeFeo 2016). Additionally, TNG people often have limited resources to support them after they experience violence, or they face additional discrimination when trying to access services (e.g., a trans woman being denied access to a women's shelter) (Barrett and Sheridan 2017).

Rejection is characterized by others distancing or ending a relationship with a TNG person because of prejudice against TNG people. Research shows that one of the most harmful forms of rejection is familial rejection, parental rejection in particular (Klein and Golub 2016).

Among TNG people, family acceptance or rejection is a prominent—possibly the most prominent—predictor of mental health outcomes (Puckett et al. 2019; Simons et al. 2013). Parental rejection may be particularly harmful to TNG youth who may be financially dependent on their parents and have less autonomy and resources than adults. Additionally, parental rejection may lead to TNG youth being kicked out of their homes and prevented from socially or medically affirming their gender (Ashley 2019). In addition to family rejection, many TNG people report experiencing rejection when dating (Gamarel et al. 2022) and exclusion from religious communities (Exline et al. 2021).

Nonaffirmation and invalidation. Testa et al. (2015) added a unique distal stressor experienced by TNG people to the minority stress model: *nonaffirmation*, which occurs when "one's internal sense of gender identity is not affirmed by others" (p. 66). Nonaffirmation is associated with higher odds of experiencing depressive symptoms, suicidal ideation (Parr and Howe 2019), and PTSD symptoms (Barr et al. 2022) among TNG people. Many TNG people experience nonaffirmation on a daily basis (Puckett et al. 2021), and nonbinary people appear to experience the highest levels of nonaffirmation, compared with trans men and trans women (Goldberg et al. 2019). A common form of nonaffirmation is misgendering (the use of incorrect gendered language or pronouns), which has been linked to increased psychological distress (McLemore 2018).

Identity invalidation, which is similar to but distinct from nonaffirmation, has been highlighted as a unique distal stressor among TNG people, nonbinary people in particular (Johnson et al. 2020). Identity invalidation is defined as the refusal to accept someone's identity as "real" or "true." Invalidation appears to be particularly relevant to the experiences of nonbinary people, because it occurs when the legitimacy of one's gender identity is called into question altogether. Many people acknowledge the legitimacy of trans men and trans women's gender identities, as they exist within the gender binary, but may challenge the legitimacy of nonbinary identities. Other qualitative studies have similarly found that nonbinary people have frequent experiences of invalidation that likely contribute to negative mental health outcomes (Matsuno et al. 2021).

Proximal Stressors

Internalized stigma, expectations of rejection, and concealment. Proximal stressors result from distal stressors and reflect how stigma influences a person's sense of self, expectations for the future, and identity concealment versus disclosure. TNG people internalize negative messages about their gender identity that create distress and are associated with other negative mental health outcomes (Breslow et al. 2015). A qualitative study by Rood et al. (2017a) found that TNG people often received social messages that labeled their identity as abnormal, unnatural, and immoral; participants also internalized messages that TNG people are not real or are being deceptive, are sexually deviant or predators, and are mentally ill. TNG BIPOC received additional messages such as that TNG BIPOC are less valuable than white TNG people or that their culture and gender cannot coexist (Rood et al. 2017b). Another qualitative study found that nonbinary people internalized beliefs that their identity was not valid and that they were a burden or inconvenience to others (Matsuno et al. 2021).

Expectations of rejection (also known as negative expectations of the future) refers to a TNG person's anticipation of stigma being enacted in a given situation (Hendricks and Testa 2012). Rood et al. (2016) identified expectations of rejection as a prevalent daily stressor for TNG people that was influenced by past experiences of distal minority stressors and knowledge of society's stance toward TNG individuals. TNG participants' expectations of experiencing stigma were increased in gendered spaces (e.g., bathrooms), around people who knew their TNG status, and when they believed they did not "pass" as cisgender (Rood et al. 2016). TNG BIPOC reported increased expectations of rejection based on race and ethnicity but also identified feeling more prepared to cope with rejection (Rood et al. 2016). A qualitative study found that *bodily vigilance* (i.e., alertness to how other people are reading one's gender or gender expression) is a closely related but distinct proximal stressor associated with heightened anxiety and self-monitoring as a product of marginalization (Puckett et al. 2021). However, this stressor has yet to be tested quantitatively.

Concealment (not disclosing one's TNG status) differs in significant ways among TNG people compared with cisgender lesbian, gay, bisexual, queer, plus (LGBQ+) people (Testa et al. 2015). Testa et al. (2015) highlighted how a TNG individual's ability to conceal their identity may depend on physical factors, gender expression, and access to gender-affirming medical interventions. Additionally, some scholars question whether concealment is truly a proximal stressor, given that its consequences can be both positive, by providing protection from distal stressors, and negative, by blocking authenticity (Martinez et al. 2017; Rood et al. 2017a). Concealment of sex assigned at birth appears to have a different impact from concealing one's gender identity; indeed, it can actually function to affirm one's gender identity (Rood et al. 2017a). Concealment may also function differently among nonbinary people, who are rarely identified by others as nonbinary without disclosing their identity (Matsuno et al. 2021). In fact, one study found that nonbinary adults who had high levels of concealment had less distress compared with low-level concealers (Flynn and Smith 2021).

Gender dysphoria, vicarious stress, and mental/emotional labor. Recent research has expanded the original minority stress model to include additional proximal stressors found among TNG individuals. The feeling or experience of *gender dysphoria* refers to the distress or discomfort experienced as a result of an incongruence or branching of one's gender identity and one's body or presentation (Lindley and Galupo 2020), not to be conflated with gender dysphoria as a clinical diagnosis in DSM-5-TR (American Psychiatric Association 2022). Both qualitative and quantitative research studies have supported the conceptualization of gender dysphoria as a proximal stressor for TNG people because it can be triggered by distal stressors (e.g., nonaffirmation), is correlated with other proximal stressors (e.g., internalized stigma), and is related to negative mental health outcomes (Lindley and Galupo 2020). Understanding gender dysphoria within the minority stress framework allows opportunities for tailored interventions to reduce gender dysphoria.

Recent qualitative research has offered new insights on two additional proximal stressors experienced by TNG individuals: vicarious stress and mental/emotional labor. *Vicarious stress* refers to the "emotional toll of exposure to stress narratives from other TNG people or social representations of TNG people," such as learning about another TNG person experiencing a hate crime (Puckett et al. 2021). *Mental/emotional labor* is defined as the additional cognitive and affective energy used as a result of experiencing distal stressors and is often compounded by stress related to additional marginalized identities (Matsuno et al. 2021). For example, TNG people may expend extra cognitive and affective energy in educating others about their identity and feeling the need to defend or prove their identity to others. More quantitative research is needed to confirm whether these constructs fit as proximal stressors within the minority stress framework.

Resilience and Well-Being

Research about TNG resilience has lagged behind research on minority stress. Quantitative studies have typically conceptualized resilience as the ability to "bounce back" from challenges and hardships. Although this definition may fit with traditional psychological definitions of the construct of resilience, it has limitations when applied to TNG people.

Qualitative research shows that TNG people experience resilience in unique and novel ways. For instance, some TNG people describe their resilience as self-defining their gender experience and rejecting narratives that have been imposed on them by society (e.g., Shelton et al. 2018; Singh et al. 2014). Other studies indicate that TNG people live out their own resilience through connections to the TNG community (e.g., Nicolazzo 2016; Singh et al. 2011). In addition, specific to resisting marginalization, TNG people describe resilience as developing critical consciousness, developing pride and a positive sense of self, and engaging in social activism (Bockting et al. 2020; Bowling et al. 2019; Nicolazzo 2016; Singh 2013; Singh and Mckleroy 2011; Singh et al. 2011, 2014). It is important to note that engaging in social activism to resist marginalization may simultaneously be associated with more exposure to stressors, complicating the quantitative assessment of this resilience factor (Breslow et al. 2015).

Research using general assessments of resilience has shown that it is associated with less depression, anxiety, and psychological distress (Breslow et al. 2015; Puckett et al. 2019; Testa et al. 2015). Research using TNG-specific conceptualizations of resilience has found that identity pride is inversely associated with psychological distress (Bockting et al. 2013). Findings in relation to community connectedness are mixed: some research has shown that it is associated with less depression and anxiety (Testa et al. 2015); other research has found only weak associations or failed to find significant associations with mental health (Puckett et al. 2019).

A small body of literature has examined *belongingness* specifically as a predictor of well-being and found significant associations between TNG community belongingness and increased positive psychological outcomes, and also between general community belongingness (e.g., campus belonging) and reduced distress (Barr et al. 2016; Budge et al. 2020). Thus connection to community alone may be insufficient as a source of resilience, and factors affecting belongingness within TNG communities (including race/ethnicity) may be relevant (BrckaLorenz et al. 2021). Resilience has also been shown to buffer the effects of alienation on anxiety (Scandurra et al. 2018) and of enacted stigma on depression and suicidal ideation (Scandurra et al. 2017). However, research examining buffering effects has typically failed to find significant results with either generic or TNG-specific resilience variables (Breslow et al. 2015; Jäggi et al. 2018). For instance, identity pride was not found to buffer the effects of enacted stigma on mental health (Bockting et al. 2013).

Sociopolitical Context

All these minority stress and resilience factors are experienced primarily at the individual or interpersonal level, within a person's microsystem and mesosystem. Research and community narratives also consistently implicate macrosystem factors in TNG people's community or larger sociopolitical context as important contributors to health and well-being (e.g., DuBois and Juster 2022). Structural stigma—the manifestation of stigma in society-level conditions, cultural norms, and institutional policies or practices (Hatzenbuehler 2016)—can be considered a source of minority stress. TNG people encounter structural stigma in myriad ways, including negative media portrayals of TNG people, psychopathologization, cissexist and binary gender norms, difficulty accessing affirming care (owing to, for instance, low clinician competency or insurance denials), hostile sociocultural climates (e.g., transnegative views), and discriminatory laws and policies (Puckett et al. 2021; White Hughto et al. 2015), which have been on the rise in the United States (Sonoma 2022). Research has demonstrated that structural stigma increases TNG people's risk for negative mental and physical health (DuBois and Juster 2022; Valentine and Shipherd 2018) and is associated with decreased life satisfaction (Bränström and Pachankis 2021).

Additionally, the broader sociopolitical context shapes how people experience these distal and proximal minority stressors, as well as their opportunities for accessing resilience factors. For example, TNG people are more likely to conceal their TNG identity in countries with high sociopolitical stigma (Bränström and Pachankis 2021) and conversely face less stigma, discrimination, and violence in areas where legislation and community mores condemn anti-trans bias (Gleason et al. 2016). The support TNG people experience in their microsystems is affected by sociocultural norms in complex ways (Katz-Wise et al. 2022). The broader sociopolitical context also influences who is more likely to experience minority stress and who has more access to resilience factors. For example, because of pervasive structural racism as well as intersectional stigma (e.g., transmisogyny and transmisogynoir), some TNG BIPOC and transfeminine BIPOC face particularly high rates of discrimination, violence, and related distress (Millar and Brooks 2021; Reisner et al. 2016).

Limitations

Although it is a helpful starting place, the minority stress model that is often applied to TNG samples was initially meant to describe the lived experiences of cisgender LGBQ+ people. As such, this model is inherently constrained in its capacity to describe TNG experiences and needs modifications to ensure that TNG-specific stressors are reflected. Recent advances, as outlined earlier, have begun to address this limitation, including the integration of gender dysphoria (Lindley and Galupo 2020) as a proximal stressor and the identification of other minority stressors, such as vicarious stress, bodily vigilance (Puckett et al. 2021), and mental/emotional labor (Matsuno et al. 2021).

Important critiques also apply to resilience. General frameworks that view resilience as an ability to bounce back or other similar descriptions may miss unique ways that resilience is lived out by TNG individuals and communities. Traditional individualistic frameworks of psychology may overlook gender-specific forms of resilience, like self-defining one's gender (Singh 2013), or communal/group-level forms of resilience, like connecting with others with a shared identity (Singh et al. 2011).

Regarding both minority stress and resilience, the literature is limited in terms of representation. Much of the existing literature about TNG people has included primarily white subjects, so it is debatable how well these advances reflect the lives of TNG BIPOC. Limited research has examined variability in experiences of minority stress and resilience across gender subgroups within TNG populations. Given these limitations, we believe it is crucial for TNG voices to lead efforts to create models that aim to describe these communities' experiences. This means integrating TNG people into research in ways that prioritize their input, perhaps through participatory research designs. TNG researchers are also leading these studies, given their insights from lived experience. Through these types of practices, we can move beyond models that were developed for cisgender people and envision a research base that more accurately and fully reflects TNG lives.

IMPLICATIONS FOR INTERVENTIONS

Minority stress theory can help structure and guide the ways clinicians work to improve TNG mental health and well-being. First, MST can be incorporated into individual- and community-level psychoeducation to help individuals experiencing gender minority stress understand their experiences within this framework, and thus receive validation. Multiple articles have discussed ways of bringing this approach into psychotherapy (Austin and Craig 2015; Budge et al. 2021).

Second, by grounding understanding of clients' mental health in the concept of minority stress, clinicians underscore the importance of prevention and harm reduction regarding distal stressors. This means that mental health clinicians must work as advocates—both for clients within their specific systems (e.g., school, family, work) and at the sociopolitical level (Ashley and Domínguez 2021; Dickey and Singh 2017; Puckett 2019). Clinicians can also help clients process experiences of minority stressors in an emotionally safe holding environment, just as we would approach facilitated trauma processing. Third, clinicians can adopt individual and systemic interventions targeting proximal stressors. Such interventions might include attending to internalized stigma in psychotherapy (Puckett and Levitt 2015) and working with a client to reduce and manage gender dysphoria (Austin et al. 2022). Finally, efforts must include those that strengthen both client and community resilience. A helpful model for integrating resilience into clinical practice is the Transgender Resilience Intervention Model (TRIM; Matsuno and Israel 2018). As ever, clinicians should use approaches that best fit their clients' existing strengths and idiosyncratic needs.

CONCLUSION

Understanding minority stress is critical to culturally responsive care when working with TNG people. The research clearly demonstrates that these stressors play a key role in health disparities (James et al. 2016; Valentine and Shipherd 2018). Without taking these contextual factors into account, clinicians may misattribute mental health issues to a person's gender experience or pathologize TNG identities. Furthermore, TNG people's lives consist of more than just the stressors they experience: resilience must also be considered. Research in these areas has grown in recent years, and TNG people should lead future work in these areas to ensure that future efforts best reflect the lived experiences of TNG communities.

REFERENCES

American Psychiatric Association: Diagnostic and Statistical Manual of Mental Disorders, 5th Edition, Text Revision. Washington, DC, American Psychiatric Association, 2022

Ashley F: Puberty blockers are necessary, but they don't prevent homelessness: caring for transgender youth by supporting unsupportive parents. Am J Bioeth 19(2):87–89, 2019 30784386

Ashley F, Domínguez S Jr: Transgender healthcare does not stop at the doorstep of the clinic. Am J Med 134(2):158–160, 2021 33228952

Austin A, Craig SL: Transgender affirmative cognitive behavioral therapy: clinical considerations and applications. Prof Psychol Res Pr 46(1):21–29, 2015

Austin A, Holzworth J, Papciak R: Beyond diagnosis: "Gender dysphoria feels like a living hell, a nightmare one cannot ever wake up from." Psychol Sex Orientat Gend Divers 9(1):12–20, 2022

Bardales N: Finding a job in "a beard and a dress": evaluating the effectiveness of transgender anti-discrimination laws. Unpublished thesis, University of California, San Diego, 2013

Barr SM, Budge SL, Adelson JL: Transgender community belongingness as a mediator between strength of transgender identity and well-being. J Couns Psychol 63(1):87–97, 2016 26751157

Barr SM, Roberts D, Thakkar KN: Psychosis in transgender and gender non-conforming individuals: a review of the literature and a call for more research. Psychiatry Res 306:114272, 2021 34808496

Barr SM, Snyder KE, Adelson JL, Budge SL: Posttraumatic stress in the trans community: the roles of anti-transgender bias, non-affirmation, and internalized transphobia. Psychol Sex Orientat Gend Divers 9(4):410–421, 2022

Barrett BJ, Sheridan DV: Partner violence in transgender communities: what helping professionals need to know. J GLBT Fam Stud 13(2):137–162, 2017

Bockting WO, Miner MH, Swinburne Romine RE, et al: Stigma, mental health, and resilience in an online sample of the US transgender population. Am J Public Health 103(5):943–951, 2013 23488522

Bockting W, Barucco R, LeBlanc A, et al: Sociopolitical change and transgender people's perceptions of vulnerability and resilience. Sex Res Soc Policy 17(1):162–174, 2020 32742526

Bowling J, Baldwin A, Schnarrs PW: Influences of health care access on resilience building among transgender and gender non-binary individuals. Int J Transgend 20(2-3):205–217, 2019 32999607

Bränström R, Pachankis JE: Country-level structural stigma, identity concealment, and day-to-day discrimination as determinants of transgender people's life satisfaction. Soc Psychiatry Psychiatr Epidemiol 56(9):1537–1545, 2021 33582826

BrckaLorenz A, Duran A, Fassett K, Palmer D: The within-group differences in LGBQ+ college students' belongingness, institutional commitment, and outness. J Divers High Educ 14(1):135–146, 2021

Breslow AS, Brewster ME, Velez BL, et al: Resilience and collective action: exploring buffers against minority stress for transgender individuals. Psychol Sex Orientat Gend Divers 2(3):253–265, 2015

Brooks VR: Minority Stress and Lesbian Women. Lexington, MA, Lexington Books, 1981

Budge SL, Domínguez S Jr, Goldberg AE: Minority stress in nonbinary students in higher education: the role of campus climate and belongingness. Psychol Sex Orientat Gend Divers 7(2):222–229, 2020

Budge SL, Sinnard MT, Hoyt WT: Longitudinal effects of psychotherapy with transgender and nonbinary clients: a randomized controlled pilot trial. Psychotherapy (Chic) 58(1):1–11, 2021 32567869

Davy Z: The DSM-5 and the politics of diagnosing transpeople. Arch Sex Behav 44(5):1165–1176, 2015 26054486

Dickey LM, Singh AA: Social justice and advocacy for transgender and gender-diverse clients. Psychiatr Clin North Am 40(1):1–13, 2017 28159137

Downing JM, Przedworski JM: Health of transgender adults in the U.S., 2014–2016. Am J Prev Med 55(3):336–344, 2018 30031640

DuBois LZ, Juster R-P: Lived experience and allostatic load among transmasculine people living in the United States. Psychoneuroendocrinology 143:105849, 2022 35797839

Exline JJ, Przeworski A, Peterson EK, et al: Religious and spiritual struggles among transgender and gender-nonconforming adults. Psychol Relig Spiritual 13(3):276–286, 2021

Flynn S, Smith NG: Interactions between blending and identity concealment: effects on non-binary people's distress and experiences of victimization. PLoS One 16(3):e0248970, 2021 33740032

Gamarel KE, Jadwin-Cakmak L, King WM, et al: Stigma experienced by transgender women of color in their dating and romantic relationships: implications for gender-based violence prevention programs. J Interpers Violence 37(9–10):NP8161–NP8189, 2022 33256510

Gleason HA, Livingston NA, Peters MM, et al: Effects of state nondiscrimination laws on transgender and gender-nonconforming individuals' perceived community stigma and mental health. J Gay Lesbian Ment Health 20(4):350–362, 2016

Goldberg AE, Kuvalanka K, dickey l: Transgender graduate students' experiences in higher education: a mixed-methods exploratory study. J Divers High Educ 12(1):38–51, 2019

Hatzenbuehler ML: Structural stigma: research evidence and implications for psychological science. Am Psychol 71(8):742–751, 2016 27977256

Hendricks ML, Testa RJ: A conceptual framework for clinical work with transgender and gender nonconforming clients: an adaptation of the Minority Stress Model. Prof Psychol Res Pr 43(5):460–467, 2012

Human Rights Campaign: Fatal violence against the transgender and gender nonconforming community in 2021. HRC, 2021. https://www.hrc.org/resources/fatal-violence-against-the-transgender-and-gender-non-conforming-community-in-2021. Accessed July 17, 2023.

Jäggi T, Jellestad L, Corbisiero S, et al: Gender minority stress and depressive symptoms in transitioned Swiss transpersons. BioMed Res Int 2018:8639263, 2018 29850581

James SE, Herman JL, Rankin S, et al: The Report of the 2015 U.S. Transgender Survey. Washington, DC, National Center for Transgender Equality, 2016. Available at: https://transequality.org/sites/default/files/docs/usts/USTS-Full-Report-Dec17.pdf. Accessed June 25, 2023.

Johnson AH: Transnormativity: a new concept and its validation through documentary film about transgender men. Sociol Inq 86(4):465–491, 2016

Johnson KC, LeBlanc AJ, Deardorff J, Bockting WO: Invalidation experiences among non-binary adolescents. J Sex Res 57(2):222–233, 2020 31070487

Kattari SK, Begun S: On the margins of marginalized: transgender homelessness and survival sex. Affilia 32(1):92–103, 2017

Katz-Wise SL, Godwin EG, Parsa N, et al: Using family and ecological systems approaches to conceptualize family and community-based experiences of transgender and/or nonbinary youth from the Trans Teen and Family Narratives Project. Psychol Sex Orientat Gend Divers 9(1):21–36, 2022 35755166

Klein A, Golub SA: Family rejection as a predictor of suicide attempts and substance misuse among transgender and gender nonconforming adults. LGBT Health 3(3):193–199, 2016 27046450

Lefevor GT, Boyd-Rogers CC, Sprague BM, Janis RA: Health disparities between genderqueer, transgender, and cisgender individuals: an extension of minority stress theory. J Couns Psychol 66(4):385–395, 2019 30896208

Lindley L, Galupo MP: Gender dysphoria and minority stress: support for inclusion of gender dysphoria as a proximal stressor. Psychol Sex Orientat Gend Divers 7(3):265–275, 2020

Martinez LR, Sawyer KB, Thoroughgood CN, et al: The importance of being "me": the relation between authentic identity expression and transgender employees' work-related attitudes and experiences. J Appl Psychol 102(2):215–226, 2017 27786497

Matsuno E, Israel T: Psychological interventions promoting resilience among transgender individuals: transgender resilience intervention model (TRIM). Couns Psychol 46(5):632–655, 2018

Matsuno E, Balsam KF, Bricker NL, Savarese E: The Enby Project: understanding minority stress and resilience among nonbinary people, in Gender Out of the Box: New Directions in Research With Nonbinary Populations (symposium). Chaired by Balsam KF. Presented at the annual convention of the American Psychological Association, online, August 2021

McLemore KA: A minority stress perspective on transgender individuals' experiences with misgendering. Stigma Health 3(1):53–64, 2018

McNeil J, Ellis SJ, Eccles FJR: Suicide in trans populations: a systematic review of prevalence and correlates. Psychol Sex Orientat Gend Divers 4(3):341–353, 2017

Meyer IH: Prejudice, social stress, and mental health in lesbian, gay, and bisexual populations: conceptual issues and research evidence. Psychol Bull 129(5):674–697, 2003 12956539

Millar K, Brooks CV: Double jeopardy: Minority stress and the influence of transgender identity and race/ethnicity. Int J Transgender Health 23(1-2):133–148, 2021 35403114

Murad MH, Elamin MB, Garcia MZ, et al: Hormonal therapy and sex reassignment: a systematic review and meta-analysis of quality of life and psychosocial outcomes. Clin Endocrinol (Oxf) 72(2):214–231, 2010 19473181

Nicolazzo Z: "Just go in looking good": the resilience, resistance, and kinship-building of trans* college students. J Coll Student Dev 57(5):538–556, 2016

Parr NJ, Howe BG: Heterogeneity of transgender identity nonaffirmation microaggressions and their association with depression symptoms and suicidality among transgender persons. Psychol Sex Orientat Gend Divers 6(4):461–474, 2019

Price SF, Puckett JA, Mocarski R: The impact of the 2016 presidential elections on transgender and gender diverse people. Sex Res Soc Policy 18(4):1094–1103, 2021 34925634

Puckett JA: An ecological approach to therapy with gender minorities. Cognit Behav Pract 26(4):647–655, 2019

Puckett JA, Levitt HM: Internalized stigma within sexual and gender minorities: change strategies and clinical implications. J LGBT Issues Couns 9(4):329–349, 2015

Puckett JA, Cleary P, Rossman K, et al: Barriers to gender-affirming care for transgender and gender nonconforming individuals. Sex Res Soc Policy 15(1):48–59, 2018 29527241

Puckett JA, Matsuno E, Dyar C, et al: Mental health and resilience in transgender individuals: what type of support makes a difference? J Fam Psychol 33(8):954–964, 2019 31318262

Puckett JA, Aboussouan AB, Ralston AL, et al: Systems of cissexism and the daily production of stress for transgender and gender diverse people. Int J Transgender Health 24(1):113–126, 2021 36713141

Reisner SL, White Hughto JM, Gamarel KE, et al: Discriminatory experiences associated with posttraumatic stress disorder symptoms among transgender adults. J Couns Psychol 63(5):509–519, 2016 26866637

Rood BA, Reisner SL, Surace FI, et al: Expecting rejection: understanding the minority stress experiences of transgender and gender-nonconforming individuals. Transgend Health 1(1):151–164, 2016 29159306

Rood BA, Maroney MR, Puckett JA, et al: Identity concealment in transgender adults: a qualitative assessment of minority stress and gender affirmation. Am J Orthopsychiatry 87(6):704–713, 2017a 29154610

Rood BA, Reisner SL, Puckett JA, et al: Internalized transphobia: exploring perceptions of social messages in transgender and gender-nonconforming adults. Int J Transgend 18(4):411–426, 2017b

Scandurra C, Amodeo AL, Valerio P, et al: Minority stress, resilience, and mental health: a study of Italian transgender people. J Soc Issues 73(3):563–585, 2017

Scandurra C, Bochicchio V, Amodeo AL, et al: Internalized transphobia, resilience, and mental health: applying the psychological mediation framework to Italian transgender individuals. Int J Environ Res Public Health 15(3):508, 2018 29534023

Schulz SL: The informed consent model of transgender care: an alternative to the diagnosis of gender dysphoria. J Humanist Psychol 58(1):72–92, 2018

Serano J: Psychology, sexualization and trans-invalidations. Presented at the 8th Annual Philadelphia Trans-Health Conference, 2009. Available at: https://www.juliaserano.com/av/Serano-TransInvalidations.pdf. Accessed June 25, 2023.

Shelton J, Wagaman MA, Small L, Abramovich A: I'm more driven now: resilience and resistance among transgender and gender expansive youth and young adults experiencing homelessness. Int J Transgend 19(2):144–157, 2018

Simons L, Schrager SM, Clark LF, et al: Parental support and mental health among transgender adolescents. J Adolesc Health 53(6):791–793, 2013 24012067

Singh AA: Transgender youth of color and resilience: negotiating oppression and finding support. Sex Roles 68:690–702, 2013

Singh AA, Mckleroy VS: "Just getting out of bed is a revolutionary act": the resilience of transgender people of color who have survived traumatic life events. Traumatology 17(2):34–44, 2011

Singh AA, Hays DG, Watson LS: Strength in the face of adversity: resilience strategies of transgender individuals. J Couns Dev 89(1):20–27, 2011

Singh AA, Meng SE, Hansen AW: "I am my own gender": resilience strategies of trans youth. J Couns Dev 92(2):208–218, 2014

Smith E, Pössel P: Exploring the relation between adolescents' number of perceived reasons for discrimination and depressive symptoms. Res Child Adolesc Psychopathol 50(4):549–560, 2022 34633601

Sonoma S: Guide for Media Covering State Legislation Targeting LGBTQ People. New York, GLAAD, 2022. Available at: https://www.glaad.org/blog/guide-media-covering-state-legislation-targeting-lgbtq-people. Accessed June 25, 2023.

Testa RJ, Habarth J, Peta J, et al: Development of the Gender Minority Stress and Resilience measure. Psychol Sex Orientat Gend Divers 2(1):65–77, 2015

Testa RJ, Michaels MS, Bliss W, et al: Suicidal ideation in transgender people: gender minority stress and interpersonal theory factors. J Abnorm Psychol 126(1):125–136, 2017 27831708

Thoma BC, Salk RH, Choukas-Bradley S, et al: Suicidality disparities between transgender and cisgender adolescents. Pediatrics 144(5):e20191183, 2019 31611339

Valentine SE, Shipherd JC: A systematic review of social stress and mental health among transgender and gender non-conforming people in the United States. Clin Psychol Rev 66:24–38, 2018 29627104

White Hughto JM, Reisner SL: A systematic review of the effects of hormone therapy on psychological functioning and quality of life in transgender individuals. Transgend Health 1(1):21–31, 2016 27595141

White Hughto JM, Reisner SL, Pachankis JE: Transgender stigma and health: a critical review of stigma determinants, mechanisms, and interventions. Soc Sci Med 147:222–231, 2015 26599625

Wirtz AL, Poteat TC, Malik M, Glass N: Gender-based violence against transgender people in the United States: a call for research and programming. Trauma Violence Abuse 21(2):227–241, 2020 29439615

Yerke AF, DeFeo J: Redefining intimate partner violence beyond the binary to include transgender people. J Fam Violence 31(8):975–979, 2016

CHAPTER 3

(Rethinking) the Neuroscience of Gender Identity

Simón(e) Sun, Ph.D.
Teddy G. Goetz, M.D., M.S.
Kristen Eckstrand, M.D., Ph.D.

WHEN considering the role of psychiatry and mental health in the provision of mental health care for transgender, non-binary, and/or gender-expansive (TNG) individuals, it is natural to wonder what role the brain may play and what clues neuroscience may offer. For some, this interest may be driven by questions of "what makes me, me?"; others may wonder about how to harness the incredible power of the brain to address the mental health disparities plaguing TNG communities.

Despite its vast implications, the intersection between gender and neuroscience is only recently an area of inquiry, owing to the siloed histories of sex and gender in science, particularly across genetics, endocrinology, neuroscience, and psychiatry. Additionally, the concept of gender is tied to its origin in the psychiatrists and physicians who, when providing gender-affirming care, used gender to isolate psychological variation tied to sexual characteristics and maintain a cisheteronormative binary understanding of sex. In this chapter, we describe the history of the neuroscience of sex and gender, current knowledge within neuroscience about sex and gender, and clinical applications of this knowledge.

Because the neuroscience literature has commonly (and incorrectly) conflated sex and gender (see later section, "The History of Gender in Neuroscience"), we introduce the following framework and approach, informed by numerous studies and commentaries (Figure 3–1) (Eliot and Richardson 2016; Fausto-Sterling 2019; Holmes and Monks 2019; Hyde et al. 2019; Llaveria Caselles 2021; Maney 2016; Miyagi et al. 2021).

1. *Sex* refers to biological components of an individual directly involved in sexual reproduction and the development thereof. Terms such as *female, intersex*, and *male* are used to describe characteristics of an individual—not individuals themselves. When referring to the sexual categorization of an individual, sex assigned at birth (male, female, intersex) is presumed.

2. *Gender/sex* refers to physiological and psychological aspects of an individual that are not directly related to but nonetheless are dependent on, interact with, or are influenced by sexual reproduction and its development. This aligns with a fieldwide shift toward precise language to distinguish when a phenomenon of study cannot be exclusively tied to either biological or sociological origin (Fausto-Sterling 2012; Kaiser et al. 2007; van Anders and Dunn 2009). Many studies that report sex differences in the brain are in this domain. Thus, we use *gender/sex* instead of *sex* when interpreting such findings. For example, a report on sex variability in a particular neuroanatomical region is referred to as a *gender/sex difference*. Terms such as *masculine, androgynous, ambiguous*, and *feminine* are used to describe gender/sex characteristics.

3. *Gender* refers to psychosocial and sociocultural aspects of an individual and their environment that relate to the perception by and of that individual as belonging to a sociocultural category with expected sex-, gender/sex-, and gender-related characteristics. As it is a unique aspect to human culture, the study of gender in animal models is inappropriate and inaccurate. Animal research that purports to study gender is relegated to category 2, gender/sex. Terms such as *non-binary, agender, man*, and *woman* are used to describe genders and their characteristics.

This framework recenters the question "what is the neuroscience of gender?" from unidimensional and static neuroanatomical correlations to the nonlinear interactions between biological, psychological, and sociological mechanisms at work (Llaveria Caselles 2021). It emphasizes the importance of the contextual dependence of sex labels (male, female, intersex) (Richardson 2022). In their scientific, medical, and cultural usage, these labels are often assigned based on one variable (e.g., in laboratory rodent studies, animals are often sexed by cursory visual estimation of anogenital distance and external genitalia). This is in contrast to the many biological contributors to sexual traits such as genetic and chromosomal makeup, hormone

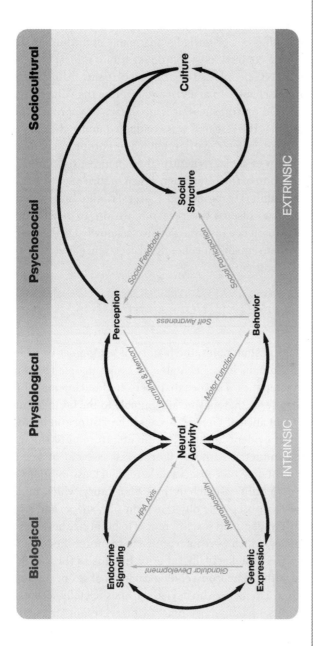

FIGURE 3–1. A framework for understanding the neuroscience of gender.

Schematic illustrating different components of gender (*bold words*) and known interactions between specific components (*black arrows*, indicating directionality). Examples of mechanisms that enable one component to influence another shown with *gray arrows*, indicating directionality. For example, the hypothalamic-pituitary-adrenal (HPA) axis is the site of a mechanism by which neural activity converging at the hypothalamus leads to endocrine changes. This release is in turn able to inhibit or excite neurons that express glucocorticoid receptors (represented by the *bidirectional arrow*). Intrinsic components of gender are represented on the left and extrinsic components on the right, with interactions between intrinsic and extrinsic mechanisms intersecting in the center.

fluctuations, developmental stage, age, environment, and social status. These contributors act as nodes of influence (bold words in Figure 3–1), in which specific mechanisms of study can reveal their influence on sex/gender-related characteristics.

Throughout this chapter, we acknowledge that many of the human studies we describe here were conducted with little regard for ethical considerations when involving TNG people as research participants. Although it is beyond the scope of this chapter to analyze and critique the failures of research programs centered on transness, it is necessary to approach these studies understanding that the research was conducted under the contexts emerging from normative cisheteropatriarchal white European colonialist gender norms. As a form of social structure, these neurosexist and racist norms affect the perception of the researcher, which in turn affects data acquisition and interpretation (Duchesne and Kaiser Trujillo 2021; Schmitz and Höppner 2014). As we discuss this research, we aim to discuss these common pitfalls in neuroscience research yet also acknowledge the significant amount of work that remains to generate neuroscience literature that actually benefits TNG communities.

THE HISTORY OF GENDER IN NEUROSCIENCE

From a phenomenological standpoint, the history of sex/gender in science dates back as long as humans have been able to assign people to groups based on shared characteristics. The idea that there are fundamental differences between (binary) sexes that may be attributable to the brain is found in scientific writing from ancient Greece. Because the distinction between sex and gender was not evident in the scientific literature until the mid-1900s, studies were conducted without rigorous assessment of sex and assuming the existence of only two observable sexes. Such assumptions are evident in early neuroscientific research in the 19th century, which studied the brain based on visibly observable differences in size, shape, and structure. This research falsely identified sex differences in brain size between assumed females and males, which were interpreted to reinforce the societally held belief that males were intellectually superior to females (Broca 1861). This research aligned with the neuropsychological ideas of sex prevailing at the time, according to which males who deviated from societally acceptable behaviors and emotions—particularly males who were not "masculine enough" or who engaged in same-sex relationships—were deemed "sexual inverts" (Ellis 1897). As the groundwork for modern neuroscience was not begun until the 20th century, critical scientific exploration about sex/gender in neuroscience did not occur until the 1950s.

The early 1900s brought advancements to the use of medicine to modify sex characteristics in what is now considered gender-affirming care, but the distinction between sex and gender identity was not described until the 1950s/60s (Stoller 1968). Researchers at the time hypothesized that sex and gender both existed on a binary, but that they were two nonoverlapping categories (Holmes and Monks 2019; Woolley 1910). Similarly, medical providers used the sex/gender distinction to support the emphasis on cisheteronormative outcomes for intersex and transgender individuals seeking care (Gill-Peterson 2018). The result of this siloed biomedical discourse was an emphasis on sex as a product of nature and gender as a product of nurture or culture.

Unfortunately, the consequences of early definitions of sex as a biological variable and gender as a cultural influence affected which construct was deemed "scientific" and thus important to study in neuroscience. As a result, the majority of modern neuroscience has focused entirely on sex differences and sexual dimorphisms, albeit through flawed methodology that assessed neither sex nor gender clearly. Under such persistent neurosexist assumptions in research, neuroanatomists examined animal and human brains, concluding that there are macro- and micro-level sexual dimorphisms (Swaab and Hofman 1984), with the implications of these conclusions persisting today. For example, based on early (unreplicated) findings of differences in brain hemispheric laterality, popular culture pundits mused that men are more "right-brained" and women more "left-brained" to explain differences in emotionality. Despite recent meta-analyses demonstrating that assumed sex accounts for < 1% of the variation in the brain (Eliot et al. 2021), one need only look to contemporary culture to find hundreds of books and articles falsely explaining, and reinforcing, binary social gender assumptions through poorly sourced neuroanatomical studies.

Although much of the fanfare over sexual dimorphisms is unwarranted, there are notable sexual dimorphisms in the brain, and beginning in the 1980s, these regions became the key focus for identifying the etiology of TNG identities. In contrast to emerging social and philosophical theories of the time suggesting that gender is not binary (Butler 1990), neuroscience applied century-old hypotheses of sexual inversion to develop the "cross-sex shift hypothesis" of the brain. Under this antiquated hypothesis, brains exposed to various factors (e.g., genetics, prenatal hormones) could develop to become more "male-like" or "female-like," and these cross-sex shifts were supposed to explain why someone assigned one sex at birth may have an incongruent gender (Swaab et al. 2021) or even exhibit same-sex sexual behavior (Abé et al. 2021).

After nearly 30 years of neuroscience research, such ideas persist today in the scientific literature across domains of sexual orientation, gender identity, and gender expression (Abé et al. 2021; Folkierska-Żukowska et al. 2020; Garcia-Sifuentes and Maney 2021) despite small samples, small effect sizes, failure to replicate effects in larger samples (Ganna et al. 2019; Lambert 2019), and repeated calls for methodological improvements and reconsiderations (Clayton and Tannenbaum 2016; Miyagi et al. 2021; Woitowich and Woodruff 2019). Essentialist assumptions regarding the etiology of gender identity have led to overinterpretation of results, including attempts to use research to describe negative health trends in lesbian, gay, bisexual, transgender, queer, intersex, asexual, and more (LGBTQIA+) populations (Li et al. 2021). These conclusions are incompatible with data demonstrating that adequate social support and gender affirmation results in significant improvements in the mental health of TNG people (Colizzi et al. 2013; Durwood et al. 2017; Nobili et al. 2018).

The history of gender in neuroscience has not yet led to appreciable benefits for TNG communities, but there is now a robust evidence base debunking a singular neural theory for sex, gender expression, or gender identity. Such evidence continues to support sex and gender as having complex, multifactorial, individual characteristics that are not amenable to simple explanation. Further, based on the lack of meaningful findings from the last 150 years, one could argue that the primary lesson we have learned from neuroscience is that continued application of binary assumptions of sex and gender in neuroscience will be exceedingly unlikely to lead to scientific advancement for people of any gender, much less those who are TNG (Aghi et al. 2022).

A NEUROSCIENCE OF GENDER: INTEGRATING NEUROENDOCRINOLOGY

With these considerations in mind, the overlap of different conditions relating to gender and sex in transgender and intersex populations suggests that two particular biological and physiological factors—genes and hormones—significantly contribute to an individual's sense of gender.

The prevalence of gender dysphoria in intersex individuals is on average higher than in the general population. Importantly, intersex individuals with alterations in genes encoding for hormone steroidogenesis (5α-reductase deficiency and 17β-hydroxysteroid dehydrogenase deficiency) have among the highest incidence of gender dysphoria (Babu and Shah 2021; Furtado et al. 2012). Conversely, transgender persons who have sought medical treatments for gender dysphoria are more likely to have atypical karyotypes (chromosomal profiles), with differences presenting in both sex chromosomes and autosomes (Inoubli et al. 2011). Recent studies have found preliminary evidence that transgender individuals have genetic variants in genes related to hormone signaling, including hormone receptors, steroidogenesis enzymes, and related cofactors (Fernández et al. 2020; Foreman et al. 2019; Theisen et al. 2019); however, the replicability of these data remains to be seen. Nevertheless, these preliminary findings, in conjunction with the success of gender-affirming hormone therapy (GAHT) for TNG populations (Aghi et al. 2022), suggest that intrinsic physiological aspects of gender/sex (Figure 3–1, left section) emerge in part from the interaction of steroid hormones, gene expression, and neural circuitry in the brain.

A large proportion of gender/sex characteristics in the brain are established and regulated by the "gonadal" or "sex" hormones: the estrogens (estrone, estradiol, estriol), progesterone, and testosterone. All derived from cholesterol, steroid hormones circulate in the bloodstream and can freely cross the blood–brain barrier. Primarily produced by gonads, adrenal cortex, and placenta, they are also synthesized locally in the brain (Do Rego et al. 2009). The extent to which neuronally synthesized hormones contribute to neurological development, differentiation, and function is still underexplored. Several populations of neurons also express aromatase and locally convert circulating and neuron-synthesized testosterone into estrogen to mediate their effects (Naftolin and Ryan 1975). Some prohormones are found at much higher levels in the brain than in the plasma (Corpéchot et al. 1981; Ebner et al. 2006; Labrie et al. 2005), and the steroidogenic enzymes or their mRNAs have been found in both neurons and glial cells in various brain regions (Do Rego et al. 2009).

Steroidal hormones are ligands that readily pass through cellular and nuclear membranes. Each hormone has a set of receptors that it can bind to, each encoded by its own gene: estrogens bind to estrogen receptor alpha (ERα, encoded by *Esr1*) and/or beta (ERβ, encoded by *Esr2*), progesterone to progesterone receptor (PR, encoded by *Pgr*), and testosterone to androgen receptor (AR, encoded by *Ar*). Thus, the expression of these nuclear receptors determines whether a brain region can respond to the presence of its corresponding hormone.

When a hormone-receptor complex is formed, it acts as a transcription factor to regulate the expression of target genes. The hormone-receptor complex interacts with other nuclear receptor coregulators (Sun and Xu 2020) and transcriptional machinery that bind directly to DNA at specific nucleotide sequences called *response elements*: estrogen-ERα/ERβ at estrogen response element (ERE) and testosterone-AR at androgen response element (ARE). Testosterone can also bind to glucocorticoid response elements (GREs), which typically are bound by corticosteroids. Glucocorticoid receptors can also bind to AREs (Manoli and Tollkuhn 2018). These receptors can also tether to other DNA-binding proteins and can regulate gene expression without interacting directly with the genome. Hormone receptor action through DNA binding is known as *canonical* hormone signaling. *Noncanonical* hormone signaling, the effects of which are only partially understood, is known to occur through pathways that do not involve receptors interacting with DNA or other transcription factors (Davey and Grossmann 2016; Heldring et al. 2007). Because they have similar structures, progesterone is also able to bind to androgen receptors (Bardin et al. 1983) and glucocorticoid receptors (Rupprecht et al. 1993); dihydrotestosterone (DHT) is an even more potent AR agonist than testosterone (Tóth and Zakár 1982).

In addition to binding to DNA, hormone receptors can regulate the epigenome to control gene expression. *Epigenetics* refers to the control of gene expression by molecular changes to DNA and/or its 3D structure, without changing the DNA sequence itself. There are two primary ways in which epigenetic changes can occur: DNA methylation and chromatin remodeling.

DNA methylation involves the addition of a methyl group onto a cytosine nucleotide that is upstream of a guanine to activate or repress gene expression. In the brain, DNA methylation is mediated by DNA methyltransferases.

Epigenetic control also occurs through *chromatin remodeling*. Chromatin is a mixture of DNA and proteins that form chromosomes. DNA wraps around proteins known as histones, forming units of chromatin known as *nucleosomes*. The accessibility of chromatin controls whether a gene can be expressed. *Heterochromatin*, tightly packed chromatin, prevents gene expression machinery from accessing genes. In contrast, *euchromatin* is open and loosely packed, exposing DNA sites for gene expression machinery to bind to and initiate gene transcription. Control of chromatin accessibility occurs through posttranslational modifications (PTMs) to histone proteins, which affect the electrostatic interactions between DNA and histones. PTMs such as acetylation, methylation, and phosphorylation dynamically change in response to neural activity.

It is hypothesized that sex differentiation of neural tissue is mediated by permanent epigenomic effects of perinatal hormonal surges. Indeed, several studies have identified genes that are differentially expressed by sex (Kurian et al. 2010; Nugent and McCarthy 2011; Westberry et al. 2010), as well as genomewide sex variability (Ghahramani et al. 2014; Nugent et al. 2015). These results, along with recent work identifying neuronal gene regulation by ERα (Gegenhuber et al. 2022), illustrate the dynamic nature of epigenetic regulation by hormones, suggesting that some aspects of early life organization are not completely permanent. The functional consequences of hormonal regulation of gene expression, as well as hormonal alterations to the activity of neural networks, remain poorly understood.

Contemporary understanding of the pattern and development of gonadal hormone receptor expression in the mammalian central nervous system is incomplete. Postmortem human tissue studies have revealed the presence of hormone receptors in the brain; studies in animals, particularly rodents, have provided a map of neuronal hormone receptor expression at a relatively high spatiotemporal resolution. The four canonical gonadal hormone receptors—ERα, ERβ, PR, and AR—are highly expressed in the limbic system—medial amygdala, bed nucleus of the stria terminalis, medial preoptic area of the hypothalamus, and ventromedial hypothalamus—irrespective of gonadal or chromosomal sex, although there is notable sex variability. These brain areas are core components of numerous neural circuits that mediate reproductive, territorial, aggressive, parenting, and social behaviors, commonly referred to as the social behavior network (Li and Dulac 2018; Newman 1999; Petrulis et al. 2017; Wei et al. 2021). The broadly successful outcomes of combined social and medical gender affirmation suggest that these regions mediate important components of gender identity.

ERα, AR, and PR mediate feeding and energy homeostasis (Mauvais-Jarvis et al. 2013), and are found in the arcuate nucleus as well as in the midbrain regions such as the periaqueductal gray, raphe nucleus, substantia nigra, and ventral tegmental areas (Creutz and Kritzer 2004; Mitra et al. 2003; Purves-Tyson et al. 2012; Quadros et al. 2008; Quesada et al. 2007; Shughrue et al. 1997). These receptors are also found in the neocortex (important for sensory processing, motor execution, and cognitive functions) and the hippocampus (involved in learning and memory) (Cara et al. 2021; Mitra et al. 2003; Nuñez et al. 2003; Sar et al. 1990; Shughrue et al. 1997). Individual neurons can express varying combinations of receptors.

Hormone receptor expression is known to change with age, which further complicates understanding the implications of spatiotemporal distribution. The mechanisms by which gonadal hormones act on the brain have been explored primarily in the context of how long-lasting neurobehavioral sex differences develop. The earliest of these experiments, reported by Phoenix and colleagues in 1959, demonstrated that testosterone administration to pregnant guinea pigs resulted in a reduction in female-typical sexual behavior (lordosis) and an increase in male-typical sexual behavior (mounting) in female offspring (Phoenix et al. 1959). Based on their results, they proposed the Organization-Activation Model (OAM) of hormone-mediated neurobehavioral sex differentiation. The OAM posits that hormones sexually differentiate behaviors by permanently organizing brain tissue during early critical periods of development; in adulthood, these hormones play an activating role on the differentiated brain, resulting in sex variability of behavior. Since then, similar results have been reported in mice, rats, nonhuman primates, and humans, mediated by prenatal or perinatal exposure to androgens (or in the case of rodents, estrogens by way of aromatization of testosterone) (Hines 2011; McCarthy et al. 2009).

This research is broadly related to gender, but the attempts to translate such theories for TNG and intersex health care (Diamond 2009; Guillamon et al. 2016; Shirazi et al. 2020; Zucker et al. 1996) have been detrimental and exploitative to the very populations purported to benefit from the work (Colapinto 2006; Gill-Peterson 2018). Additionally, the OAM cannot capture changes outside development and the continual necessity of gonadal hormones to maintain sexual differentiation (Gegenhuber et al. 2022; Knoedler et al. 2022), which makes necessary a more refined dynamic model of neuroendocrine function to untangle the neurological mechanisms related to gender.

CONCLUSION: WHAT DOES THIS MEAN FOR PSYCHIATRY IN PRACTICE?

Even in a test tube, gender is messy! Considering real patients, in all of their life experiences, only underscores this messiness. Thus, in the final portion of the chapter, we ask you to think about gender with intentionality, as a multidimensional factor for each of your patients.

• *Hormonal milieu:* How does your patient's dominant hormonal milieu influence their evidence-informed psychiatric care? How would initiating or ceasing GAHT change treatment?

• *Societal (il)legibility and associated stress:* When and how does your patient experience minority stress related to their gender? Expressing their gender presentation at home, with roommates, with family, at work, walking down the street? Seeking a legal name or gender marker change? Seeking medical care? How is their societal legibility changing over time? How can these answers guide psychotherapy interventions?

• *Gender dysphoria and its impact on psychiatric diagnoses:* If applicable, how is your patient's gender dysphoria affecting their mental health? How can you work within an interdisciplinary treatment paradigm to best support gender-affirming care, in conjunction with psychiatric interventions? (See Chapters 4, 15, and 21 for information on psychopharmacology, eating disorders, and surgery evaluations.)

• *History of trauma and microtraumas:* What kinds of traumas and microtraumas has your patient experienced and do they currently experience? How do these stressors affect their psychiatric illness? How can this knowledge, along with hormonal milieu, inform their treatment?

All of these experiences affect the brain on multiple levels—genetics, neural connectivity, neural activity—and all are intrinsically rooted in the way that a patient experiences their gender within society. This means that when we are making psychopharmacological decisions for patients, we should be thinking about how to best work responsively with regard to all layers of a patient's gender, including their gender-affirming health care and the ways in which minority stress might be impeding the molecular actions of the drugs we prescribe (see Chapters 2 and 11 for information on minority stress and trauma). During psychotherapy with a patient, we must keep in mind both how their hormonal milieu may influence their neurotransmitter functioning and how their anxiety about their gendered legibility might be distracting them and preventing them from engaging fully with the therapy process, or from forming memories and making connections as you would typically expect from such an interaction.

Most of these clinical considerations, while intuitive, remain hypothetical in the sense that historically, research time, funding, and resources have not been devoted to exploring how to provide equitable mental health care for all genders. We imagine the potential power of future clinical trials focused on developing drugs that work synergistically with a specific hormonal milieu, designed for and tested in TNG patients. We hope that the discussion in this chapter inspires future work to advance equity and justice in pharmacotherapy.

Recognizing this profound opportunity for future research—rethinking the neuroscience of gender identity and how to apply it to psychiatric care for TNG patients—we propose a few particular areas in which we hope to see the research literature expand over the next few years (for more specific discussion, please see Aghi et al. 2022):

- *Impact of hormonal milieu on affect and behavior:* Because estrogens, androgens, and progestogens cross the blood–brain barrier and have receptor targets present in the central nervous system, absolute and relative hormonal levels likely affect mood, arousal, and responses to stimuli. This area of research would be fruitful for better predicting affective and behavioral changes associated with GAHT, beyond the psychological impact of greater congruence between self-understanding and embodiment (Hughto et al. 2020; Murad et al. 2010). These areas should also be studied for individuals who undergo pubertal blockade to halt endogenous puberty before initiating GAHT.
- *Possibilities of modulating GAHT outcomes:* Gender-affirming care is far from one-size-fits-all (e.g., Beek et al. 2015), and GAHT is capable of driving a variety of embodied changes, some desired by an individual and others adamantly unwanted. Methods for modulating specific hormonal effects through more selective hormone therapy and/or neuromodulation mechanisms have the potential to revolutionize GAHT and

allow TNG people to more directly pursue their affirmation goals and seek gender euphoria.

- *Impact of dominant hormonal milieu on psychiatric medication efficacy:* In light of the receptor distribution for estrogens, androgens, and progestogens in the brain, it is possible (perhaps likely) that psychiatric medication efficacy may be modulated by the hormonal environment. Some medications may be more likely to achieve the clinically desired results for certain individuals, based on their hormonal milieu, and the success of these medications may change over time. Research on differential responses to psychiatric medications between groups stratified by dominant hormonal milieu may offer improved guidelines for first-line medication selection on an individual basis.

- *Impact of chronic stress from gender-related micro- and macroaggressions on neurochemistry, psychiatric illness, and response to mental health treatment:* Physiological and psychological impacts of chronic stress are well characterized (Agorastos and Chrousos 2022), and TNG people are subject to elevated levels of chronic stress because of marginalization related to gender identity and gender modality (see Chapters 2 and 11 for information on minority stress and trauma). Accordingly, experiences of discrimination and harassment may affect neurochemistry and mental health, as well as how an individual responds to a given treatment. Such areas warrant further investigation.

- *Impact of gender-affirming surgery on neurochemistry, psychiatric illness, and response to mental health treatment:* As discussed earlier, exposure to chronic stressors is known to increase risk of psychiatric illness; a chronic sense of incongruent embodiment could qualify as such a stimulus. Indeed, improvements in mood, anxiety, and suicidality have been demonstrated following gender-affirming surgery (e.g., Akhavan et al. 2021; Hughto et al. 2020). This effect may be mediated by induced alterations in neurochemistry, which could even change how an individual responds to specific medications. These areas have not yet been explored.

REFERENCES

Abé C, Lebedev A, Zhang R, et al: Cross-sex shifts in two brain imaging phenotypes and their relation to polygenic scores for same-sex sexual behavior: a study of 18,645 individuals from the UK Biobank. Hum Brain Mapp 42(7):2292–2304, 2021 33635603

Aghi K, Goetz TG, Pfau DR, et al: Centering the needs of transgender, nonbinary, and gender-diverse populations in neuroendocrine models of gender-affirming hormone therapy. Biol Psychiatry Cogn Neurosci Neuroimaging 7(12):1268–1279, 2022 35863692

Agorastos A, Chrousos GP: The neuroendocrinology of stress: the stress-related continuum of chronic disease development. Mol Psychiatry 27(1):502–513, 2022 34290370

Akhavan AA, Sandhu S, Ndem I, Ogunleye AA: A review of gender affirmation surgery: what we know, and what we need to know. Surgery 170(1):336–340, 2021 33741180

Babu R, Shah U: Gender identity disorder (GID) in adolescents and adults with differences of sex development (DSD): a systematic review and meta-analysis. J Pediatr Urol 17(1):39–47, 2021 33246831

Bardin CW, Brown T, Isomaa VV, Jänne OA: Progestins can mimic, inhibit and potentiate the actions of androgens. Pharmacol Ther 23(3):443–459, 1983 6371845

Beek TF, Kreukels BPC, Cohen-Kettenis PT, Steensma TD: Partial treatment requests and underlying motives of applicants for gender affirming interventions. J Sex Med 12(11):2201–2205, 2015 26553507

Broca P: Sur le volume et la forme du cerveau suivant les individus et suivant les races. Bull Soc Anthropol 2:139–204, 1861

Butler J: Gender Trouble: Feminism and the Subversion of Identity. Abingdon, UK, Routledge, 1990

Cara AL, Henson EL, Beekly BG, Elias CF: Distribution of androgen receptor mRNA in the prepubertal male and female mouse brain. J Neuroendocrinol 33(12):e13063, 2021 34866263

Clayton JA, Tannenbaum C: Reporting sex, gender, or both in clinical research? JAMA 316(18):1863–1864, 2016 27802482

Colapinto J: As Nature Made Him: The Boy Who Was Raised as a Girl, 2nd Edition. New York, Harper Perennial, 2006

Colizzi M, Costa R, Pace V, Todarello O: Hormonal treatment reduces psychobiological distress in gender identity disorder, independently of the attachment style. J Sex Med 10(12):3049–3058, 2013 23574768

Corpéchot C, Robel P, Axelson M, et al: Characterization and measurement of dehydroepiandrosterone sulfate in rat brain. Proc Natl Acad Sci USA 78(8):4704–4707, 1981 6458035

Creutz LM, Kritzer MF: Mesostriatal and mesolimbic projections of midbrain neurons immunoreactive for estrogen receptor beta or androgen receptors in rats. J Comp Neurol 476(4):348–362, 2004 15282710

Davey RA, Grossmann M: Androgen receptor structure, function and biology: from bench to bedside. Clin Biochem Rev 37(1):3–15, 2016 27057074

Diamond M: Clinical implications of the organizational and activational effects of hormones. Horm Behav 55(5):621–632, 2009 19446079

Do Rego JL, Seong JY, Burel D, et al: Neurosteroid biosynthesis: enzymatic pathways and neuroendocrine regulation by neurotransmitters and neuropeptides. Front Neuroendocrinol 30(3):259–301, 2009 19505496

Duchesne A, Kaiser Trujillo A: Reflections on neurofeminism and intersectionality using insights from psychology. Front Hum Neurosci 15:684412, 2021 34658813

Durwood L, McLaughlin KA, Olson KR: Mental health and self-worth in socially transitioned transgender youth. J Am Acad Child Adolesc Psychiatry 56(2):116–123.e2, 2017 28117057

Ebner MJ, Corol DI, Havlíková H, et al: Identification of neuroactive steroids and their precursors and metabolites in adult male rat brain. Endocrinology 147(1):179–190, 2006 16223859

Eliot L, Richardson SS: Sex in context: limitations of animal studies for addressing human sex/gender neurobehavioral health disparities. J Neurosci 36(47):11823–11830, 2016 27881769

Eliot L, Ahmed A, Khan H, Patel J: Dump the "dimorphism": comprehensive synthesis of human brain studies reveals few male-female differences beyond size. Neurosci Biobehav Rev 125:667–697, 2021 33621637

Ellis H: Studies in the Psychology of Sex, Vol I: Sexual Inversion. Watford, UK, University Press, 1897

Fausto-Sterling A: Sex/Gender: Biology in a Social World. Abingdon, UK, Routledge, 2012

Fausto-Sterling A: Gender/sex, sexual orientation, and identity are in the body: how did they get there? J Sex Res 56(4-5):529–555, 2019 30875248

Fernández R, Delgado-Zayas E, Ramírez K, et al: Analysis of four polymorphisms located at the promoter of the estrogen receptor alpha ESR1 gene in a population with gender incongruence. Sex Med 8(3):490–500, 2020 32409288

Folkierska-Żukowska M, Rahman Q, Marchewka A, et al: Male sexual orientation, gender nonconformity, and neural activity during mental rotations: an fMRI study. Sci Rep 10(1):18709, 2020 33127919

Foreman M, Hare L, York K, et al: Genetic link between gender dysphoria and sex hormone signaling. J Clin Endocrinol Metab 104(2):390–396, 2019 30247609

Furtado PS, Moraes F, Lago R, et al: Gender dysphoria associated with disorders of sex development. Nat Rev Urol 9(11):620–627, 2012 23045263

Ganna A, Verweij KJH, Nivard MG, et al; 23andMe Research Team: Large-scale GWAS reveals insights into the genetic architecture of same-sex sexual behavior. Science 365(6456):eaat7693, 2019 31467194

Garcia-Sifuentes Y, Maney DL: Reporting and misreporting of sex differences in the biological sciences. eLife 10:e70817, 2021 34726154

Gegenhuber B, Wu MV, Bronstein R, Tollkuhn J: Gene regulation by gonadal hormone receptors underlies brain sex differences. Nature 606(7912):153–159, 2022 35508660

Ghahramani NM, Ngun TC, Chen P-Y, et al: The effects of perinatal testosterone exposure on the DNA methylome of the mouse brain are late-emerging. Biol Sex Differ 5(1):8, 2014 24976947

Gill-Peterson J: Histories of the Transgender Child. Minneapolis, MN, University of Minnesota Press, 2018

Guillamon A, Junque C, Gómez-Gil E: A review of the status of brain structure research in transsexualism. Arch Sex Behav 45(7):1615–1648, 2016 27255307

Heldring N, Pike A, Andersson S, et al: Estrogen receptors: how do they signal and what are their targets. Physiol Rev 87(3):905–931, 2007 17615392

Hines M: Gender development and the human brain. Annu Rev Neurosci 34:69–88, 2011 21438685

Holmes MM, Monks DA: Bridging sex and gender in neuroscience by shedding a priori assumptions of causality. Front Neurosci 13:475, 2019 31143099

Hughto JMW, Gunn HA, Rood BA, Pantalone DW: Social and medical gender affirmation experiences are inversely associated with mental health problems in a U.S. non-probability sample of transgender adults. Arch Sex Behav 49(7):2635–2647, 2020 32215775

Hyde JS, Bigler RS, Joel D, et al: The future of sex and gender in psychology: five challenges to the gender binary. Am Psychol 74(2):171–193, 2019 30024214

Inoubli A, De Cuypere G, Rubens R, et al: Karyotyping, is it worthwhile in transsexualism? J Sex Med 8(2):475–478, 2011 21114769

Kaiser A, Kuenzli E, Zappatore D, Nitsch C: On females' lateral and males' bilateral activation during language production: a fMRI study. Int J Psychophysiol 63(2):192–198, 2007 16797758

Knoedler JR, Inoue S, Bayless DW, et al: A functional cellular framework for sex and estrous cycle-dependent gene expression and behavior. Cell 185(4):654–671.e22, 2022 35065713

Kurian JR, Olesen KM, Auger AP: Sex differences in epigenetic regulation of the estrogen receptor-alpha promoter within the developing preoptic area. Endocrinology 151(5):2297–2305, 2010 20237133

Labrie F, Luu-The V, Bélanger A, et al: Is dehydroepiandrosterone a hormone? J Endocrinol 187(2):169–196, 2005 16293766

Lambert J: No 'gay gene': Massive study homes in on genetic basis of human sexuality. Nature 573(7772):14–15, 2019 31481774

Li H, Fernández-Guasti A, Xu Y, Swaab D: Sexual orientation, neuropsychiatric disorders and the neurotransmitters involved. Neurosci Biobehav Rev 131:479–488, 2021 34597715

Li Y, Dulac C: Neural coding of sex-specific social information in the mouse brain. Curr Opin Neurobiol 53:120–130, 2018 30059820

Llaveria Caselles E: Epistemic injustice in brain studies of (trans)gender identity. Front Sociol 6:608328, 2021 33869551

Maney DL: Perils and pitfalls of reporting sex differences. PhilosTrans R Soc London Ser B Biol Sci 371(1688):20150119, 2016

Manoli DS, Tollkuhn J: Gene regulatory mechanisms underlying sex differences in brain development and psychiatric disease. Ann NY Acad Sci 1420(1):26–45, 2018

Mauvais-Jarvis F, Clegg DJ, Hevener AL: The role of estrogens in control of energy balance and glucose homeostasis. Endocr Rev 34(3):309–338, 2013 23460719

McCarthy MM, Wright CL, Schwarz JM: New tricks by an old dogma: mechanisms of the Organizational/Activational Hypothesis of steroid-mediated sexual differentiation of brain and behavior. Horm Behav 55(5):655–665, 2009 19682425

Mitra SW, Hoskin E, Yudkovitz J, et al: Immunolocalization of estrogen receptor beta in the mouse brain: comparison with estrogen receptor alpha. Endocrinology 144(5):2055–2067, 2003 12697714

Miyagi M, Guthman EM, Sun SED: Transgender rights rely on inclusive language. Science 374(6575):1568–1569, 2021 34941389

Murad MH, Elamin MB, Garcia MZ, et al: Hormonal therapy and sex reassignment: a systematic review and meta-analysis of quality of life and psychosocial outcomes. Clin Endocrinol (Oxf) 72(2):214–231, 2010 19473181

Naftolin F, Ryan KJ: The metabolism of androgens in central neuroendocrine tissues. J Steroid Biochem 6(6):993–997, 1975 809621

Newman SW: The medial extended amygdala in male reproductive behavior. A node in the mammalian social behavior network. Ann NY Acad Sci 877:242–257, 1999

Nobili A, Glazebrook C, Arcelus J: Quality of life of treatment-seeking transgender adults: a systematic review and meta-analysis. Rev Endocr Metab Disord 19(3):199–220, 2018 30121881

Nugent BM, McCarthy MM: Epigenetic underpinnings of developmental sex differences in the brain. Neuroendocrinology 93(3):150–158, 2011 21411982

Nugent BM, Wright CL, Shetty AC, et al: Brain feminization requires active repression of masculinization via DNA methylation. Nat Neurosci 18(5):690–697, 2015 25821913

Nuñez JL, Huppenbauer CB, McAbee MD, et al: Androgen receptor expression in the developing male and female rat visual and prefrontal cortex. J Neurobiol 56(3):293–302, 2003 12884268

Petrulis A, Fiber JM, Swann JM: The medial amygdala, hormones, pheromones, social behavior network, and mating behavior, in Hormones, Brain and Behavior, 3rd Edition. Edited by Pfaff DW, Joëls M. Cambridge, MA, Academic Press, 2017, pp 329–343

Phoenix CH, Goy RW, Gerall AA, Young WC: Organizing action of prenatally administered testosterone propionate on the tissues mediating mating behavior in the female guinea pig. Endocrinology 65:369–382, 1959 14432658

Purves-Tyson TD, Handelsman DJ, Double KL, et al: Testosterone regulation of sex steroid-related mRNAs and dopamine-related mRNAs in adolescent male rat substantia nigra. BMC Neurosci 13:95, 2012 22867132

Quadros PS, Schlueter LJ, Wagner CK: Distribution of progesterone receptor immunoreactivity in the midbrain and hindbrain of postnatal rats. Dev Neurobiol 68(12):1378–1390, 2008 18712784

Quesada A, Romeo HE, Micevych P: Distribution and localization patterns of estrogen receptor-beta and insulin-like growth factor-1 receptors in neurons and glial cells of the female rat substantia nigra: localization of ERbeta and IGF-1R in substantia nigra. J Comp Neurol 503(1):198–208, 2007 17480015

Richardson SS: Sex contextualism. Philos Theory Pract Biol 14(2), 2022

Rupprecht R, Reul JM, van Steensel B, et al: Pharmacological and functional characterization of human mineralocorticoid and glucocorticoid receptor ligands. Eur J Pharmacol 247(2):145–154, 1993 8282004

Sar M, Lubahn DB, French FS, Wilson EM: Immunohistochemical localization of the androgen receptor in rat and human tissues. Endocrinology 127(6):3180–3186, 1990 1701137

Schmitz S, Höppner G: Neurofeminism and feminist neurosciences: a critical review of contemporary brain research. Front Hum Neurosci 8:546, 2014 25120450

Shirazi TN, Self H, Cantor J, et al: Timing of peripubertal steroid exposure predicts visuospatial cognition in men: evidence from three samples. Horm Behav 121:104712, 2020 32059854

Shughrue PJ, Lane MV, Merchenthaler I: Comparative distribution of estrogen receptor-alpha and -beta mRNA in the rat central nervous system. J Comp Neurol 388(4):507–525, 1997 9388012

Stoller RJ: Sex and Gender: The Development of Masculinity and Femininity. Abingdon, UK, Routledge, 1968

Sun Z, Xu Y: Nuclear receptor coactivators (NCOAs) and corepressors (NCORs) in the brain. Endocrinology 161(8):bqaa083, 2020 32449767

Swaab DF, Hofman MA: Sexual differentiation of the human brain: a historical perspective. Prog Brain Res 61:361–374, 1984 6396708

Swaab DF, Wolff SEC, Bao A-M: Sexual differentiation of the human hypothalamus: relationship to gender identity and sexual orientation. Handb Clin Neurol 181:427–443, 2021 34238476

Theisen JG, Sundaram V, Filchak MS, et al: The use of whole exome sequencing in a cohort of transgender individuals to identify rare genetic variants. Sci Rep 9(1):20099, 2019 31882810

Tóth M, Zakár T: Relative binding affinities of testosterone, 19-nortestosterone and their 5 alpha-reduced derivatives to the androgen receptor and to other androgen-binding proteins: a suggested role of 5 alpha-reductive steroid metabolism in the dissociation of "myotropic" and "androgenic" activities of 19-nortestosterone. J Steroid Biochem 17(6):653–660, 1982 6891012

van Anders SM, Dunn EJ: Are gonadal steroids linked with orgasm perceptions and sexual assertiveness in women and men? Horm Behav 56(2):206–213, 2009 19409392

Wei D, Talwar V, Lin D: Neural circuits of social behaviors: innate yet flexible. Neuron 109(10):1600–1620, 2021 33705708

Westberry JM, Trout AL, Wilson ME: Epigenetic regulation of estrogen receptor alpha gene expression in the mouse cortex during early postnatal development. Endocrinology 151(2):731–740, 2010 19966177

Woitowich NC, Woodruff TK: Opinion: Research community needs to better appreciate the value of sex-based research. Proc Natl Acad Sci USA 116(15):7154–7156, 2019 30971497

Woolley HT: A review of the recent literature on the psychology of sex. Psychol Bull 7(10):335–342, 1910

Zucker KJ, Bradley SJ, Oliver G, et al: Psychosexual development of women with congenital adrenal hyperplasia. Horm Behav 30(4):300–318, 1996 9047259

Psychopharmacological Considerations for Transgender, Non-binary, and/or Gender-Expansive (TNG) People

Hyun-Hee "Heather" Kim, M.D.
Teddy G. Goetz, M.D., M.S.
Victoria Grieve, Pharm.D.

PSYCHIATRIC diagnoses and serious psychological distress are especially common within TNG communities (James et al. 2016; Matsuno and Budge 2017; Reisner et al. 2016b; Rimes et al. 2017; Veale et al. 2017; Wanta et al. 2019), specifically depression and anxiety (Reisner et al. 2016a); substance use disorders (Kidd et al. 2021; Rimes et al. 2017); eating disorders (Jones et al. 2018; Nagata et al. 2020; Sequeira et al. 2017); bipolar disorder, schizophrenia, and obsessive-compulsive disorder (Warrier et al. 2020); self-harm (Rimes et al. 2017); and suicidality (Perez-Brumer et al. 2017; Rimes et al. 2017). TNG communities also experience increased incidence of neurodevelopmental conditions such as autism and ADHD (Warrier et al. 2020). This increased prevalence predominantly results from the psychosocial stressors associated with having to exist within a cisheteronormative society (e.g., Kattari et al. 2019; Kidd et al. 2021; Timmins et al. 2017; Warren et al. 2016), as described by the Minority Stress Model (see Chapter 2, "Stigma and Mental Health Inequities") (e.g., Breslow et al. 2015; Hendricks and Testa 2012; Lefevor et al. 2019; McLemore 2018). Psychiatric care for TNG people with these conditions often includes a combination of psychotherapy and psychopharmacology, integrated with gender-affirming health care. When patients who take psychiatric medications consider starting gender-affirming hormone therapy (GAHT), certain interactions need to be considered. Symptoms of psychiatric illness (including anxiety, depression, suicidality, and disordered eating [Testa et al. 2017]) may significantly improve with initiation of GAHT, but other psychiatric conditions may need direct and concurrent treatment.

We focus on the most commonly used medications, and our recommendations are limited by the current research landscape. Concern for drug interactions and side effects is largely extrapolated from analyzing multiple studies on varied compounds (e.g., estradiol and E2 vs. modified forms) and dosing regimens (e.g., oral, subcutaneous, intramuscular, transdermal), despite their distinct pharmacological activity and risk profiles. Few studies specifically look at medication interactions in TNG persons taking GAHT. As gender-affirming medical care becomes increasingly available, it will become even harder to extrapolate risk (e.g., cardiovascular disease, metabolic disorders, osteoporosis) across this heterogeneous group. We eagerly await more comprehensive research to improve these recommendations.

GONADOTROPIN-RELEASING HORMONE ANALOGS/AGONISTS

Leuprolide and Histrelin

Case Example: Rosie

Rosie is a 10-year-old trans girl with a history of ADHD and gender dysphoria. For 2 years, methylphenidate has been effective for her ADHD. She is well adjusted at home and at school, but she is increasingly worried about her body changing: she is starting to experience pubertal changes and sees the same in her friends. Her endocrinologist recommends starting a puberty blocker. Her parents are concerned about potential side effects and interactions with her current medication regimen, and they would like to speak with you before making any changes to medications.

Gonadotropin-releasing hormone analogs/agonists (GnRHas), popularly referred to as *puberty blockers*, have been in use since the 1980s. They have been used safely in children of all genders for the treatment of central precocious puberty; in adults to treat prostate carcinoma; and during in vitro fertilization to induce controlled ovarian stimulation. Endogenously, pulsatile release of GnRH stimulates the release of follicle-stimulating hormone and luteinizing hormone, which act on the ovaries and testes to produce estrogen and testosterone, leading to development of secondary sex characteristics during puberty (Grumbach 2002). When exogenous GnRHas are continuously present, GnRH receptors are desensitized over time, inhibiting the release of luteinizing hormone. GnRHas are now commonly used to suppress pubertal changes in patients with gender dysphoria at Tanner Stage 2. In TNG adults, GnRHas may be more effective than spironolactone in suppressing serum testosterone (Angus et al. 2021).

Use of GnRHas in pubertal suppression is a fully reversible intervention that allows young patients time to mature, explore their gender identity, and understand better the risks and benefits of GAHT. This often leads to improvement in psychiatric symptoms, behavioral problems (de Vries et al. 2011), and suicidal ideation (Turban et al. 2020). Appropriate use of pubertal suppression may decrease the dosages of GAHT needed for desired physiological changes (Jensen et al. 2019) and prevent the need for surgical procedures, such as hair removal, facial reconstruction, or chest reconstruction (Shumer et al. 2016). Beginning pubertal suppression later in puberty, but before full chest tissue development, may enable a patient to undergo less-extensive chest reconstruction surgery (Shumer et al. 2016). The most commonly used GnRHas are leuprolide acetate (intramuscular injection) and histrelin acetate (subcutaneous implant). GnRHas appear to be consistently effective for preventing pubertal changes regardless of sex assigned at birth (Mejia-Otero et al. 2021). Such medications are generally well tolerated, and adverse events are rare (Cohen-Kettenis and Klink 2015). In the United States, the choice of specific agent is primarily driven, unfortunately, by health insurance coverage and availability.

Side Effects

Aside from injection or surgical site–related reactions, the most reported side effects of GnRHas are hot flashes and mood swings, as would be expected with a decrease in endogenous hormone levels. Weight gain has been reported in TNG youth on GnRHas (Jensen et al. 2019), and increases in body mass index (BMI) and metabolic changes have been reported in patients with central precocious puberty treated with GnRHas (De Sanctis et al. 2019). Although these effects on weight and metabolism are not reported consistently, clinicians should be mindful of potential overlap with psychiatric medications known to cause weight gain and metabolic changes (e.g., antipsychotics, lithium, valproic acid, mirtazapine). Leuprolide has been associated with prolonged QT interval, including at least one documented case of torsades de pointes (Abbasi et al. 2020). This is also a potential effect of many psychotropic medications, including stimulants; selective serotonin reuptake inhibitors

(SSRIs), particularly citalopram; and antipsychotics, particularly thioridazine, ziprasidone, and IV haloperidol. Clinicians should be cautious of polypharmacy and individual risk factors for arrhythmias (Beach et al. 2013).

In the literature, impaired bone health is the most discussed theoretical risk of GnRHas. Age at which pubertal suppression is initiated appears to be negatively correlated with bone mineral density (BMD) Z score (Lee et al. 2020). Bone mass accrual and BMD are determined by a number of static factors (genetics, comorbidities, malabsorption) and modifiable factors (calcium/Vitamin D intake, physical exercise, hormones). Lower BMD Z scores have been described in TNG adults and children, but in particular, children and adolescents assigned male sex at birth and receiving pubertal suppression have increased prevalence of low Z scores (Lee et al. 2020).

Puberty is important for bone mass accrual and linear bone growth, with most adult bone mass formed by age 20 and peaking by the early 30s (Rice et al. 2018). Low BMD generally predicts osteoporosis later in life. It is unclear whether lower BMD found in TNG patients is clinically meaningful, but clinicians should be aware of the potential impact of GnRHas, as well as numerous psychiatric medications, on bone health in this crucial developmental period. Studies show an increase in BMD or decrease in bone turnover once GAHT is started after pubertal suppression (Mahfouda et al. 2019), indicating that the risk related to bone health can be mitigated by timely initiation of GAHT or allowing endogenous puberty to proceed.

Among psychiatric medications, SSRIs, stimulants, benzodiazepines, anti-epileptic drugs, and antipsychotics have been linked to various measures of bone health outcomes, particularly in adults. SSRIs have been linked to osteoporosis and lower BMD in older populations (Zhou et al. 2018); this is confounded by the association between depression/depressive symptoms and poor bone health (Bab and Yirmiya 2010; Gebara et al. 2014). How SSRIs affect developing bones is less clear (Rice et al. 2018). SSRIs can have opposing actions on bone health centrally and peripherally. Increased central nervous system serotonin may decrease sympathetic tone, thus increasing bone formation, whereas peripheral serotonin may decrease osteoblasts, decreasing bone formation (Ducy and Karsenty 2010). Data assessing how SSRIs influence bone health among children and adolescents are inconsistent. Although SSRIs may have a negative impact on BMD among youth with eating disorders or those taking SSRIs for longer periods of time (>24 months), BMD improves with treatment of depression (Rice et al. 2018).

Although stimulant medications clearly decrease growth velocity, especially early in treatment, their long-lasting effect on bone health is controversial (Rice et al. 2018). Stimulants often suppress appetite, leading to decreased nutritional intake, which is detrimental to bone mass accrual. Weight itself is an additional factor in BMD: loading effects on weight-bearing bones increase BMD (van Leeuwen et al. 2017). Additionally, increased sympathetic tone increases osteoclast activation, and leptin mediates bone formation/resorption (Ducy 2011). Per data gathered in the National Health and Nutrition Examination Survey, children on stimulants for >3 months had lower BMD than controls; however, they were also found to have a lower weight than controls and lower weight for their age (Feuer et al. 2016). No specific guidelines exist for children on stimulants for monitoring of bone health, but clinicians should monitor for excessive weight loss, poor appetite, and overall growth.

Use of benzodiazepines has been linked to increased risk of fractures, especially in older cisgender women, a relationship that is only partially explained by sedation leading to increased incidence of falls (Rice et al. 2018). Benzodiazepines have been linked to reduced BMD, decreased Vitamin D, and increased serum alkaline phosphatase (ALP) (Fan et al. 2016). No data exist regarding intermittent use of benzodiazepines in children and effects on bone health.

Anti-epileptic drugs (AEDs), used for various indications in psychiatry, may affect bone health in several ways. Enzyme-inducing AEDs (e.g., carbamazepine) increase Vitamin D metabolism, which reduces calcium absorption from the gastrointestinal tract and can cause secondary hyperparathyroidism (Fan et al. 2016). Valproic acid depletes carnitine, which is important for bone formation. Carbamazepine, gabapentin, oxcarbazepine, and topiramate have been linked to decreased BMD Z scores. In contrast, lithium may increase osteogenesis (Wong et al. 2020). Although valproic acid has been linked to decreased linear growth and decreased BMD in children, it has not been found to alter Vitamin D levels. Baseline and periodic monitoring of Vitamin D levels with Vitamin D supplementation is recommended for all pediatric patients on AEDs (Rice et al. 2018).

Antipsychotics have also been linked to bone loss, although the data are confounded in the adult literature because schizophrenia is independently linked to decreased bone health, as is cigarette smoking (Rice et al. 2018). In adults and pubertal adolescents taking antipsychotics, the primary concern for bone health has been hyperprolactinemia causing hypogonadism and leading to bone loss (Naidoo et al. 2003). Antipsychotics may also affect bone directly through the inhibitory action of prolactin on osteoblasts and indirectly by causing sedation and decreased activity (Calarge et al. 2013). Like SSRIs, atypical antipsychotics may induce serotonergic effects on bone (Calarge et al. 2013). Strong D2 antagonists (e.g., risperidone) are most likely to cause hyperprolactinemia, whereas quetiapine, ziprasidone, and clozapine tend to spare prolactin (Roke et al. 2009; Wu et al. 2013). Switching to aripiprazole from risperidone or olanzapine has been shown to reduce prolactin levels (Byerly et al. 2009), and aripiprazole has been used as an adjunct to reduce side effects related to hyperprolactinemia in adults (Besag et al. 2021).

It may not be possible or safe to avoid using GnRHas or psychiatric medications, so clinicians should remain cognizant of medication considerations specific to youth undergoing pubertal suppression. TNG children and adolescents in psychiatric treatment are more likely to experience certain factors that may additionally adversely impact growth and bone health, such as inadequate dietary calcium and Vitamin D (Lee et al. 2020), lack of exercise (Lee et al. 2020), disordered eating (Nagata et al. 2020; Parker et al. 2010), and substance misuse (Kidd et al. 2021). Clinicians should work with patients and families to address such risk factors and comorbidities, considering Vitamin D supplementation, nutritional counseling when appropriate, incorporation of physical activity, and avoiding the use of tobacco products.

HORMONES

Estrogen and Estradiol

Case Example: Luna

Luna (they/she) is a 20-year-old non-binary patient you have been treating for bipolar disorder in your outpatient practice. They are currently doing well on lamotrigine and aripiprazole. They occasionally take sumatriptan for their migraines and albuterol as needed for exercise-induced asthma. Luna recently had their first visit at the trans health clinic to discuss starting E2 patches for gender-affirming hormone therapy. Their internist raised concerns about potential interaction between the mood stabilizer and estrogen and would like Luna to discuss with you possible alternatives to treat their bipolar disorder.

The use of organ extracts for hypogonadism and dysmenorrhea has been described in Chinese medical literature since the 600s, and even earlier descriptions of ingesting pregnant mare urine may have been for hormonal effects, as hypothesized by archaeologist Timothy Taylor (Zurada et al. 2018). Estrogen therapy was first introduced to Western medicine in the late 1800s (Santen and Simpson 2019). Emmenin, the first bioidentical estrogen derived from urine of pregnant people, was marketed in 1933, followed by several other forms of estrogen (ethinyl E2, diethylstilbestrol). In 1941, Premarin (conjugated estrogens derived from the urine of pregnant mares) was introduced. Estrogen began to be used in GAHT in the 1950s by endocrinologists Harry Benjamin (United States) and Christian Hamburger (Denmark) (Zurada et al. 2018). Synthetic and organ-derived estrogens are used in numerous clinical applications: GAHT, oral contraceptive pills, menopause hormone therapy, and treatment of hypogonadism, prostate cancer, and breast cancer. In the 1970s, a study found increased risk of endometrial cancer from estrogens, causing a significant decrease in use of estrogen therapy for cisgender women. That trend slackened in the 1980s when it was found that addition of progestin mitigated the risk of endometrial cancer (Kohn et al. 2021).

TNG patients seeking GAHT receive frequent counseling on numerous risks. Much of the data, however, are extrapolated from the use of estrogens in patients who had gone through estrogenic puberty. Historical use of conjugated estrogens (e.g., Premarin) or synthetic estrogens (e.g., ethinyl E2), neither of which are commonly used in GAHT, further complicates the existing evidence. Even the data that are more specific to transgender women may not be fully applicable to transfeminine young adults receiving estrogen after puberty blockade, as opposed to starting estrogen after undergoing androgenic puberty. E2, a bioidentical estrogen most commonly used in GAHT, is the most important endogenously produced estrogen. Prodrug esters of E2 (e.g., E2 valerate or cypionate) may be injected subcutaneously or intramuscularly. All estrogens exert their physiological effects via nuclear estrogen receptors alpha and beta (ERα and ERβ) and via extracellular G protein–coupled receptors (Kuhl 2005). Different types of estrogen lead to different physiological changes (Kuhl 2005).

Psychiatric Medications and Metabolism of Estrogen

Estrogens undergo hepatic metabolism mostly by cytochrome P450 enzymes (predominantly CYP1A2 and 3A4) (Tsuchiya et al. 2005), although they are also metabolized by enzymes in other tissues into metabolites with variable estrogenic activity. Considerable individual variation in estrogen metabolism results from genetic factors and external factors (e.g., diet, alcohol/substance use, smoking, physical activity) (Kuhl 2005). Any medications that induce or inhibit the relevant enzymes may affect E2 levels. Among psychotropic medications, nefazodone and suboxone are important CYP3A4 inhibitors (Preskorn 2020), which may cause higher-than-anticipated E2 serum levels. Carbamazepine, oxcarbazepine, topiramate, phenobarbital, and St. John's wort are CYP3A4 inducers (Preskorn 2020) and, conversely, may lead to serum E2 levels that are lower than expected. Fluvoxamine is an inhibitor of CYP1A2 and 3A4 (Preskorn 2020), whereas tobacco is an inducer. Modafinil induces both CYP3A4 and CYP1A2 (Preskorn 2020).

E2 is also highly protein-bound by albumin, corticosteroid-binding globulin (CBG), and sex hormone–binding globulin (SHBG) (Hammond 2016). Only the unbound hormone is active, and the proportion of free E2 is inversely related to the level of SHBG (Hammond 2016). Carbamazepine and phenytoin increase SHBG by inducing the hepatic cytochrome P450 system (Isojärvi et al. 1995b), thereby reducing estrogenic action (Isojärvi et al. 1988, 1995b). E2 also may decrease serum lamotrigine levels by increasing hepatic glucuronidation (Chen et al. 2009).

Whenever possible, it is beneficial to opt for medications that do not have a significant impact on the metabolism of E2, such as lithium, which bypasses liver metabolism entirely, or oxcarbazepine (Isojärvi et al. 1995a) rather than carbamazepine. When alternatives are not feasible (because, for instance, other mood stabilizers fail to improve symptoms), closer monitoring of serum E2 levels and clinical effects may be indicated.

Side Effects

GAHT appears to be overwhelmingly safe and linked with positive outcomes (D'hoore and T'Sjoen 2022; Mahfouda et al. 2019). Potential cardiovascular and venous thromboembolism (VTE) risks of E2 GAHT have received particular attention, given the prothrombotic effects of E2 found in studies of primarily cisgender women (Tchaikovski and Rosing 2010).

The literature on actual cardiovascular and VTE risk in TNG patients is mixed (D'hoore and T'Sjoen 2022). In the Behavioral Risk Factor Surveillance System data from 2014 to 2017, transgender women had a twofold increase in odds of myocardial infarction compared with cisgender women, but their odds were comparable to those of cisgender men when controlled for age, smoking status, and comorbidities (Alzahrani et al. 2019). Limits to data generalizability include changes in hormonal regimens over time (D'hoore and T'Sjoen 2022), variability in regional practices, and whether GAHT was medically monitored or self-managed (Alzahrani et al. 2019).

Cardiovascular disease is more common among TNG than non-TNG people, but its prevalence—like that of other disproportionate health burdens affecting TNG patients—is highly influenced by social determinants of health and not wholly attributable to GAHT. Per data from the Behavioral Risk Factor Surveillance System, transgender respondents were less likely than cisgender respondents to follow CDC exercise recommendations (Alzahrani et al. 2019). Contributing factors to this observation may include discomfort related to dysphoria (e.g., being more acutely aware of one's body during exercise; physical limitations when wearing a shaper/corset or binder), gender-based discrimination (e.g., lack of gender-inclusive changing and shower facilities; legal or practical inability to safely use gender-congruent facilities), and societal discrimination and exclusion based on other facets of identity. TNG respondents in that survey were more likely to be young and of an ethnic minority group, both factors that are associated with lack of economic access to healthy foods and safe spaces for exercise.

Metabolically, estrogen GAHT may be correlated with increased body fat, decreased lean body mass, increased BMI, and increased overall body weight (T'Sjoen et al. 2019); "unfavorable changes in lipid profiles" (Elamin et al. 2010); and increased triglyceride levels, without any other significant changes in LDL or HDL cholesterol (Maraka et al. 2017). Yet very few clinically significant negative events (e.g., myocardial infarction, stroke, VTE, or death) were noted in those studies (Maraka et al. 2017). Current data support the overall safety of estrogen GAHT with appropriate medical monitoring, despite statistically significant changes in metabolic parameters.

Whereas the literature is inconclusive on the potential negative metabolic effects of E2, the side effects of psychotropic medications are clear. Antipsychotics, especially clozapine and olanzapine, are well known for causing weight gain and dyslipidemia (Hasnain et al. 2012; Hirsch et al. 2017). Antipsychotics also seem to be associated with an increased risk of VTE (the mechanism is unclear; Jönsson et al. 2018). Of the antidepressants, amitriptyline, mirtazapine, and paroxetine carry an increased risk of weight gain, whereas fluoxetine and bupropion are linked to weight loss (Alonso-Pedrero et al. 2019; Serretti et al. 2010). Lithium and valproic acid are both linked to weight gain (Baptista et al. 1995; Grootens et al. 2018); carbamazepine and lamotrigine have a lower risk of weight gain than other AEDs (Grootens et al. 2018). Antipsychotics present an additional challenge when prescribed concurrently with estrogen GAHT, as they share the risk of hyperprolactinemia (T'Sjoen et al. 2019), which may complicate interpretation of prolactin levels. Prolactin-sparing antipsychotics such as quetiapine and clozapine are also linked with significant weight gain (Hasnain et al. 2012; Hirsch et al. 2017), so ziprasidone (a prolactin-sparing option) or aripiprazole (linked with reducing prolactin levels) may be a better option, given concurrent metabolic considerations and prolactin levels.

Progesterone

The use of progesterone in feminizing GAHT has been controversial historically. The World Professional Association for Transgender Health (WPATH) and University of California, San Francisco, guidelines on gender affirmation state that the side effects of progesterone are considered too harsh given its limited benefits, but those conclusions were drawn from evidence on medroxyprogesterone and other synthetic progesterones rather than bioequivalent micronized progesterone. To date, there has been no large-scale study of the effects of micronized progesterone on TNG people. There is reason to believe that micronized progesterone can help with the following: sped-up feminization (by reducing conversion of testosterone to 5α-dihydrotestosterone); suppressed endogenous testosterone production; optimal breast maturation to Tanner Stage 5; improved sleep cycles; resolution of menstrual-like symptoms such as hot flashes and morning sickness; and increasing BMD while reducing cardiovascular disease and breast cancer risk from estradiol supplementation (Prior 2019). However, owing to the paucity of data related to the effects of micronized progesterone, it is challenging to anticipate interactions with psychopharmacological agents.

Clinicians are encouraged to try progesterone in patients who are interested in adding it to their GAHT while taking special care to work with the patient on evaluating challenges as they occur. As more individuals use progesterone as part of GAHT, more data will become available.

Testosterone

Case Example: Alex

Alex (he/him) is a 30-year-old trans man who has been referred to you for medication evaluation and management. He has been diagnosed with social anxiety and major depressive disorder. He notes that his social anxiety significantly improved after he started taking testosterone a year ago and started working at his new job in a more affirming and supportive professional environment.

Unfortunately, he has continued to have episodes of depression that have not improved despite consistent weekly psychotherapy. He is open to antidepressant medication to see if it could help with his symptoms, but he wants to make sure that it will not interfere with the effectiveness of his hormone therapy. He asks you for recommendations.

Although testosterone was not isolated and purified until the 20th century, the function of testes and their bodily effects have been known since antiquity from observing humans and animals after testes loss (Nieschlag and Nieschlag 2019). Through the Victorian era, as with estrogens, commercially available thyroid and testis-derived preparations were popularly consumed for broad indications such as "rejuvenation" and virility (Borell 1976). Although organotherapy found an enthusiastic consumer market (Borell 1976), it was eventually replaced with more chemically refined hormone therapy, made possible through the isolation of testosterone in 1935 (Handelsman 2020).

Testosterone induces variable expression of androgen-responsive genes by binding to the androgen receptor, a steroid nuclear receptor (Handelsman 2020). Aromatase converts testosterone to E2 (Handelsman 2020), and 5α-hydroxylase converts testosterone to 5α-dihydrotestosterone (DHT), a much more potent androgen with greater binding affinity for the androgen receptor (Srinivas-Shankar and Wu 2006). Because of concern about peripheral aromatase conversion of testosterone to estrogen, especially in adipose tissue, some clinicians have considered prescribing aromatase inhibitors to TNG patients (Carswell and Roberts 2017; Chan et al. 2018); research suggests, however, that transmasculine patients taking testosterone typically have E2 levels within the reference range for cisgender men (Chan et al. 2018).

Psychiatric Medications and Metabolism of Testosterone
Testosterone undergoes hepatic metabolism, with CYP3A4 being the most important (and abundant) liver enzyme (Usmani et al. 2003), and additional

minor pathways via CYP2C19, CYP2C9, and CYP2D6 (Yamazaki and Shimada 1997). CYP3A4 inhibitors such as nefazodone and suboxone may lead to higher testosterone levels by inhibiting its metabolism, whereas oxcarbazepine, modafinil, topiramate, phenobarbital, and St. John's wort are CYP3A4 inducers (Preskorn 2020) and may, conversely, lower testosterone levels. Progesterone and fluvoxamine are CYP2C19 inhibitors (Preskorn 2020). Carbamazepine induces CYP3A4, CYP2C19, and CYP2C9 (Preskorn 2020). Fluoxetine inhibits CYP2C9 (Preskorn 2020). CYP2D6 is inhibited by bupropion, fluoxetine, and paroxetine (Preskorn 2020). Like estrogen, testosterone is highly protein-bound in serum by albumin, CBG, and sex hormone–binding globulin (SBHG). One to two percent of testosterone remains as a free fraction in serum (Wheeler 1995).

Side Effects

For the vast majority of patients, medically monitored testosterone for gender affirmation is safe and effective, yielding significant improvements in overall functioning (Mahfouda et al. 2019). A systematic review by Velho et al. (2017) reported no severe adverse effects. Body composition changes were common: an increase in total body weight, a decrease in body fat, and an increase in lean body mass. A low risk of clinically significant hypertension has been reported, which in two cases resolved with cessation of testosterone.

Existing studies primarily focused on adult transgender men, around age 30, living in Europe or the United States (Velho et al. 2017). As with estrogen, findings from adults who have initiated testosterone after endogenous puberty may be difficult to apply to adolescents and young adults who have only gone through androgenic puberty with exogenous testosterone. Regardless, when prescribing any one of the numerous psychiatric medications known for metabolic side effects (such as antipsychotics, amitriptyline, mirtazapine, paroxetine, lithium, or valproic acid) along with testosterone, patients should be counseled for such overlapping risks and undergo regular monitoring of metabolic parameters.

Formulations in current use for testosterone GAHT appear to be generally safe for liver function. None of the studies in a 2017 systematic review reported a clinically significant increase in liver enzymes (Velho et al. 2017). For most psychiatric medications, serious hepatotoxicity tends to be idiosyncratic and rare (Sedky et al. 2012). Although all of the antidepressants on the market appear to have the potential for rare, idiosyncratic, unpredictable cases of hepatotoxicity, they generally are safe (Todorović Vukotić et al. 2021). Monoamine oxidase inhibitors (MAOIs) and tricyclics seem to have a slightly higher risk than SSRIs (Sedky et al. 2012). An exception is nefazodone, which carries a well-established risk of hepatotoxicity (DeSanty and Amabile 2007). Antipsychotics can be associated with a transient, benign elevation in liver enzymes and are rarely associated with severe hepatotoxicity (Todorović Vukotić et al. 2021). Benign elevation of liver enzymes can occur in ≤20% of patients on phenothiazines, such as chlorpromazine, but clinically significant hepatotoxicity is much rarer, at 0.1%–1% (Sedky et al. 2012). Clozapine can be associated with asymptomatic elevated liver enzymes in 30%–50% of patients, and risperidone in ≤50% of patients (Sedky et al. 2012). Of the mood stabilizers, carbamazepine, divalproate, and lamotrigine have all been linked to liver pathology, from benign elevations in liver enzymes and hyperammonemia to rare cases of fulminant liver failure (Dols et al. 2013; Sedky et al. 2012). Oxcarbazepine is safer than carbamazepine in terms of hepatotoxicity (Sedky et al. 2012). Especially when a patient has additional risk factors, such as polypharmacy or type 2 diabetes, testosterone treatment concurrent with antipsychotics or AEDs should include routine monitoring of liver function (Dols et al. 2013; Todorović Vukotić et al. 2021).

Erythrocytosis is a common side effect of testosterone GAHT; yet, unlike erythrocytosis in myeloproliferative neoplasms, it does not seem to be correlated with other clinically significant events (such as thromboembolism) in the vast majority of patients (Shatzel et al. 2017). The potentially compounded increased risk of VTE with antipsychotics (Hägg et al. 2009; Jönsson et al. 2018), however, may be of particular consideration for patients with heightened risk profiles (e.g., having multiple risk factors, previous VTE, or strong family history of VTE), as antipsychotics have been identified as a predictor of recurrent VTE (Liu et al. 2021), even when controlling for other risk factors (Parker et al. 2010). New neurological symptoms in such patients may warrant further workup.

Androgen-induced skin changes (e.g., sebocyte growth, sebum production, infundibular keratinization) increase the risk of acne in patients on testosterone (Motosko et al. 2019; Yeung et al. 2020). Acne is a well-known side effect of lithium (Dunner 2003), although not via an androgenic pathway, and has been noted as a rare potential side effect of tricyclic antidepressants, sertraline, escitalopram, and quetiapine (Kazandjieva and Tsankov 2017). For patients on testosterone, retinoids are typically the acne treatment of choice (Kazandjieva and Tsankov 2017). Most hormonal treatments for acne (estrogens or spironolactone) are likely to interfere with the effects of testosterone but may be an option for those who have reached maximal effects of testosterone, typically after 2 years (Motosko et al. 2019). For severe acne, isotretinoin may be an option for patients without additional risks for hepatotoxicity and with careful monitoring (Motosko et al. 2019). Testosterone has not been evaluated for its efficacy as a contraceptive, and all patients on isotretinoin require appropriate history-taking and counseling regarding the teratogenicity of isotretinoin and pregnancy-related risks (Singer and Keuroghlian 2020).

PERIOPERATIVE MEDICATIONS

Case Example: Leo

Leo (he/they) is a 26-year-old non-binary transmasculine person with depression and anxiety, which have been managed chronically with escitalopram for the past 2 years. He has been on testosterone GAHT for a year as well, with blood work consistently showing physiological levels. As they approach phalloplasty, they ask you about whether they will need to stop their GAHT or SSRI. What do you tell him?

Acknowledging the many interactions and potential side effects discussed thus far, one must carefully consider decisions about continuing medications in the perioperative period of gender-affirming surgery. Ultimately, clinicians should defer to the surgeon's guidance, as the surgical team is most familiar with specific intraoperative and postoperative medication regimens and the particular risk profile of a given surgical procedure. With this caveat, we offer some general considerations based on the literature (as limited as it is with regard to high-quality data) and our own clinical experience (Table 4–1).

First, with regard to GAHT, the most prominent theoretical concern is for patients on E2 therapy, which can increase risk of VTE (Goldstein et al. 2019). One way to reduce risk is to consider the medication formulation. In general, oral estradiol has been robustly shown to present a higher risk for VTE than transdermal E2, because of the first-pass metabolism (e.g., Tangpricha and den Heijer 2017), so transdermal E2 is generally preferred (e.g., Hembree et al. 2017). Based on data in cisgender women on oral estradiol replacement, some surgeons recommend holding estrogen GAHT for 2–4 weeks after surgery (e.g., Ellsworth and Colon 2006), although this is far from a universal recommendation. For suitable surgical candidates who lack established VTE risk factors, the most recent literature on the topic suggests that surgeons engage in shared decision-making with patients regarding possible GAHT continuation throughout the perioperative period, on a case-by-case basis, considering their Caprini Risk Assessment and the planned procedure (Blasdel et al. 2021; Haveles et al. 2021; Hontscharuk et al. 2021; Kozato et al. 2021). Other possible VTE risk factors—both modifiable (e.g., smoking, sedentary lifestyle, alcohol consumption [e.g., Lindqvist et al. 2009]) and nonmodifiable (e.g., hereditary clotting disorders, antiphospholipid antibody syndrome [e.g., Kerrebrouck et al. 2022; Ott et al. 2010])—are not contraindications to surgery but do factor into perioperative management. It is essential to optimize modifiable risk factors as much as possible (stop smoking, increase exercise, decrease alcohol consumption) before and after surgery. Patients with underlying medical conditions may

TABLE 4–1.　Medication use during the perioperative period

Anticonvulsants, SSRIs,[a] antipsychotics,[b] benzodiazepines, methadone, modafinil	Usually can be continued in the perioperative period
Lithium[c]	Probably can be continued for minor surgery, but usually should be stopped before major surgery
Tricyclic antidepressants	Case by case: balance significant drug-drug interactions with withdrawal symptoms
MAOIs[d]	Stop before elective surgery

[a]SSRIs can increase bleeding risk when combined with nonsteroidal anti-inflammatory drugs, so it is important to consider each patient's risk profile.

[b]For patients taking clozapine, there are significant risks of anesthesia reactions, including hypotension and vital sign instability (Doherty et al. 2006). Decisions about continuation should also consider potential risks of psychotic symptoms worsening in the perioperative period. We recommend consulting with an anesthesia colleague if unsure about how to proceed.

[c]In the case of cessation, we recommend monitoring serum electrolytes before resuming lithium after surgery.

[d]MAOIs should be stopped ≥10 days before surgery to allow for a suitable washout period, facilitating synthesis of sufficient monoamine oxidase.

require a different prophylaxis plan or even surgical method for certain procedures; management decisions should be made in conjunction with the patient's hematologist and surgeon. Prospective studies are needed to more fully evaluate VTE risk for patients on E2, based on age, medication regimen, type of surgery, and operating time.

Possible side effects from testosterone—erythrocytosis, liver dysfunction, and lipid elevations—that could impact surgical readiness should be monitored with routine outpatient lab tests. Brief, temporary cessation of GAHT perioperatively is unlikely to decrease the risks of such adverse events. While there has been a suggestion that individuals on testosterone could exhibit increased perioperative cardiovascular risks, no conclusive evidence has yet been published. TNG people taking testosterone as GAHT may experience myocardial infarction at one-third the rate of age-matched cisgender men (but note that these data are >20 years old [van Kesteren et al. 1997]). Just as GAHT has been robustly shown to improve mental health (e.g., Hughto et al. 2020; Murad et al. 2010), the potential mental health ramifications of GAHT cessation cannot be understated. Anecdotally, shifting to an estrogen-predominant hormonal milieu or experiencing plummeting hormone levels, for those who have previously undergone gonadectomy, can exacerbate preexisting psychiatric illness and cause psychological distress. Although limited data exist for TNG patients undergoing GAHT, this intuitively follows observed psychiatric ramifications of menopause in cisgender women (e.g., Hoyt and Falconi 2015). Individuals who have not undergone hysterectomy could additionally experience resumption of menses (e.g., Light et al. 2014); minimal existing data characterize this experience, but based on the psychological benefits of menstrual cessation (e.g., Murad et al. 2010; Schwartz et al. 2022), resumption of periods likely carries a high risk of inducing dysphoria and distress. As there are no data supporting the benefit of stopping testosterone before gender-affirming surgery, surgeons are increasingly allowing patients to continue testosterone perioperatively, although individual surgeons may have distinct practices and protocols for specific patients with comorbid health conditions.

We emphasize that all decisions should defer to the surgeon's guidance, but here we summarize general considerations and expert consensus, per Oprea et al. (2022) and Jenkins and Kontos (2015) unless otherwise noted. With regard to the timing of stopping medications before surgery: except for MAOIs, the general rule is to stop five half-lives before surgery.

REFERENCES

Abbasi D, Faiek S, Shetty S, Khan E: Shock from twisting peaks: a rare case of recurrent torsades de pointes secondary to leuprolide-induced prolonged QT. Cureus 12(7):e9041, 2020 32782861

Alonso-Pedrero L, Bes-Rastrollo M, Marti A: Effects of antidepressant and antipsychotic use on weight gain: a systematic review. Obes Rev 20(12):1680–1690, 2019 31524318

Alzahrani T, Nguyen T, Ryan A, et al: Cardiovascular disease risk factors and myocardial infarction in the transgender population. Circ Cardiovasc Qual Outcomes 12(4):e005597, 2019 30950651

Angus LM, Nolan BJ, Zajac JD, Cheung AS: A systematic review of antiandrogens and feminization in transgender women. Clin Endocrinol (Oxf) 94(5):743–752, 2021 32926454

Bab IA, Yirmiya R: Depression and bone mass. Ann N Y Acad Sci 1192(1):170–175, 2010 20392233

Baptista T, Teneud L, Contreras Q, et al: Lithium and body weight gain. Pharmacopsychiatry 28(2):35–44, 1995 7624385

Beach SR, Celano CM, Noseworthy PA, et al: QTc prolongation, torsades de pointes, and psychotropic medications. Psychosomatics 54(1):1–13, 2013 23295003

Besag FMC, Vasey MJ, Salim I: Is adjunct aripiprazole effective in treating hyperprolactinemia induced by psychotropic medication? A narrative review. CNS Drugs 35(5):507–526, 2021 33880739

Blasdel G, Shakir N, Parker A, et al: Letter to the editor from Blasdel et al: "No venous thromboembolism increase among transgender female patients remaining on estrogen for gender-affirming surgery." J Clin Endocrinol Metab 106(9):e3783–e3784, 2021 33846750

Borell M: Organotherapy, British physiology, and discovery of the internal secretions. J Hist Biol 9(2):235–268, 1976 11610067

Breslow AS, Brewster ME, Velez BL, et al: Resilience and collective action: exploring buffers against minority stress for transgender individuals. Psychol Sex Orientat Gend Divers 2(3):253–265, 2015

Byerly MJ, Marcus RN, Tran QV, et al: Effects of aripiprazole on prolactin levels in subjects with schizophrenia during cross-titration with risperidone or olanzapine: analysis of a randomized, open-label study. Schizophr Res 107(2-3):218–222, 2009 19038534

Calarge CA, Ivins SD, Motyl KJ, et al: Possible mechanisms for the skeletal effects of antipsychotics in children and adolescents. Ther Adv Psychopharmacol 3(5):278–293, 2013 24167704

Carswell JM, Roberts SA: Induction and maintenance of amenorrhea in transmasculine and nonbinary adolescents. Transgend Health 2(1):195–201, 2017 29142910

Chan KJ, Jolly D, Liang JJ, et al: Estrogen levels do not rise with testosterone treatment for transgender men. Endocr Pract 24(4):329–333, 2018 29561193

Chen H, Yang K, Choi S, et al: Up-regulation of UDP-glucuronosyltransferase (UGT) 1A4 by 17β-estradiol: a potential mechanism of increased lamotrigine elimination in pregnancy. Drug Metab Dispos 37(9):1841–1847, 2009 19546240

Cohen-Kettenis PT, Klink D: Adolescents with gender dysphoria. Best Pract Res Clin Endocrinol Metab 29(3):485–495, 2015 26051304

De Sanctis V, Soliman AT, Di Maio S, et al: Long-term effects and significant adverse drug reactions (ADRs) associated with the use of gonadotropin-releasing hormone analogs (GnRHa) for central precocious puberty: a brief review of literature. Acta Biomed 90(3):345–359, 2019 31580327

DeSanty KP, Amabile CM: Antidepressant-induced liver injury. Ann Pharmacother 41(7):1201–1211, 2007 17609231

de Vries AL, Steensma TD, Doreleijers TA, Cohen-Kettenis PT: Puberty suppression in adolescents with gender identity disorder: a prospective follow-up study. J Sex Med 8(8):2276–2283, 2011 20646177

D'hoore L, T'Sjoen G: Gender-affirming hormone therapy: an updated literature review with an eye on the future. J Intern Med 291(5):574–592, 2022 34982475

Doherty J, Bell PF, King DJ: Implications for anaesthesia in a patient established on clozapine treatment. Int J Obstet Anesth 15(1):59–62, 2006 16256331

Dols A, Sienaert P, van Gerven H, et al: The prevalence and management of side effects of lithium and anticonvulsants as mood stabilizers in bipolar disorder from a clinical perspective: a review. Int Clin Psychopharmacol 28(6):287–296, 2013 23873292

Ducy P: The role of osteocalcin in the endocrine cross-talk between bone remodelling and energy metabolism. Diabetologia 54(6):1291–1297, 2011 21503740

Ducy P, Karsenty G: The two faces of serotonin in bone biology. J Cell Biol 191(1):7–13, 2010 20921133

Dunner DL: Drug interactions of lithium and other antimanic/mood-stabilizing medications. J Clin Psychiatry 64(Suppl 5):38–43, 2003 12720483

Elamin MB, Garcia MZ, Murad MH, et al: Effect of sex steroid use on cardiovascular risk in transsexual individuals: a systematic review and meta-analyses. Clin Endocrinol (Oxf) 72(1):1–10, 2010 19473174

Ellsworth WA IV, Colon GA: Management of medical morbidities and risk factors before surgery: smoking, diabetes, and other complicating factors. Semin Plast Surg 20(4):205–213, 2006

Fan HC, Lee HS, Chang KP, et al: The impact of anti-epileptic drugs on growth and bone metabolism. Int J Mol Sci 17(8):1242, 2016 27490534

Feuer AJ, Thai A, Demmer RT, Vogiatzi M: Association of stimulant medication use with bone mass in children and adolescents with attention-deficit/hyperactivity disorder. JAMA Pediatr 170(12):e162804, 2016 27695823

Gebara MA, Shea ML, Lipsey KL, et al: Depression, antidepressants, and bone health in older adults: a systematic review. J Am Geriatr Soc 62(8):1434–1441, 2014 25039259

Goldstein Z, Khan M, Reisman T, Safer JD: Managing the risk of venous thromboembolism in transgender adults undergoing hormone therapy. J Blood Med 10:209–216, 2019 31372078

Grootens KP, Meijer A, Hartong EG, et al: Weight changes associated with antiepileptic mood stabilizers in the treatment of bipolar disorder. Eur J Clin Pharmacol 74(11):1485–1489, 2018 30083876

Grumbach MM: The neuroendocrinology of human puberty revisited. Horm Res 57(Suppl 2):2–14, 2002 12065920

Hägg S, Jönsson AK, Spigset O: Risk of venous thromboembolism due to antipsychotic drug therapy. Expert Opin Drug Saf 8(5):537–547, 2009 19569978

Hammond GL: Plasma steroid-binding proteins: primary gatekeepers of steroid hormone action. J Endocrinol 230(1):R13–R25, 2016 27113851

Handelsman DJ: Androgen physiology, pharmacology, use and misuse. Endotext. October 5, 2020

Hasnain M, Vieweg WV, Hollett B: Weight gain and glucose dysregulation with second-generation antipsychotics and antidepressants: a review for primary care physicians. Postgrad Med 124(4):154–167, 2012 22913904

Haveles CS, Wang MM, Arjun A, et al: Effect of cross-sex hormone therapy on venous thromboembolism risk in male-to-female gender-affirming surgery. Ann Plast Surg 86(1):109–114, 2021 32079810

Hembree WC, Cohen-Kettenis PT, Gooren L, et al: Endocrine treatment of gender-dysphoric/gender-incongruent persons: an Endocrine Society Clinical Practice Guideline. J Clin Endocrinol Metab 102(11):3869–3903, 2017 28945902

Hendricks ML, Testa RJ: A conceptual framework for clinical work with transgender and gender nonconforming clients: an adaptation of the Minority Stress Model. Prof Psychol Res Pr 43(5):460–467, 2012

Hirsch L, Yang J, Bresee L, et al: Second-generation antipsychotics and metabolic side effects: a systematic review of population-based studies. Drug Saf 40(9):771–781, 2017 28585153

Hontscharuk R, Alba B, Manno C, et al: Perioperative transgender hormone management: avoiding venous thromboembolism and other complications. Plast Reconstr Surg 147(4):1008–1017, 2021 33776045

Hoyt LT, Falconi AM: Puberty and perimenopause: reproductive transitions and their implications for women's health. Soc Sci Med 132:103–112, 2015 25797100

Hughto JMW, Gunn HA, Rood BA, Pantalone DW: Social and medical gender affirmation experiences are inversely associated with mental health problems in a U.S. non-probability sample of transgender adults. Arch Sex Behav 49(7):2635–2647, 2020 32215775

Isojärvi JI, Pakarinen AJ, Myllylä VV: Effects of carbamazepine therapy on serum sex hormone levels in male patients with epilepsy. Epilepsia 29(6):781–786, 1988 3191895

Isojärvi JI, Laatikainen TJ, Pakarinen AJ, et al: Menstrual disorders in women with epilepsy receiving carbamazepine. Epilepsia 36(7):676–681, 1995a 7555984

Isojärvi JI, Pakarinen AJ, Rautio A, et al: Serum sex hormone levels after replacing carbamazepine with oxcarbazepine. Eur J Clin Pharmacol 47(5):461–464, 1995b DOI: 10.1007/BF00196862 7720770

James SE, Herman JL, Rankin S, et al: The Report of the 2015 U.S. Transgender Survey. Washington, DC, National Center for Transgender Equality, 2016. Available at: https://transequality.org/sites/default/files/docs/usts/USTS-Full-Report-Dec17.pdf. Accessed March 1, 2022.

Jenkins JA, Kontos N: The Maudsley Prescribing Guidelines in Psychiatry, 12th Edition. New York, Wiley-Blackwell, 2015

Jensen RK, Jensen JK, Simons LK, et al: Effect of concurrent gonadotropin-releasing hormone agonist treatment on dose and side effects of gender-affirming hormone therapy in adolescent transgender patients. Transgend Health 4(1):300–303, 2019 31663037

Jones BA, Haycraft E, Bouman WP, et al: Risk factors for eating disorder psychopathology within the treatment seeking transgender population: the role of cross-sex hormone treatment. Eur Eat Disord Rev 26(2):120–128, 2018 29318711

Jönsson AK, Schill J, Olsson H, et al: Venous thromboembolism during treatment with antipsychotics: a review of current evidence. CNS Drugs 32(1):47–64, 2018 29423659

Kattari SK, Bakko M, Hecht HK, Kattari L: Correlations between healthcare provider interactions and mental health among transgender and nonbinary adults. SSM Popul Health 10:100525, 2019 31872041

Kazandjieva J, Tsankov N: Drug-induced acne. Clin Dermatol 35(2):156–162, 2017 28274352

Kerrebrouck M, Vantilborgh A, Collet S, T'Sjoen G: Thrombophilia and hormonal therapy in transgender persons: a literature review and case series. Int J Transgender Health 23(4):1–15, 2022

Kidd JD, Goetz TG, Shea EA, Bockting WO: Prevalence and minority-stress correlates of past 12-month prescription drug misuse in a national sample of transgender and gender nonbinary adults: results from the U.S. Transgender Survey. Drug Alcohol Depend 219:108474, 2021 33360852

Kohn JR, Katebi Kashi P, Acosta-Torres S, et al: Fertility-sparing surgery for patients with cervical, endometrial, and ovarian cancers. J Minim Invasive Gynecol 28(3):392–402, 2021 33373729

Kozato A, Fox GWC, Yong PC, et al: No venous thromboembolism increase among transgender female patients remaining on estrogen for gender-affirming surgery. J Clin Endocrinol Metab 106(4):e1586–e1590, 2021 33417686

Kuhl H: Pharmacology of estrogens and progestogens: influence of different routes of administration. Climacteric 8(Suppl 1):3–63, 2005 16112947

Lee JY, Finlayson C, Olson-Kennedy J, et al: Low bone mineral density in early pubertal transgender/gender diverse youth: findings from the Trans Youth Care Study. J Endocr Soc 4(9):bvaa065, 2020 32832823

Lefevor GT, Boyd-Rogers CC, Sprague BM, Janis RA: Health disparities between genderqueer, transgender, and cisgender individuals: an extension of minority stress theory. J Couns Psychol 66(4):385–395, 2019 30896208

Light AD, Obedin-Maliver J, Sevelius JM, Kerns JL: Transgender men who experienced pregnancy after female-to-male gender transitioning. Obstet Gynecol 124(6):1120–1127, 2014 25415163

Lindqvist PG, Epstein E, Olsson H: The relationship between lifestyle factors and venous thromboembolism among women: a report from the MISS study. Br J Haematol 144(2):234–240, 2009 19036105

Liu Y, Xu J, Fang K, et al: Current antipsychotic agent use and risk of venous thromboembolism and pulmonary embolism: a systematic review and meta-analysis of observational studies. Ther Adv Psychopharmacol 11:2045125320982720, 2021 33505665

Mahfouda S, Moore JK, Siafarikas A, et al: Gender-affirming hormones and surgery in transgender children and adolescents. Lancet Diabetes Endocrinol 7(6):484–498, 2019 30528161

Maraka S, Singh Ospina N, Rodriguez-Gutierrez R, et al: Sex steroids and cardiovascular outcomes in transgender individuals: a systematic review and meta-analysis. J Clin Endocrinol Metab 102(11):3914–3923, 2017 28945852

Matsuno E, Budge SL: Non-binary/genderqueer identities: a critical review of the literature. Curr Sex Health Rep 9(3):116–120, 2017

McLemore KA: A minority stress perspective on transgender individuals' experiences with misgendering. Stigma Health 3(1):53–64, 2018

Mejia-Otero JD, White P, Lopez X: Effectiveness of puberty suppression with gonadotropin-releasing hormone agonists in transgender youth. Transgend Health 6(1):31–35, 2021 33614957

Motosko CC, Zakhem GA, Pomeranz MK, Hazen A: Acne: a side-effect of masculinizing hormonal therapy in transgender patients. Br J Dermatol 180(1):26–30, 2019 30101531

Murad MH, Elamin MB, Garcia MZ, et al: Hormonal therapy and sex reassignment: a systematic review and meta-analysis of quality of life and psychosocial outcomes. Clin Endocrinol (Oxf) 72(2):214–231, 2010 19473181

Nagata JM, Murray SB, Compte EJ, et al: Community norms for the Eating Disorder Examination Questionnaire (EDE-Q) among transgender men and women. Eat Behav 37:101381, 2020 32416588

Naidoo U, Goff DC, Klibanski A: Hyperprolactinemia and bone mineral density: the potential impact of antipsychotic agents. Psychoneuroendocrinology 28(Suppl 2):97–108, 2003 12650684

Nieschlag E, Nieschlag S: Endocrine history: the history of discovery, synthesis and development of testosterone for clinical use. Eur J Endocrinol 180(6):R201–R212, 2019 30959485

Oprea AD, Keshock MC, O'Glasser AY, et al: Preoperative management of medications for psychiatric diseases: Society for Perioperative Assessment and Quality Improvement consensus statement. Mayo Clin Proc 97(2):397–416, 2022 35120702

Ott J, Kaufmann U, Bentz EK, et al: Incidence of thrombophilia and venous thrombosis in transsexuals under cross-sex hormone therapy. Fertil Steril 93(4):1267–1272, 2010 19200981

Parker C, Coupland C, Hippisley-Cox J: Antipsychotic drugs and risk of venous thromboembolism: nested case-control study. BMJ 341:c4245, 2010 20858909

Perez-Brumer A, Day JK, Russell ST, Hatzenbuehler ML: Prevalence and correlates of suicidal ideation among transgender youth in California: findings from a representative, population-based sample of high school students. J Am Acad Child Adolesc Psychiatry 56(9):739–746, 2017 28838578

Preskorn SH: Drug-drug interactions (DDIs) in psychiatric practice, part 9: interactions mediated by drug-metabolizing cytochrome P450 enzymes. J Psychiatr Pract 26(2):126–134, 2020 32134885

Prior JC: Progesterone is important for transgender women's therapy: applying evidence for the benefits of progesterone in ciswomen. J Clin Endocrinol Metab 104(4):1181–1186, 2019 30608551

Reisner SL, Katz-Wise SL, Gordon AR, et al: Social epidemiology of depression and anxiety by gender identity. J Adolesc Health 59(2):203–208, 2016a 27267142

Reisner SL, Poteat T, Keatley J, et al: Global health burden and needs of transgender populations: a review. Lancet 388(10042):412–436, 2016b 27323919

Rice JN, Gillett CB, Malas NM: The impact of psychotropic medications on bone health in youth. Curr Psychiatry Rep 20(11):104, 2018 30246221

Rimes KA, Goodship N, Ussher G, et al: Non-binary and binary transgender youth: comparison of mental health, self-harm, suicidality, substance use and victimization experiences. Int J Transgend 20(2-3):230–240, 2017 32999609

Roke Y, van Harten PN, Boot AM, Buitelaar JK: Antipsychotic medication in children and adolescents: a descriptive review of the effects on prolactin level and associated side effects. J Child Adolesc Psychopharmacol 19(4):403–414, 2009 19702492

Santen RJ, Simpson E: History of estrogen: its purification, structure, synthesis, biologic actions, and clinical implications. Endocrinology 160(3):605–625, 2019 30566601

Schwartz BI, Effron A, Bear B, et al: Experiences with menses in transgender and gender nonbinary adolescents. J Pediatr Adolesc Gynecol 35(4):450–456, 2022 35123055

Sedky K, Nazir R, Joshi A, et al: Which psychotropic medications induce hepatotoxicity? Gen Hosp Psychiatry 34(1):53–61, 2012 22133982

Sequeira GM, Miller E, McCauley H, et al: Impact of gender expression on disordered eating, body dissatisfaction and BMI in a cohort of transgender youth. J Adolesc Health 60(2)(Suppl. 1):S87, 2017

Serretti A, Mandelli L, Laura M: Antidepressants and body weight: a comprehensive review and meta-analysis. J Clin Psychiatry 71(10):1259–1272, 2010 21062615

Shatzel JJ, Connelly KJ, DeLoughery TG: Thrombotic issues in transgender medicine: a review. Am J Hematol 92(2):204–208, 2017 27779767

Shumer DE, Reisner SL, Edwards-Leeper L, Tishelman A: Evaluation of Asperger syndrome in youth presenting to a gender dysphoria clinic. LGBT Health 3(5):387–390, 2016 26651183

Singer S, Keuroghlian AS: A call for gender identity data collection in iPLEDGE and increasing the number of isotretinoin prescribers among transgender health providers. LGBT Health 7(5):216–219, 2020 32456537

Srinivas-Shankar U, Wu FC: Drug insight: testosterone preparations. Nat Clin Pract Urol 3(12):653–665, 2006 17149382

Tangpricha V, den Heijer M: Oestrogen and anti-androgen therapy for transgender women. Lancet Diabetes Endocrinol 5(4):291–300, 2017 27916515

Tchaikovski SN, Rosing J: Mechanisms of estrogen-induced venous thromboembolism. Thromb Res 126(1):5–11, 2010 20163835

Testa RJ, Rider GN, Haug NA, Balsam KF: Gender confirming medical interventions and eating disorder symptoms among transgender individuals. Health Psychol 36(10):927–936, 2017 28368143

Timmins L, Rimes KA, Rahman Q: Minority stressors and psychological distress in transgender individuals. Psychol Sex Orientat Gend Divers 4(3):328–340, 2017

Todorović Vukotić N, Đorđević J, Pejić S, et al: Antidepressants- and antipsychotics-induced hepatotoxicity. Arch Toxicol 95(3):767–789, 2021 33398419

T'Sjoen G, Arcelus J, Gooren L, et al: Endocrinology of transgender medicine. Endocr Rev 40(1):97–117, 2019 30307546

Tsuchiya Y, Nakajima M, Yokoi T: Cytochrome P450-mediated metabolism of estrogens and its regulation in human. Cancer Lett 227(2):115–124, 2005 16112414

Turban JL, King D, Carswell JM, Keuroghlian AS: Pubertal suppression for transgender youth and risk of suicidal ideation. Pediatrics 145(2):e20191725, 2020 31974216

Usmani KA, Rose RL, Hodgson E: Inhibition and activation of the human liver microsomal and human cytochrome P450 3A4 metabolism of testosterone by deployment-related chemicals. Drug Metab Dispos 31(4):384–391, 2003 12642463

van Kesteren PJM, Asscheman H, Megens JAJ, Gooren LJG: Mortality and morbidity in transsexual subjects treated with cross-sex hormones. Clin Endocrinol (Oxf) 47(3):337–342, 1997 9373456

van Leeuwen J, Koes BW, Paulis WD, van Middelkoop M: Differences in bone mineral density between normal-weight children and children with overweight and obesity: a systematic review and meta-analysis. Obes Rev 18(5):526–546, 2017 28273691

Veale JF, Watson RJ, Peter T, Saewyc EM: Mental health disparities among Canadian transgender youth. J Adolesc Health 60(1):44–49, 2017 28007056

Velho I, Fighera TM, Ziegelmann PK, Spritzer PM: Effects of testosterone therapy on BMI, blood pressure, and laboratory profile of transgender men: a systematic review. Andrology 5(5):881–888, 2017 28709177

Wanta JW, Niforatos JD, Durbak E, et al: Mental health diagnoses among transgender patients in the clinical setting: an all-payer electronic health record study. Transgend Health 4(1):313–315, 2019 31701012

Warren JC, Smalley KB, Barefoot KN: Psychological well-being among transgender and genderqueer individuals. Int J Transgend 17(3–4):114–123, 2016

Warrier V, Greenberg DM, Weir E, et al: Elevated rates of autism, other neurodevelopmental and psychiatric diagnoses, and autistic traits in transgender and gender-diverse individuals. Nat Commun 11(1):3959, 2020 32770077

Wheeler MJ: The determination of bio-available testosterone. Ann Clin Biochem 32(Pt 4):345–357, 1995 7486793

Wong SK, Chin KY, Ima-Nirwana S: The skeletal-protecting action and mechanisms of action for mood-stabilizing drug lithium chloride: current evidence and future potential research areas. Front Pharmacol 11:430, 2020 32317977

Wu TC, Chen HT, Chang HY, et al: Mineralocorticoid receptor antagonist spironolactone prevents chronic corticosterone induced depression-like behavior. Psychoneuroendocrinology 38(6):871–883, 2013 23044404

Yamazaki H, Shimada T: Progesterone and testosterone hydroxylation by cytochromes P450 2C19, 2C9, and 3A4 in human liver microsomes. Arch Biochem Biophys 346(1):161–169, 1997 9328296

Yeung H, Ragmanauskaite L, Zhang Q, et al: Prevalence of moderate to severe acne in transgender adults: a cross-sectional survey. J Am Acad Dermatol 83(5):1450–1452, 2020 32109538

Zhou C, Fang L, Chen Y, et al: Effect of selective serotonin reuptake inhibitors on bone mineral density: a systematic review and meta-analysis. Osteoporos Int 29(6):1243–1251, 2018 29435621

Zurada A, Salandy S, Roberts W, et al: The evolution of transgender surgery. Clin Anat 31:878–886, 2018

CHAPTER 5

Affirming and Intersectional Psychiatric Care for Two-Spirit People

Adaptation, Cultural Resilience, and Indigenous Identities

Jack Bruno, M.S.W.
Emerson J. Dusic, M.P.H.
Henri M. Garrison-Desany, Ph.D., M.S.P.H.
Fiona (Fí) Fonseca, M.D., Ph.D.
Arjee Javellana Restar, Ph.D., M.P.H.

DISCUSSION OF DIVERSE INDIGENOUS GENDERS AND SEXUALITIES, AS DISTINCT FROM COLONIAL BINARIES

The term *Two Spirit* (sometimes abbreviated *2S*) is used by some Indigenous people native to the land generally known today as Turtle Island, or North America, to indicate a sexual orientation or gender identity that exists outside of/apart from Western, colonial, categorical (i.e., binary) understandings of identity. Some Two-Spirit people, but not all, may consider themselves members of the transgender, nonbinary, and/or gender-diverse (TNG) or broader lesbian, gay, bisexual, transgender, queer, intersex, asexual, and more (LGBTQIA+) communities. In addition, not all LGBTQIA+ Indigenous people identify as Two Spirit. Indigenous people may identify as

Two Spirit in some contexts, using a tribally specific term in one setting, and identify as a member of LGBTQIA+ communities in another, to negotiate belonging, as a protective strategy, or to communicate different relational stances within various spaces.

These nuances often reflect significant cultural differences in how individuals and communities conceptualize identity, roles, and responsibilities within family, community systems, spirituality, and ceremony (Ansloos et al. 2021). In addition, Indigenous genders are often heavily linked to a people's land, languages, resources, and web of relations (Robinson 2020). The term *Two Spirit* is often embraced by those embodying elements of both masculinity and femininity, those walking between and through gendered positions, those holding expansive understandings of their gender or sexuality, and those resisting Western binarism. In the National Transgender Discrimination Survey, 15% of respondents identified themselves as Two Spirit (Grant et al. 2011).

The sociohistorical context in which *Two Spirit* was coined gestures to the dynamics surrounding usage of the term. In 1990, Indigenous activists from many tribal identities gathered at the Native American, First Nations, Gay and Lesbian American Conference and created *Two Spirit* as a way to refer to Indigenous people who did not identify as cisgender or heterosexual (Anguksuar 1997). By coining this identity label, they worked to create a pantribal identity that accounts for their unique experiences as Indigenous people with expansive genders and sexualities. The label also allows them to claim a specific intersectional identity distinct from 1) cisgender and heterosexual Indigenous people and 2) LGBTQIA+ people who are not Indigenous. It holds space to address the ways in which Two-Spirit people experience oppressive stressors specifically as Indigenous people, and as people with minoritized genders or sexualities. These efforts also opened the door for Two-Spirit political organization and community building.

The creation of a pantribal identity—one not specific to a single tribe or language group—also opened opportunities to embody, explore, or reclaim tribally specific ways of gendered or sexual belonging. Importantly, there is no monolithic "Native American culture." There are >570 federally recognized tribes and >200 nonrecognized Indigenous communities in the United States alone (Balsam et al. 2004; Thomas et al. 2022). They speak >300 languages and represent an incredible diversity of cultures, beliefs, and practices, including those related to sexuality and gender (Balsam et al. 2004). Many tribal cultures have included community members who occupy sociocultural/spiritual roles that, throughout history, fall outside of Western understandings of the gender binary. It is outside of the scope of this chapter to address the long history and varied expression of genders in Indigenous communities; ample historical and contemporary accounts from multiple Indigenous perspectives are available for additional information.

Individuals may carry the knowledge of these identities specific to their communities of origin and use language that reflects their own understandings of gender and sexuality, in addition to or instead of identifying as Two Spirit or LGBTQIA+. However, ongoing genocidal projects targeting Indigenous languages and ways of knowing have led to the suppression of those traditional worldviews. During the past 200 years, forced or coerced education and Christian conversion in residential and boarding schools in Canada and the United States have pressured Indigenous people to adopt gender and sexual binaries as part of assimilationist violence against Indigenous communities (Robinson 2020). Thousands of children were taken from their families and kin networks by colonial agents, were stripped of their clothing, had their hair cut, were brutally punished for speaking their languages or practicing ceremonies, and often were taught outdated vocational skills (Evans-Campbell et al. 2012). As part of this process, children were physically segregated into boys and girls, erasing and violating children with genders not adhering to colonial, cisheterosexual expectations (Ellasante 2021). In response to being punished for the use of Indigenous languages in the schools, children were forced to distance themselves from their cultures and languages or find ways to practice and maintain their cultural knowledge away from the eyes of school personnel. Because languages were targeted, encoded knowledge such as Indigenous understandings of gender and gendered practices was threatened. Two-Spirit people who survived the boarding schools reported that they were more likely to use alcohol at higher rates, experience thoughts of suicide, or attempt suicide (Evans-Campbell et al. 2012).

Because of this history, generational or spiritual differences may exist relating to expansive genders and sexualities, wherein older or more culturally connected members have a more accepting view of nonbinary or expansive identities based on their interactions with colonial structures. Whether or not one experienced the boarding or residential school systems may also impact views on more traditional understandings of gender and sexuality or Two-Spirit identities (Cameron 2005).

ROLE OF HISTORICAL AND INTERGENERATIONAL TRAUMA

The colonial projects of assimilation included suppression and punishment of those who occupied social, spiritual, occupational, and sexual roles that did not conform to colonial understandings of heterosexuality or binary gender expression (Benson 2020). The ongoing violence of forced assimilation and cultural genocide contributed to ruptures in intergenerational transmission of tribal knowledge, including the roles of gender-expansive and sexually expansive members. Thus a sense of cultural loss surrounds this knowledge that distinguishes Two-Spirit and other Indigenous identities from colonial systems of gender and sexuality. Rather than claiming power for LGBTQIA+ communities, Two-Spirit and Indigenous people outside of colonial structures are working to reclaim that which was suppressed (Ristock et al. 2017). The ongoing effects of the boarding and residential schools are prime examples of the multiple forms of violence that constitute historical oppression—that is, experiences of oppression since initial colonial efforts, which continue to impact generations by operating through systemic, structural inequities (Burnette 2015). Importantly, boarding school experiences had negative impacts on the next generation of Two-Spirit people as well. Two-Spirit people raised by boarding school survivors were themselves more likely to experience negative outcomes such as suicidality, PTSD, and general anxiety (Evans-Campbell et al. 2012).

Colonialism and genocidal policies affect Indigenous people holistically. For example, the suppression of Indigenous spiritual practices undercuts the role that Two-Spirit people play in their community's spiritual life, which may negatively impact the individual's sense of belonging and responsibility to their community. In addition, actions that target Indigenous languages work to erase tribal understandings of gender and sexual diversity. The well-being of Two-Spirit people is intrinsically linked to the well-being of the community, as well as the language, spirituality, and land rights of the people. In this context, disruptions in the ability to connect to one's culture, relationships, and land affect the psychosocial well-being of Indigenous LGBTQIA+ and Two-Spirit people (Ansloos et al. 2021; Hardy et al. 2020).

The set of policies related to blood quantum and tribal enrollment creates a burden of proof for individuals and tribal communities to claim their identities as Indigenous people. Failure to meet the externally imposed requirements for membership can invalidate an entire community's claim to treaty rights and access to tribally based services, essentially writing groups out of existence (Ellasante 2021). In addition, biracial or multiracial people may be deemed ineligible for tribal membership, regardless of their standing in the community. These factors highlight the complexity of Indigenous identities as legal and political constructs as well as cultural, ethnic, or racial identities. In short, genocidal practices have affected many communities' relationships with members who have expansive genders and sexualities, as well as the structure of the community itself. Belongingness as Two-Spirit people exists within a larger, somewhat uneasy terrain of belonging because of the ongoing colonial projects attempting to disempower and dismantle Indigenous communities.

Contemporary nonnative LGBTQIA+ communities and organizations may romanticize Indigenous peoples' historical understandings of gender and sexuality and the concept of a Two-Spirit identity. Nonetheless they are often unaware of, or not inclusive of, Indigenous people in their activism and priorities. In addition, non-Indigenous use of the term *Two Spirit* to identify oneself is considered cultural appropriation (Cameron 2005).

Two Spirit was coined in response to the intersectional oppressions facing Indigenous people who are minoritized based on their gender identity, expression, or sexuality and against settler colonialism in particular (Ellasante 2021). The use of Two Spirit, rather than another term under the LGBTQIA+ umbrella, may also be an important way for members to centralize the importance of their Indigeneity or tribal identity, signaling their own sociopolitical alignments and responsibilities to their communities (Ansloos et al. 2021). In addition, Two-Spirit identities are created and interpreted within Indigenous epistemologies (Robinson 2020). The act of self-naming as Two Spirit may be seen as an act of resistance against ongoing colonial efforts to eradicate Indigenous understandings of gender (Ellasante 2021).

SOCIAL DETERMINANTS OF HEALTH FOR INDIGENOUS TWO-SPIRIT AND TNG PEOPLE

Unfortunately, research on mental health outcomes for Two-Spirit and TNG Indigenous people is limited by the marginalization of these intersecting identities in health care. Much of what does exist is centered solely on health disparities. From 1980 to 2019, only five articles addressed mental health and Two-Spirit people (Thomas et al. 2022).

In general, well-being for Indigenous people should be considered holistically, including elements of the spiritual and emotional along with the physical and mental. Additionally, the health and well-being of an individual's community context, family, and kinship networks and other extended membership structures may be intrinsically and reciprocally linked (Ansloos et al. 2021; Hardy et al. 2020). The individual's relational and community network is a crucial context for understanding determinants of health, barriers to health, potential interventions, and strengths—especially in the context of intersecting structural discrimination and active resistance.

When considering the social determinants of health for Two-Spirit people, it is important to attend to the intersecting forces of racism, colonialism, cisgenderism, and heterosexism. Colonialism, in particular, produces negative outcomes from the systemic, material, interpersonal, and intrapersonal violence that has affected tribal nations, communities, families, and individuals. Across multiple domains of social determinants of health, Two-Spirit people and Indigenous LGBTQIA+ people report higher rates of experiences of discrimination, barriers to access, and violence than their non-Indigenous peers.

According to the 2015 U.S. Transgender Survey Report, 23% of Indigenous respondents were unemployed, compared with 5% of non-Indigenous participants. Twenty-one percent of Indigenous TNG people said they had lost a job owing to their gender identity, whereas the rate among non-Indigenous TNG participants was 13% (James et al. 2016). Fifty-five percent of Indigenous TNG people reported being discriminated against in hiring practices, compared with 42% of white TNG people (Grant et al. 2011). Thirty-one percent had been denied promotion, a higher rate than that of their white peers at 21% (Grant et al. 2011). Relatedly, 41% of Indigenous people surveyed were considered to be living in poverty, compared with just 12% of non-Indigenous respondents. The rate for those experiencing homelessness was also higher for Indigenous people, at 21%, versus 12% for non-Indigenous TNG people (James et al. 2016). These economic and environmental factors may also contribute to the finding that Indigenous Two-Spirit and TNG people experience five subtypes of intimate partner violence—physical, psychological, trans-related, stalking, and forced sex—at rates significantly higher than among other groups of TNG people (King et al. 2021).

Rates of childhood physical abuse by caretakers are also high for Two-Spirit participants, nearly double those of Indigenous people who are not Two Spirit (Balsam et al. 2004), and have been linked to significant mental health outcomes for Indigenous people, more so than other forms of childhood trauma (Hobfoll et al. 2002). In K–12 educational settings, 61% of Two-Spirit and Indigenous TNG people reported identity-related abuse, including harassment, bullying, suspension, and sexual assault at the hands of peers as well as adults (Grant et al. 2011). Because of combined stressors, Two-Spirit and Indigenous TNG students reported leaving school owing to harassment (28%), transition-related financial reasons (40%), and discriminatory financial aid and scholarship practices (33%) (Grant et al. 2011). Transphobic and racist practices have also been documented in juvenile justice settings, wherein Two-Spirit and Indigenous youth are not affirmed in their gender throughout their involvement with that system (Benson 2020). Inequities in education have lasting implications for career training, housing, insurance coverage, and employment opportunities.

In the realm of incarceration, one study found that 30% of Two-Spirit or Indigenous TNG people had been jailed for any reason, suggesting that Two-Spirit communities are also affected by mental and physical aspects of incarceration, including physical and sexual harassment and assault and denial of health care while in custody (Grant et al. 2011). Among Indigenous adults of all gender identities, 9.2% reported experiencing serious psychological distress in the past 30 days, a rate three times that of white participants (National Center for Health Statistics 2018). Accumulated historical, intergenerational, and personal traumas, as well as chronic and acute stressors, contribute to Two-Spirit and Indigenous TNG people reporting an alarmingly high prevalence of at least one suicide attempt in their lives (56% in one study [Grant et al. 2011]), high prevalence of posttraumatic stress symptoms, and high prevalence of substance use over their lifetimes (Balsam et al. 2004).

There is a need for additional research regarding the impact that historical oppression and the chronic stressors of colonialism, heterosexism, and cissexism have on the well-being and mental health outcomes of Two-Spirit and LGBTQIA+ Indigenous people. Many studies that address mental health among Indigenous populations do not describe specific outcomes for their Two-Spirit or LGBTIQA+ participants, and studies of LGBTQIA+ mental health often omit Indigenous participants because of small sample sizes (Balsam et al. 2004).

BARRIERS TO CARE

In addition to pressures such as unemployment, abuse, impoverishment, and forced migration, the lack of accessible and culturally responsive care is a barrier for Two-Spirit and Indigenous TNG people (Teengs and Travers 2006). Historical oppression and ongoing inequities influence Two-Spirit people to distrust clinicians and other health services (Substance Abuse and Mental Health Services Administration 2006).

Colonialism shapes the dominant systems that provide for the delivery of health care and may revictimize Indigenous community members with expansive genders (Hunt 2016). Two-Spirit clients may struggle to access mental health services in general owing to concerns around the lack of availability of Indian Health Services in urban areas, minimal transportation in more rural settings, lack of insurance coverage (24% of Indigenous people), or the paucity of Indigenous clinicians (Substance Abuse and Mental Health Services Administration 2006).

Interactions with providers were cited as sources of negative experiences, with 50% of Indigenous respondents to the 2015 U.S. Transgender Survey reporting they experienced at least one negative interaction with a health care provider related to their gender identity, versus 33% of non-Indigenous TNG people (James et al. 2016). Medical neglect has also been reported, with 36% of Two-Spirit and Indigenous TNG respondents reporting having been denied health care altogether, versus 17% of white TNG people (Grant et al. 2011). Thirty-seven percent of Two-Spirit and Indigenous LGBTQIA+ people surveyed also avoided seeing a provider out of fear of gender identity–based mistreatment, versus 23% of non-Indigenous people (James et al. 2016). Research has found that Indigenous Two-Spirit and TNG people who were assigned male at birth experienced high levels of inequities in accessing gender-affirming mental health care, and that Two-Spirit and Indigenous LGBTQIA+ people reported high rates of severe distress (47.4%) (Lett et al. 2022). This gap may be the result of limited services that resonate with Indigenous people within LGBTQIA+ spaces and of Indigenous spaces that provide limited resources and visibility for Two-Spirit and LGBTQIA+ members (Ansloos et al. 2021).

ROLE OF COMMUNITY STRENGTHS, RESILIENCE, AND CULTURAL CONTINUITY

More research is needed to support the protective factors, social supports, relationships, strengths, and practices of resilience used by Two-Spirit people and their communities. A continued focus on health disparities and disease-prevention interventions has yet to address this gap in understanding Two-Spirit health and wellness holistically (Thomas et al. 2022). Emerging research has begun to highlight the protective effects of cultural connectedness, engagement in community spiritual life and ceremony, language use, relationships with Elders, and understandings of the negative impacts of colonialism. A study of Indigenous people conducted in an urban setting found no difference in cultural variables between Two-Spirit participants and those who did not identify as such. Most Two-Spirit respondents reported that they considered their cultural practices, traditional ways, and spiritual beliefs to be very important (Balsam et al. 2004). This finding reinforces the importance of community connectedness and cultural identification when conceptualizing strengths and resiliency for many Two-Spirit people. Assumptions should not be made that a Two-Spirit person is or is not connected to their community, that a community as a monolith is accepting or not accepting of Two-Spirit people, or that a person or community has maintained or reclaimed a tribally specific understanding of genders outside of Western heterosexist gender binaries.

Relationships with community Elders may act as sources of affirmation, strength, and support for Two-Spirit people (Walters et al. 2006). This may especially be the case when Two-Spirit Elders are able to share community knowledge and cultivate a sense of belonging for Two-Spirit youth (Ansloos et al. 2021). The transmission of knowledge, community wisdom, and tribal cultures paired with a strong sense of connectedness and understanding of colonization has been shown to decrease Two-Spirit people's experiences of suicidality and other mental health concerns (Hunt 2016); this effect is frequently referred to as *culture as treatment*. Culture as treatment seeks to connect or reconnect Indigenous people to their communities to address feelings of alienation, loneliness, disconnection, or other concerns related to holistic well-being. The use of traditional healing practices, often in conjunction with mainstream therapies, has been linked with improvements in health outcomes (Buchwald et al. 2000).

Two-Spirit youth may find that participating in their community's ceremonial life serves as a protective factor that supports their sense of health and well-being, if they are able to do so in a community that is affirming and are not limited by heterosexist or cissexist barriers (Laing 2018). In fact, cultural connectedness appears to be a primary protective determinant of health for Indigenous people (Snowshoe et al. 2017). Indigenous youth's mental wellness appears to be promoted through high levels of connection to their identity, integration in their community, and feelings of personal and political efficacy (Kirmayer et al. 2003). Efforts that support a tribal community's self-determination, political efficacy, sovereignty, spiritual life, language use, and cultural practices also serve as protective factors for Two-Spirit people with a high level of cultural connectedness (Ansloos et al. 2021).

Of course, an exploration of strengths, resources, and supports also includes the individual's personality, skills, talents, motivations, and experiences. These individual-level considerations should not be downplayed or ignored when working with Two-Spirit people. Considering family, kinship networks, community memberships, and additional micro-level factors is a critical component of affirming care for Two-Spirit people.

REFERENCES

Anguksuar: A postcolonial colonial perspective on Western [mis]conceptions of the cosmos and the restoration of indigenous taxonomies, in Two-Spirit People: Native American Gender Identity, Sexuality, and Spirituality. Edited by Jacobs S-E, Thomas W, Lang S. Urbana, IL, University of Illinois Press, 1997, pp 217–222

Ansloos J, Zantingh D, Ward K, et al: Radical care and decolonial futures: conversations on identity, health, and spirituality with Indigenous queer, trans, and Two-Spirit youth. Int J Child Youth Family Stud 12(3–4):74–103, 2021

Balsam KF, Huang B, Fieland KC, et al: Culture, trauma, and wellness: a comparison of heterosexual and lesbian, gay, bisexual, and two-spirit Native Americans. Cultur Divers Ethnic Minor Psychol 10(3):287–301, 2004 15311980

Benson K: What's in a pronoun? The ungovernability and misgendering of trans Native kids in juvenile justice in Washington state. J Homosex 67(12):1691–1712, 2020 31116672

Buchwald D, Beals J, Manson SM: Use of traditional health practices among Native Americans in a primary care setting. Med Care 38(12):1191–1199, 2000 11186298

Burnette CE: Disentangling Indigenous women's experiences with intimate partner violence in the United States. Crit Soc Work 16(1):1–20, 2015

Cameron M: Two-Spirited Aboriginal people: continuing cultural appropriation by non-Aboriginal society. Can Womens Stud 24(2,3):123–127, 2005

Ellasante IK: Radical sovereignty, rhetorical borders, and the everyday decolonial praxis of Indigenous peoplehood and Two-Spirit reclamation. Ethn Racial Stud 44(9):1507–1526, 2021

Evans-Campbell T, Walters KL, Pearson CR, Campbell CD: Indian boarding school experience, substance use, and mental health among urban two-spirit American Indian/Alaska natives. Am J Drug Alcohol Abuse 38(5):421–427, 2012 22931076

Grant JM, Mottet LA, Tanis J, et al: Injustice at Every Turn: A Report of the National Transgender Discrimination Survey. Washington, DC, National Center for Transgender Equality and National Gay and Lesbian Task Force, 2011

Hardy B-J, Lesperance A, Foote I, et al; Native Youth Sexual Health Network (NYSHN): Meeting Indigenous youth where they are at: knowing and doing with 2SLGBTTQQIA and gender non-conforming Indigenous youth: a qualitative case study. BMC Public Health 20(1):1871, 2020 33287787

Hobfoll SE, Bansal A, Schurg R, et al: The impact of perceived child physical and sexual abuse history on Native American women's psychological well-being and AIDS risk. J Consult Clin Psychol 70:252–257, 2002

Hunt S: An Introduction to the Health of Two-Spirit People: Historical, Contemporary and Emergent Issues. Prince George, British Columbia, Canada, National Collaborating Centre for Aboriginal Health, 2016

James SE, Herman JL, Rankin S, et al: The Report of the 2015 U.S. Transgender Survey. Washington, DC, National Center for Transgender Equality, 2016. Available at: https://transequality.org/sites/default/files/docs/usts/USTS-Full-Report-Dec17.pdf. Accessed March 20, 2023.

King WM, Restar A, Operario D: Exploring multiple forms of intimate partner violence in a gender and racially/ethnically diverse sample of transgender adults. J Interpers Violence 36(19-20):NP10477–NP10498, 2021 31526070

Kirmayer L, Simpson C, Cargo M: Healing traditions: culture, community, and mental health promotion with Canadian Aboriginal peoples. Australas Psychiatry 11:15–23, 2003

Laing M: Conversations With Young Two-Spirit, Trans and Queer Indigenous People About the Term Two-Spirit. Doctoral dissertation, University of Toronto, Toronto, ON, Canada, 2018. Available at: https://tspace.library.utoronto.ca/handle/1807/91455. Accessed March 7, 2023.

Lett E, Abrams MP, Gold A, et al: Ethnoracial inequities in access to gender-affirming mental health care and psychological distress among transgender adults. Soc Psychiatry Psychiatr Epidemiol 57(5):963–971, 2022 35137246

National Center for Health Statistics: Serious Psychological Distress in the Past 30 Days Among Adults Aged 18 and Over, by Selected Characteristics: United States, Average Annual, Selected Years 1997–1998 Through 2015–2016. Atlanta, GA, Centers for Disease Control and Prevention, 2018. Available at: https://www.cdc.gov/nchs/data/hus/2017/046.pdf.

Ristock J, Zoccole A, Passante L, Potskin J: Impacts of colonization on Indigenous Two-Spirit/LGBTQ Canadians' experiences of migration, mobility and relationship violence. Sexualities 22(5–6):767–784, 2017

Robinson M: Two-Spirit identity in a time of gender fluidity. J Homosex 67(12):1675–1690, 2020 31125297

Substance Abuse and Mental Health Services Administration: Culture, Race, and Ethnicity—A Supplement to Mental Health: A Report of the Surgeon General. Rockville, MD, U.S. Department of Health and Human Services, 2006

Snowshoe A, Crooks CV, Tremblay PF, Hinson RE: Cultural connectedness and its relation to mental wellness for First Nations youth. J Prim Prev 38(1-2):67–86, 2017 27807659

Teengs DO, Travers R: "River of life, rapids of change": understanding HIV vulnerability among Two-Spirit youth who migrate to Toronto. Can Aborig J Commun Based HIV/AIDS Res 1:17–28, 2006

Thomas M, McCoy T, Jeffries I, et al: Native American Two Spirit and LGBTQ health: a systematic review of the literature. J Gay Lesbian Ment Health 26(4):1–36, 2022

Walters KL, Evans-Campbell T, Simoni J, et al: "My Spirit in My Heart": Identity experiences and challenges among American Indian Two-Spirit Women. J Lesbian Stud 10(1/2):125–149, 2006

CHAPTER 6

Intersectional Approaches to Affirming Mental Health Care for Black Transgender, Nonbinary, and/or Gender-Expansive (TNG) People in North America

Henri M. Garrison-Desany, Ph.D., M.S.P.H.
Emerson J. Dusic, M.P.H.
Jack Bruno, M.S.W.
Fiona (Fí) Fonseca, M.D., Ph.D.
Arjee Javellana Restar, Ph.D., M.P.H.

BLACK TNG individuals face extremely high rates of violence, stigma, and discrimination in the United States, compared with both Black cisgender and white TNG counterparts. Such experiences contribute to disproportionate, severe burdens of mental, behavioral, and physical health disorders for this population. Yet current research underrepresents and underreports Black TNG experiences, because such projects simply group mental health issues for Black TNG people within HIV research or collapse categories of trans feminine individuals with cisgender men who have sex with men (MSM). Such work fails to describe the multiple forms of marginalization that Black TNG people face, including from within the Black community. This marginalization is the result not only of slavery in the United States, structural racism, and ongoing traumatization resulting from those events, but also of cisnormativity and forced gender expectations. Approaches to improve the mental health of Black TNG individuals must acknowledge and address the complex factors that influence their health and well-being, including diversity within the Black TNG community, social determinants of health, and structural and interpersonal barriers to health care. Additionally, the positive impact of social support through queer family structures, *ballroom culture* (an underground African American and Latino lesbian, gay, bisexual, transgender, queer, and more (LGBTQ+) subculture of drag queen pageants), spirituality, and engagement in mutual aid and community activism should be levied when considering potential pathways to address existing disparities. All these issues together should be considered compounding factors under an intersectional model of minority stress theory, wherein Black TNG people face experiences of violence and mental health disparities because they are Black, because they are TNG, and because they are Black and TNG.

PREVALENCE OF MENTAL AND BEHAVIORAL HEALTH DISORDERS

Black TNG people experience higher rates (vs. white peers) of a broad range of mental health disorders, including depression (Jefferson et al. 2013) and serious mental illness such as schizophrenia (Brown and Jones 2014). Notably, in one recent year, an estimated 59% of Black TNG youth seriously considered attempting suicide, and 32% attempted suicide (The Trevor Project 2020). Yet there remains a dearth of studies specifically focused on Black TNG people's experiences. Many TNG mental health studies have been underpowered to estimate the Black TNG community's prevalence of mental health disorders, because of insufficient recruitment of Black participants. Researchers often group Black transgender women with Black cisgender MSM, which precludes differentiating the mental health disorder burden between these groups, despite large differences in the gender-based discrimination and violence they face (Poteat et al. 2016, 2021; Restar et al. 2021).

The Impact of Violence and Victimization

Black TNG people face staggering rates of abuse and victimization, which exacerbate mental health challenges. For example, a study of Black and Latinx transgender women in Baltimore, Maryland, and Washington, D.C., found that 91.4% of participants had faced at least one form of violence, and 86.8% had experienced multiple forms of violence (Sherman et al. 2020).

Intergroup comparisons are subject to methodological challenges; e.g., a study that reports differences compared with white TNG people only, or Black cisgender people only, misses the potential interactive effects of being both Black and TNG. Additionally, intersectional studies of the violence TNG people face often have relatively small sample sizes and may be underpowered to look at multiple axes of identity. Black TNG people, particularly transgender women, experience strikingly more frequent violence than non-Black TNG people and Black cisgender LGBQ+ people. In 2021, 36 (63%) of the 57 TNG people violently killed in the United States were Black (Human Rights Campaign 2021). There is consistent evidence that Black TNG people are more likely to experience transphobia-related violence than white counterparts (Dinno 2017; Klemmer et al. 2021). There is also some evidence that Black TNG people, and specifically Black trans women, experience higher rates of intimate partner violence (including psychological, physical, and sexual violence) compared with both white TNG and Black cisgender people (Whitfield et al. 2021); however, that association is not consistent across all cohort studies (King et al. 2021).

Violence against TNG people can also manifest in direct relation to their gender identity and transition, such as threatening to disclose someone's transgender status, withholding their medical care such as hormones, or belittling a partner specifically because they are TNG (Garthe et al. 2018; James et al. 2016). This can be exacerbated among Black TNG communities who already experience greater barriers to accessing medical care and may feel socially isolated by the smaller community dynamics compared with the overall TNG or LGBTQ+ community.

Historic Lineages Affecting Black Trans Mental Health

The robust challenges facing Black TNG communities and their effects on community members' mental health stem from centuries of white supremacy and anti-Blackness. In addition to contending with historical traumas (e.g., centuries of the slave trade and colonization), Black TNG people are subject to contemporary gender policing that such oppressive powers continue to exact (Rogers and Bryant-Davis 2022). The United States has been built on structural racism, resulting in a multigenerational and systemic discrimination that limits access to housing, employment, health services, and other resources (Bailey et al. 2017). Such insults accumulate and often additionally disrupt historic family structures and mutual aid networks (Rogers and Bryant-Davis 2022; Spade 2020). This is detrimental to child and adolescent growth and development, let alone gender exploration and self-acceptance. The issues facing one Black TNG person cannot be divorced from the legacies of slavery and forced migration (Adewale et al. 2016; Wilkins et al. 2013), Jim Crow–era laws including disenfranchisement (Thomas 2011), redlining and housing discrimination (Lynch et al. 2021; Noelke et al. 2022), and other racist practices that are embedded in societal attitudes, government programs, and institutional norms. Further, Black TNG communities contend with ongoing oppression from political, economic, and societal authorities, including over- and underpolicing and disproportionate deaths at the hands of law enforcement (DeAngelis 2021), legislation (e.g., the War on Drugs) leading to mass incarceration (Fornili 2018), and the daily struggles of "walking while Black and trans" (Edelman 2014). Intersectional care for a Black TNG person includes understanding how this myriad of forces has cultivated the environment they must negotiate today.

Notably, slavery and the subsequent oppression of Black ancestors in the United States resulted in the stripping of major cultural practices and tribal associations to reify the white-dominated Christian hegemony (Lovejoy 1997; Young 2007). With the advent of accessible genetic testing, some individuals are now able to map their genetic ancestry to specific regions or tribes; yet a genetic test cannot rectify centuries of cultural sanitization or meaningfully teach cultural practices. As a result, Black cultures have been re-formed over centuries into new rituals and praxes. This is especially true for Black TNG people, who experience multiple marginalizations, including within the Black community. As previous iterations of Black political thought and radical liberation have not considered the needs of TNG groups within the diaspora, communities have responded by creating their own spaces and modalities of social justice (Chaudhry 2019).

For instance, Kimberlé Crenshaw coined the term *intersectionality* to describe the multiple marginalizations faced by Black women, from within both white-centric feminist groups and male-centric Black liberation spaces (Crenshaw 1991). Moya Bailey built on that work in 2010 by coining the term *misogynoir* to describe the layered hatred and discrimination Black women experience that manifests under this intersectional framework (Bailey and Trudy 2018). In 2015, the term *transmisogynoir* was introduced to specifically describe the multiple marginalizations Black trans women experience in navigating the world (Wodda and Panfil 2015); transmisogynoir is likely a contributing factor to the particularly disproportionate burden of violence and victimization enacted on Black trans women and trans feminine people.

Black transgender women and trans feminine people experience both hypervisibility and hypervulnerability in much of the research around Black transgender mental health. However, Black transgender men and trans masculine people must also navigate a complicated web of gendered expectations and masculine histories as they attempt to forge pathways forward in the world (Agénor et al. 2022a, 2022b; Jourian and McCloud 2020). Multiple qualitative studies have described the challenge of their invisibility as transgender people and their increased vulnerability and visibility when they are perceived as Black cisgender men (Jourian and McCloud 2020; White et al. 2020). In a world that perceives Black masculinity as inherently threatening throughout the life course (Boyd and Mitchell 2018; Dottolo and Stewart 2008; Hall et al. 2016; Hester and Gray 2018; James 2012), Black trans masculine people must contend with their own gender histories and gendered trauma, the relative privilege they may attain in being assumed cisgender men at times ("passing"), and the continued oppression they face in the broader hegemony.

Limitations of the Current Research

Research on mental health outcomes and service utilization among Black TNG people has emerged largely within HIV research and has pertained to Black trans women and trans feminine people with MSM (Poteat et al. 2016), profoundly limiting its utility. Additionally, much of the literature on other TNG people in the United States, particularly nonbinary people, trans masculine people, trans men, and other gender-diverse groups, involves majority white samples (Cicero et al. 2020; James et al. 2016; Warren et al. 2016). Thus, Black nonbinary and trans masculine people are missing from the literature, with little information about their experiences or risk factors (Follins et al. 2014). This is especially troubling given their apparent high rates of mental health challenges, including anxiety, depression, and suicidal ideation, as reported in qualitative work (Jourian and McCloud 2020; White et al. 2020). Few articles specifically examine the challenges facing Black nonbinary people (Nicolazzo 2016), and their mental health concerns have yet to be quantitatively characterized in the literature.

DIVERSITY WITHIN THE BLACK TNG COMMUNITY

Although the Black community in the United States is often treated as a single static group, the African diaspora is varied and constantly shifting. Here, we present salient concerns for Black TNG clients and communities regarding immigration status and rurality.

Issues Facing Black Immigrants

In 2022, estimates suggested that 21% of Black people in the United States were immigrants or children of immigrants; this proportion is expected to rise each year (Tamir 2022). In the literature, Black TNG immigrants have yet to be described, indicating erasure of their pressing issues. Data suggest that the prevalence of mental health disorders and concerns among immigrant Black Caribbean communities differs from that of African American communities, and that the effect is moderated by gender. Broman et al. (2008) found that Black Caribbean men had 76% higher odds of past-year mood disorders compared with African American men, whereas Black Caribbean women had 31% lower odds of any psychiatric disorders compared with African American women; this also varied by age at immigration and by ethnic ancestry. Such work highlights the need for recognizing the heterogeneity of Black communities in mental health research and intervention (see also Chapter 10, "Caring for Displaced People").

Similarly, the literature inadequately describes stressors related to immigration status for Black immigrants lacking documentation or seeking asylum, especially regarding their intersections with Blackness. Despite often being erased from national immigration discourse, in 2016, Black immigrants made up 20.3% of people facing deportation, while accounting for only 5.4% of noncitizens in the United States (Trostle et al. 2016). Social support can foster resilience from anti-Black and cisgenderist biases and discrimination, making layered isolation especially pernicious; this is compounded by the frequency with which undocumented TNG clients seek asylum based on their gender modality (Rosati et al. 2021; Yarwood et al. 2022).

Rural Versus Urban Communities

There also remains a dearth of information around Black TNG experiences in rural areas compared with urban centers. This is likely due to broader challenges of recruiting research participants: rural communities may not be well connected to large health centers (Knutson et al. 2016; Smith et al. 2018); resources may be allocated based on urban assumptions rather than rural realities; and geography may pose challenges for outreach and transportation. One study showed that trans men living in rural areas had higher depression and global severity scores than urban trans men, as measured by the Brief Symptom Inventory (Horvath et al. 2014). As most of that sample was white, the generalizability of results to Black TNG people is unclear.

What little research has occurred shows that integration into rural communities may center around *claim to sameness*, whereby individuals are able to enact appropriate gender expressions that are legible to other rural community members; much of this may be mediated by proximity to whiteness. In a study of trans men, many participants found inclusion by belonging to communities that were primarily white; when asked to imagine how a Black TNG person might experience their communities, they anticipated difficulty integrating (Abelson 2016). Many rural white trans men in the study specifically identified their whiteness as key to their gaining social inroads and material benefits from the rural communities in which they lived.

SOCIAL DETERMINANTS OF HEALTH

Socioeconomic Status, Income, and Education

Income and socioeconomic status (SES) play a large role in Black TNG mental health outcomes. Of note, it is a common misconception that income/SES alone accounts for the health disparities between Black and white TNG communities; rather, these should be considered as compounding issues under an intersectional model of minority stress theory. Black TNG people experience reduced employment and income compared with both cisgender Black people (Russell et al. 2021) and white TNG people (Leppel 2021). In a data-driven intersectional study of SES and race, Budge et al. (2016) found stratification of both race/ethnicity and SES, with white TNG participants often having higher household incomes than non-white TNG participants, who were more likely to have high educational status but low household income; TNG participants of color also had a higher anxiety symptom burden than the white, high-income TNG group.

Education also dictates lived experience of SES. Black TNG students experience structural and interpersonal barriers to educational achievement. This manifests through programs, such as internships and community learning experiences, that disproportionately do not recruit or accept Black TNG students (Stewart and Nicolazzo 2018) and overt discrimination experienced on campus from other students, faculty, and staff (Nicolazzo 2016). Additionally, the 2015 U.S. Transgender Survey found that Black TNG people were disproportionately expelled from K–12 education if students or staff knew that they were TNG, with 10% of Black TNG people and 22% of Black trans girls being expelled, compared with 6% of all survey participants (James et al. 2016). For students, these hostile school environments create stress and opportunities for victimization and likely exacerbate mental health disparities.

Incarceration Status

For Black TNG people specifically, policing and incarceration are major risk factors for poor mental health (see also Chapter 19, "Affirming Gender Identity in the Setting of Incarceration"). In a sample of majority Black trans feminine youth in Chicago (Garofalo et al. 2006), 37% of participants had a history of incarceration; this was correlated with engaging in sex work, which 59% of participants also reported, highlighting the intersection of incarceration and employment factors in this population. Black, Latina, and mixed-race trans women are more likely, while incarcerated, to also experience victimization than white peers (Reisner et al. 2014). Additionally, a study of trans women and cis MSM found reduced social support after recent incarceration, including those spending just one night in jail, as may occur from an initial arrest (Scheidell et al. 2021). Because individuals with major mental health disorders are more likely to be incarcerated (Blank Wilson et al. 2014; Hall et al. 2019; Mulvey and Schubert 2017; White 2016), the disproportionate incarceration for Black TNG people is an important risk factor exacerbating mental health disorders in the community.

BARRIERS TO HEALTH CARE

Clinical Mistrust and Cultural Humility

The bleak history of medical experimentation on Black Americans fractured Black communities' trust of clinicians and health systems. A preeminent example is the Tuskegee Study of Untreated Syphilis in the Negro Male from 1932 to 1972, in which researchers unethically allowed syphilis infections among Black men to proceed even when treatments became available (Thomas and Quinn 1991). J. Marion Sims carries the moniker "Father of Gynecology" despite his surgical experimentation—without anesthetic—on enslaved Black people assigned female at birth, including operating on one woman 30 times before finally repairing her fistulas (Washington 2008). The long history of the medical establishment dismissing Black patients' rights endures as medical mistrust in Black communities. This mistrust has wide-reaching implications: Chen et al. (2022) found that the majority of Black trans women sampled believed conspiracy theories about COVID-19 (e.g., developed in a lab, released by the government).

Any mental health clinician who is not Black must contend with interpersonal mistrust, in addition to mistrust of clinical institutions (Suite et al. 2007; Whaley 2001a). Given the historic barriers to TNG people seeking care and lack of trust in clinicians responding positively and sensitively after disclosure of TNG identity (D'Avanzo et al. 2019; Johnson et al. 2019), Black TNG people face dual histories of oppression that impede trust. To address this, mental health clinicians should acknowledge and validate concerns about the medical establishment and address interpersonal dynamics with clients. For instance, mistrust expressed to a clinician may reflect a societal and historic mistrust rather than a personal sentiment (Whaley 2001b).

Of note, despite Black clients' high burden of distressing experiences, such exposures may not manifest as mental disorders at the same rate as for white clients (Tobin 2021). This may reflect how the diagnostic criteria and assessments were developed in other populations and not the mental health challenges and presentations of Black TNG communities, despite evidence that cross-cultural adaptation is important for treatment (Sousa and Rojjanasrirat 2011). Cultural humility in this context means addressing Black TNG clients' multifaceted concerns to establish interpersonal trust, even if institutional trust may not improve.

Cost and Insurance Barriers

The primary barrier to accessing mental health care for Black TNG people is cost. Many mental health clinicians do not accept insurance, requiring clients to pay out of pocket (Bishop et al. 2014). Even when insurance is accepted, Black TNG clients may not have comprehensive coverage. Black communities overall have lower income and SES than the population as a whole (LaVeist 2005), making cost a particular burden for Black TNG clients. No study to date has directly investigated the extent of these issues, but cost has been identified as a major barrier to health care for Black TNG people (Chen et al. 2018; Sherman et al. 2022). Patient advocates may help mitigate these obstacles by working with clients in submitting insurance claims, signing up for public insurance options, or creating payment plans. Mental health clinicians may also offer sliding-scale fees for Black TNG clients, to acknowledge and address the economic reality many potential clients face.

Anticipated Stigma for Being Transgender or Black or Both

Research robustly shows that Black clients and TNG clients often face microaggressions or discrimination when accessing mental health services (Gómez 2015; Morris et al. 2020; Nadal et al. 2016). Living at the nexus of these groups, Black TNG clients are most vulnerable. Even if a mental health clinician engages in culture- and gender-sensitive care, the therapeutic environment may be affected by a client's prior experiences with clinicians who did not. Microaggressions may manifest as statements about race (e.g., asking individuals to speak on behalf of their racial/ethnic group [Gómez 2015]) or about gender identity (e.g., assumptions about client experiences based on their gender expression [Morris et al. 2020]). Clients may experience a pernicious interaction of assumptions that being Black must lead to internalized transphobia, or that being TNG is somehow at odds with their cultural upbringing.

Siloed Treatment Modalities Lacking Intersectional Understandings

Well-intentioned mental health clinicians risk overusing a modality useful in exploring challenges related to gender identity or race/ethnicity to the detriment of interrogating other aspects of a Black TNG person's life. In physical health, *trans broken arm syndrome* refers to a clinician's focus on gender identity as the main problem to be assessed, even when a patient is presenting with an entirely unrelated concern (Oliver 2022). Mental health clinicians may fall into similar patterns. Training around TNG mental health and Black mental health often occurs in silos; it is unsurprising that clinicians default to such a framework, even if a client is discussing another area of their life. In this microaggression, an individual is reduced to one aspect of their identity, and Black TNG people are unable to explore their complex intersections or entirely separate experiences. Client-focused treatment modalities may be more useful in allowing Black TNG clients to set their own mental health agendas.

FACILITATORS TO TREATMENT AND POSITIVE MENTAL HEALTH SOCIAL SUPPORT THROUGH QUEER FAMILY STRUCTURES

Given the hostility they face from within their communities, Black TNG people have been shown in quantitative and qualitative studies to derive mental health protection from social ties and family structures. For instance, having perceived family support is a main driver for being out as TNG among Black people (Pastrana 2016). Kinship outside of biological family (fictive kin) provides key social support for many Black people (Stewart 2007).

Although the term *fictive kin* implies that the relationships are a fake imitation of biological kinship structures, nonbiological families of Black TNG people should be valued as simply that: a queer family. Sometimes called *chosen family* or *found family*, these kinship structures have the same roles and responsibilities in their relationships as biological family equivalents, as well as specialized nuances to the queer context. This is especially important for many Black TNG people who lose biological family relationships for a host of reasons, including cisgenderism/heterosexism, lack of acceptance, incarceration of biological family members related to mass incarceration more broadly, or death of biological family members related to disparities and social determinants. The dissolution of biological family relationships can reflect both interpersonal and structural injustices, buttressing the importance of other family relationships. The creation of found families is not simply due to individual relationships but rather becomes a necessity with a generational lineage dating back to slavery's dissolution of biological family ties (Rogers and Bryant-Davis 2022).

Social and Material Support in Ballroom Culture

Kin and community are especially salient for TNG people engaged in ballroom culture, which has further hierarchies around houses and the status of house mother, house father, drag mother, and similar honorifics (Bailey 2013). Whereas other spaces, such as school or work, may require self-policing of gender, ballroom can be seen as a liberatory space (Arnold and Bailey 2009; Reid 2022). Houses can extend over regional or national networks, creating long-standing lineages. The role of scene-specific parents, siblings, and children can bolster the sense of community and overall resilience in both material and social ways. In ballroom, kin labor is formalized, families may provide support during job loss or housing instability, and birthdays and milestones are celebrated (Bailey 2013). Houses and families can also function as a form of protection in areas of violence or victimization, either during a violent altercation (fighting with and for their house members) or after an incident in the form of support and shelter (Telander et al. 2017).

Complicated Religious Engagement

Religious communities also offer support. Religious Black TNG people have described their faith as, simultaneously, a source of strength and a space in which they struggle to find acceptance (Graham 2014). Families of origin may cite their faith when rejecting Black TNG people; Black TNG people may anticipate lack of acceptance because of their family's religious views. Nevertheless, personal spirituality may promote the ability to cope with societal discrimination and victimization (Golub et al. 2010; Graham 2014). Black TNG people do affiliate with and attend religious services in both affirming and nonaffirming congregations. Processing religious trauma or allowing for religious interpretations of their experiences may be helpful for some clients, and affirming congregations may offer a sense of community and a source of support.

Broader Community Activism

A major protective factor for mental health and improved treatment of mental health disorders among Black TNG people is empowerment and pride in their identity (Johnson and Rogers 2019). Additionally, support from the TNG community and involvement with peers is protective against mental distress and symptoms of mental disorders (Bariola et al. 2015; Pflum et al. 2015). There is evidence that this is especially important for transgender women and trans feminine people (Pflum et al. 2015). In light of the structural issues facing Black TNG people (Yarbrough 2021), connection to community has both psychological benefits and tangible opportunities for mutual aid. Considering the lineage of Black TNG people's involvement in broader TNG and queer, feminist, and Black organizing efforts (Carruthers 2018; Feinberg 1997; Jackson 2021; Mobley et al. 2021; Sudbury 2009), link-ing these networks and efforts can be a powerful way to connect with and draw strength from their social ancestries.

REFERENCES

Abelson MJ: "You aren't from around here": race, masculinity, and rural transgender men. Gend Place Cult 23(11):1535–1546, 2016

Adewale V, Ritchie D, Skeels SE: African-American and African perspectives on mental health: a pilot study of the pre and post colonial and slavery influences and their implications on mental health. J Commun Healthc 9(2):78–89, 2016

Agénor M, Geffen SR, Zubizarreta D, et al: Experiences of and resistance to multiple discrimination in health care settings among transmasculine people of color. BMC Health Serv Res 22(1):369, 2022a 35307008

Agénor M, Zubizarreta D, Geffen S, et al: "Making a way out of no way": understand-ing the sexual and reproductive health care experiences of transmasculine young adults of color in the United States. Qual Health Res 32(1):121–134, 2022b 34851198

Arnold EA, Bailey MM: Constructing home and family: how the ballroom commu-nity supports African American GLBTQ youth in the face of HIV/AIDS. J Gay Lesbian Soc Serv 21(2-3):171–188, 2009 23136464

Bailey MM: Butch Queens Up in Pumps: Gender, Performance, and Ballroom Cul-ture in Detroit. Ann Arbor, MI, University of Michigan Press, 2013

Bailey M, Trudy: On misogynoir: citation, erasure, and plagiarism. Fem Media Stud 18(4):762–768, 2018

Bailey ZD, Krieger N, Agénor M, et al: Structural racism and health inequities in the USA: evidence and interventions. Lancet 389(10077):1453–1463, 2017 28402827

Bariola E, Lyons A, Leonard W, et al: Demographic and psychosocial factors associ-ated with psychological distress and resilience among transgender individuals. Am J Public Health 105(10):2108–2116, 2015 26270284

Bishop TF, Press MJ, Keyhani S, Pincus HA: Acceptance of insurance by psychiatrists and the implications for access to mental health care. JAMA Psychiatry 71(2):176–181, 2014 24337499

Blank Wilson A, Draine J, Barrenger S, et al: Examining the impact of mental illness and substance use on time till re-incarceration in a county jail. Adm Policy Men-tal Health 41(3):293–301, 2014 23334515

Boyd T, Mitchell D: Black male persistence in spite of facing stereotypes in college: a phenomenological exploration. Qual Rep 23(4):893–913, 2018

Broman CL, Neighbors HW, Delva J, et al: Prevalence of substance use disorders among African Americans and Caribbean Blacks in the National Survey of American Life. Am J Public Health 98(6):1107–1114, 2008 17971551

Brown GR, Jones KT: Racial health disparities in a cohort of 5,135 transgender vet-erans. J Rac Ethn Health Dispar 1(4):257–266, 2014

Budge SL, Thai JL, Tebbe EA, Howard KAS: The intersection of race, sexual orientation, socioeconomic status, trans identity, and mental health outcomes. Couns Psychol 44(7):1025–1049, 2016

Carruthers C: Unapologetic: A Black, Queer, and Feminist Mandate for Radical Movements. Boston, MA, Beacon Press, 2018

Chaudhry VV (ed): Coalitional love-politics. Transgend Stud Q 6(4):521–538, 2019

Chen D, Matson M, Macapagal K, et al: Attitudes toward fertility and reproductive health among transgender and gender-nonconforming adolescents. J Adolesc Health 63(1):62–68, 2018 29503031

Chen Y-T, Duncan DT, Del Vecchio N, et al: COVID-19 conspiracy beliefs are not barriers to HIV status neutral care among Black cisgender sexual minority men and Black transgender women at the initial peak of the COVID-19 pandemic in Chicago, USA. AIDS Behav 26(12):3939–3949, 2022 35731308

Cicero EC, Reisner SL, Merwin EI, et al: The health status of transgender and gender nonbinary adults in the United States. PLoS One 15(2):e0228765, 2020 32084144

Crenshaw K: Mapping the margins: intersectionality, identity politics, and violence against women of color. Stanford Law Rev 43(6):1241–1299, 1991

D'Avanzo PA, Bass SB, Brajuha J, et al: Medical mistrust and PrEP perceptions among transgender women: a cluster analysis. Behav Med 45(2):143–152, 2019 31343968

DeAngelis RT: Systemic racism in police killings: new evidence from the Mapping Police Violence Database, 2013–2021. Race Justice 21533687211047944, 2021

Dinno A: Homicide rates of transgender individuals in the United States: 2010–2014. Am J Public Health 107(9):1441–1447, 2017 28727530

Dottolo AL, Stewart AJ: "Don't ever forget now, you're a Black man in America": intersections of race, class and gender in encounters with the police. Sex Roles 59(5):350–364, 2008

Edelman EA: "Walking while transgender" 1: necropolitical regulations of trans feminine bodies of colour in the nation's capital, in Queer Necropolitics. Abingdon, UK, Routledge, 2014, pp 172–190

Feinberg L: Transgender Warriors: Making History From Joan of Arc to Marsha P. Johnson and Beyond. Boston, MA, Beacon Press, 1997

Follins LD, Garrett-Walker JJ, Lewis MK: Resilience in Black lesbian, gay, bisexual, and transgender individuals: a critical review of the literature. J Gay Lesbian Ment Health 18(2):190–212, 2014

Fornili KS: Racialized mass incarceration and the war on drugs: a critical race theory appraisal. J Addict Nurs 29(1):65–72, 2018 29505464

Garofalo R, Deleon J, Osmer E, et al: Overlooked, misunderstood and at-risk: exploring the lives and HIV risk of ethnic minority male-to-female transgender youth. J Adolesc Health 38(3):230–236, 2006 16488820

Garthe RC, Hidalgo MA, Hereth J, et al: Prevalence and risk correlates of intimate partner violence among a multisite cohort of young transgender women. LGBT Health 5(6):333–340, 2018 30059268

Golub SA, Walker JJ, Longmire-Avital B, et al: The role of religiosity, social support, and stress-related growth in protecting against HIV risk among transgender women. J Health Psychol 15(8):1135–1144, 2010 20522502

Gómez JM: Microaggressions and the enduring mental health disparity: Black Americans at risk for institutional betrayal. J Black Psychol 41(2):121–143, 2015

Graham LF: Navigating community institutions: Black transgender women's experiences in schools, the criminal justice system, and churches. Sex Res Soc Policy 11(4):274–287, 2014

Hall AV, Hall EV, Perry JL: Black and blue: exploring racial bias and law enforcement in the killings of unarmed black male civilians. Am Psychol 71(3):175–186, 2016 27042881

Hall D, Lee L-W, Manseau MW, et al: Major mental illness as a risk factor for incarceration. Psychiatr Serv 70(12):1088–1093, 2019 31480926

Hester N, Gray K: For Black men, being tall increases threat stereotyping and police stops. Proc Natl Acad Sci USA 115(11):2711–2715, 2018

Horvath KJ, Iantaffi A, Swinburne-Romine R, Bockting W: A comparison of mental health, substance use, and sexual risk behaviors between rural and non-rural transgender persons. J Homosex 61(8):1117–1130, 2014 24380580

Human Rights Campaign: Fatal Violence Against the Transgender and Gender Non-Conforming Community in 2021. Washington, DC, Human Rights Campaign, 2021. Available at: https://www.hrc.org/resources/fatal-violence-against-the-transgender-and-gender-non-conforming-community-in-2021. Accessed June 24, 2022.

Jackson JM: Black feminisms, queer feminisms, trans feminisms: meditating on Pauli Murray, Shirley Chisholm, and Marsha P. Johnson against the erasure of history, in The Routledge Companion to Black Women's Cultural Histories. Abingdon, UK, Routledge, 2021, pp 284–294

James CE: Students "at risk": stereotypes and the schooling of Black boys. Urban Educ 47(2):464–494, 2012

James SE, Herman JL, Rankin S, et al: The Report of the 2015 U.S. Transgender Survey. Washington, DC, National Center for Transgender Equality, 2016. Available at: https://transequality.org/sites/default/files/docs/usts/USTS-Full-Report-Dec17.pdf. Accessed June 24, 2023.

Jefferson K, Neilands TB, Sevelius J: Transgender women of color: discrimination and depression symptoms. Ethn Inequal Health Soc Care 6(4):121–136, 2013 25346778

Johnson AH, Rogers BA: "We're the normal ones here": community involvement, peer support, and transgender mental health. Sociol Inq 90(2):271–292, 2019

Johnson AH, Hill I, Beach-Ferrara J, et al: Common barriers to healthcare for transgender people in the U.S. Southeast. Int J Transgender Health 21(1):70–78, 2019 33015660

Jourian TJ, McCloud L: "I don't know where I stand": Black trans masculine students' re/de/constructions of Black masculinity. J Coll Student Dev 61(6):733–749, 2020

King WM, Restar A, Operario D: Exploring multiple forms of intimate partner violence in a gender and racially/ethnically diverse sample of transgender adults. J Interpers Violence 36(19-20):NP10477–NP10498, 2021 31526070

Klemmer CL, Arayasirikul S, Raymond HF: Transphobia-based violence, depression, and anxiety in transgender women: the role of body satisfaction. J Interpers Violence 36(5-6):2633–2655, 2021 29528801

Knutson D, Koch JM, Arthur T, et al: "Trans broken arm": health care stories from transgender people in rural areas. J Res Women Gend 7(1):30–46, 2016

LaVeist TA: Disentangling race and socioeconomic status: a key to understanding health inequalities. J Urban Health 82(2 Suppl 3):iii26–iii34, 2005 15933328

Leppel K: Transgender men and women in 2015: employed, unemployed, or not in the labor force. J Homosex 68(2):203–229, 2021 31403900

Lovejoy P: The African Diaspora: Revisionist Interpretations of Ethnicity, Culture and Religion Under Slavery 1. Boston, MA, Massachusetts Institute of Technology, 1997. Available at: https://www.semanticscholar.org/paper/The-African-Diaspora%3A-Revisionist-Interpretations-1-Lovejoy/a81ab57a3927ea 66196205dade2bc81be9c76fc1. Accessed June 24, 2023.

Lynch EE, Malcoe LH, Laurent SE, et al: The legacy of structural racism: associations between historic redlining, current mortgage lending, and health. SSM Popul Health 14:100793, 2021 33997243

Mobley SD Jr, Johnson RW, Sewell CJP, et al: "We are not victims": unmasking Black queer and trans* student activism at HBCUs. About Campus 26(3):24–28, 2021

Morris ER, Lindley L, Galupo MP: "Better issues to focus on": transgender microaggressions as ethical violations in therapy. Couns Psychol 48(6):883–915, 2020

Mulvey EP, Schubert CA: Mentally ill individuals in jails and prisons. Crime Justice 46:231–277, 2017

Nadal KL, Whitman CN, Davis LS, et al: Microaggressions toward lesbian, gay, bisexual, transgender, queer, and genderqueer people: a review of the literature. J Sex Res 53(4-5):488–508, 2016 26966779

Nicolazzo Z: "It's a hard line to walk": Black non-binary trans* collegians' perspectives on passing, realness, and trans*-normativity. Int J Qual Stud Educ 29(9):1173–1188, 2016

Noelke C, Outrich M, Baek M, et al: Connecting past to present: examining different approaches to linking historical redlining to present day health inequities. PLoS One 17(5):e0267606, 2022 35587478

Oliver D: "Being transgender is not a medical condition": the meaning of trans broken arm syndrome. USA Today, July 27, 2022. Available at: https://www.usatoday.com/story/life/health-wellness/2021/07/27/trans-broken-arm-syndrome-what-it-how-combat-discrimination-health-care/8042475002/. Accessed June 24, 2023.

Pastrana A Jr: It takes a family: an examination of outness among Black LGBT people in the United States. J Fam Issues 37(6):765–788, 2016

Pflum SR, Testa RJ, Balsam KF, et al: Social support, trans community connectedness, and mental health symptoms among transgender and gender nonconforming adults. Psychol Sex Orientat Gend Divers 2(3):281–286, 2015

Poteat T, German D, Flynn C: The conflation of gender and sex: gaps and opportunities in HIV data among transgender women and MSM. Glob Public Health 11(7-8):835–848, 2016 26785751

Poteat TC, van der Merwe LLA, Sevelius J, Keatley J: Inclusion as illusion: erasing transgender women in research with MSM. J Int AIDS Soc 24(1):e25661, 2021 33496381

Reid S: Exploring the agency of Black LGBTQ+ youth in schools and in NYC's ballroom culture. Teach Coll Rec 124(6):01614681221111072, 2022

Reisner SL, Bailey Z, Sevelius J: Racial/ethnic disparities in history of incarceration, experiences of victimization, and associated health indicators among transgender women in the U.S. Women Health 54(8):750–767, 2014 25190135

Restar A, Jin H, Operario D: Gender-inclusive and gender-specific approaches in trans health research. Transgend Health 6(5):235–239, 2021 34993295

Rogers G, Bryant-Davis T: Historical and contemporary racial trauma among Black Americans: Black wellness matters, in Handbook of Interpersonal Violence and Abuse Across the Lifespan: A Project of the National Partnership to End Interpersonal Violence Across the Lifespan. Edited by Geffner R, White JW, Hamberger LK, et al. New York, Springer International, 2022, pp 165–199

Rosati F, Coletta V, Pistella J, et al: Experiences of life and intersectionality of transgender refugees living in Italy: a qualitative approach. Int J Environ Res Public Health 18(23):12385, 2021 34886110

Russell JS, Hickson DA, Timmins L, Duncan DT: Higher rates of low socioeconomic status, marginalization, and stress in Black transgender women compared to Black cisgender MSM in the MARI Study. Int J Environ Res Public Health 18(4):2183, 2021 33672272

Scheidell JD, Dyer TV, Hucks-Ortiz C, et al: Characterisation of social support following incarceration among black sexual minority men and transgender women in the HPTN 061 cohort study. BMJ Open 11(9):e053334, 2021 34588263

Sherman ADF, Poteat TC, Budhathoki C, et al: Association of depression and post-traumatic stress with polyvictimization and emotional transgender and gender diverse community connection among Black and Latinx transgender women. LGBT Health 7(7):358–366, 2020 32833596

Sherman ADF, Balthazar MS, Daniel G, et al: Barriers to accessing and engaging in healthcare as potential modifiers in the association between polyvictimization and mental health among Black transgender women. PLoS One 17(6):e0269776, 2022 35709158

Smith AJ, Hallum-Montes R, Nevin K, et al: Determinants of transgender individuals' well-being, mental health, and suicidality in a rural state. Rural Mental Health 42(2):116–132, 2018 30333896

Sousa VD, Rojjanasrirat W: Translation, adaptation and validation of instruments or scales for use in cross-cultural health care research: a clear and user-friendly guideline. J Eval Clin Pract 17(2):268–274, 2011 20874835

Spade D: Solidarity not charity. Soc Text 38(1):131–151, 2020

Stewart D-L, Nicolazzo Z: High impact of [whiteness] on trans* students in postsecondary education. Equity Excell Educ 51(2):132–145, 2018

Stewart P: Who is kin? Family definition in African American families. J Hum Behav Soc Environ 15(2–3):163–181, 2007

Sudbury J: Maroon abolitionists: Black gender-oppressed activists in the anti-prison movement in the U.S. and Canada. Meridians 9(1):1–29, 2009

Suite DH, La Bril R, Primm A, Harrison-Ross P: Beyond misdiagnosis, misunderstanding and mistrust: relevance of the historical perspective in the medical and mental health treatment of people of color. J Natl Med Assoc 99(8):879–885, 2007 17722664

Tamir C: Key findings about Black immigrants in the U.S. Pew Research Center, January 27, 2022. Available at: https://www.pewresearch.org/short-reads/2022/01/27/key-findings-about-black-immigrants-in-the-u-s/. Accessed June 24, 2023.

Telander K, Hosek SG, Lemos D, Jeremie-Brink G: 'Ballroom itself can either make you or break you'—Black GBT youths' psychosocial development in the house ball community. Glob Public Health 12(11):1391–1403, 2017 28278745

The Trevor Project: Black LGBTQ Youth Mental Health. West Hollywood, CA, The Trevor Project, 2020. Available at: https://www.thetrevorproject.org/research-briefs/black-lgbtq-youth-mental-health/. Accessed June 24, 2023.

Thomas KK: Deluxe Jim Crow: Civil Rights and American Health Policy, 1935–1954. Atlanta, GA, University of Georgia Press, 2011

Thomas SB, Quinn SC: The Tuskegee Syphilis Study, 1932 to 1972: implications for HIV education and AIDS risk education programs in the black community. Am J Public Health 81(11):1498–1505, 1991 1951814

Tobin CST: Distinguishing distress from disorder: Black-white patterns in the determinants of and links between depressive symptoms and major depression. J Affect Disord 279:510–517, 2021 33130551

Trostle JM, Zheng K, Lipscombe C: The State of Black Immigrants Part II: Black Immigrants in the Mass Criminalization System. Black Alliance for Just Immigration; NYU School of Law Immigrant Rights Clinic, 2016. Available at: https://nyf.issuelab.org/resource/the-state-of-black-immigrants-part-ii-black-immigrants-in-the-mass-criminalization-system.html. Accessed June 24, 2023.

Warren JC, Smalley KB, Barefoot KN: Psychological well-being among transgender and genderqueer individuals. Int J Transgend 17(3–4):114–123, 2016

Washington HA: Medical Apartheid: The Dark History of Medical Experimentation on Black Americans From Colonial Times to the Present. New York, Knopf Doubleday, 2008

Whaley AL: Cultural mistrust and mental health services for African Americans: a review and meta-analysis. Couns Psychol 29(4):513–531, 2001a

Whaley AL: Cultural mistrust: an important psychological construct for diagnosis and treatment of African Americans. Prof Psychol Res Pr 32(6):555–562, 2001b

White C: Incarcerating youth with mental health problems: a focus on the intersection of race, ethnicity, and mental illness. Youth Violence Juv Justice 14(4):426–447, 2016

White ME, Cartwright AD, Reyes AG, et al: "A whole other layer of complexity": Black transgender men's experiences. J LGBT Issues Couns 14(3):248–267, 2020

Whitfield DL, Coulter RWS, Langenderfer-Magruder L, Jacobson D: Experiences of intimate partner violence among lesbian, gay, bisexual, and transgender college students: the intersection of gender, race, and sexual orientation. J Interpers Violence 36(11–12):NP6040–NP6064, 2021 30453802

Wilkins EJ, Whiting JB, Watson MF, et al: Residual effects of slavery: what clinicians need to know. Contemp Fam Ther 35(1):14–28, 2013

Wodda A, Panfil VR: "Don't talk to me about deception": the necessary erosion of the trans-panic defense. Albany Law Rev 78(3):927–972, 2015

Yarbrough D: The carceral production of transgender poverty: how racialized gender policing deprives transgender women of housing and safety. Punishm Soc 25(1):14624745211017818, 2021

Yarwood V, Checchi F, Lau K, Zimmerman C: LGBTQI + migrants: a systematic review and conceptual framework of health, safety and wellbeing during migration. Int J Environ Res Public Health 19(2):869, 2022 35055698

Young JR: Rituals of Resistance: African Atlantic Religion in Kongo and the Lowcountry South in the Era of Slavery. Baton Rouge, LA, LSU Press, 2007

CHAPTER 7

Gender-Affirming Psychiatric Care for Asian American and Pacific Islander Communities

Arjee Javellana Restar, Ph.D., M.P.H.
Emerson J. Dusic, M.P.H.
Jack Bruno, M.S.W.
Henri M. Garrison-Desany, Ph.D., M.S.P.H.
Fiona (Fí) Fonseca, M.D., Ph.D.

TWENTY percent of adults living in the United States have been diagnosed with mental or psychiatric illness. Of all racial groups, Asian American and Pacific Islander (AAPI) adults have the lowest estimated prevalence of diagnoses and mental health service utilization (Substance Abuse and Mental Health Services Administration 2020). For instance, in 2020, only 20.8% of AAPI adults with a mental or psychiatric illness received treatment—clearly an opportunity for public intervention. Moreover, there is still very little research on transgender, nonbinary, and/or gender-expansive (TNG) AAPI adults. Despite limited yet contrasting studies with Asian American populations, there remains a lag in using intersectional approaches to address these health disparities, particularly in TNG AAPI populations who need more accessible gender-affirming mental and psychiatric care (Bith-Melander et al. 2010).

This section reviews themes from the literature on the gender-affirming mental and psychiatric care of TNG AAPI populations, with two essential caveats. First, the bulk of studies on this topic construct this population as monolithic, either by race/ethnicity (e.g., Asian Americans) or by gender/ sexual identity (e.g., lesbian, gay, bisexual, transgender, queer, and more [LGBTQ+]). Treating distinct groups as one aggregate population erases the social, economic, and political power dynamics and differences that shape the health of each specific and diverse group. Although in this chapter, as a reflection of the current literature, we often use an aggregate construction, we aim to be specific and disaggregate when possible using an intersectional lens to denote and embrace the diversity within TNG AAPI populations in the United States specific to all lines of identity (e.g., ethnicity, nationality, sexual orientation identity, migration experiences, and other identities and experiences unique to communities and groups). Second, although funding mechanisms and publications have paid increasing attention to examining the health of sexual and gender minorities across various lines of identity, the body of research specific to TNG AAPI populations is relatively new and emerging. It is therefore critical for this group's psychiatric care, including interventions and policies that shape it, to adapt as new insights fluctuate in line with the developing literature.

MENTAL HEALTH OUTCOMES AMONG TNG AAPI ADULTS

Despite scant clinic-level reports of psychiatric outcomes among TNG AAPIs, published studies on general mental health outcomes signify areas that are in need of gender-affirming psychiatric care interventions. For example, in the 2015 U.S. Transgender Survey, 39% of the TNG sample who identified as Asian and Native Hawaiian/Pacific Islander reported current, serious psychological distress. This is in stark contrast to the rates in the general population of Asians (3%) and Native Hawaiians/Pacific Islanders (5%) in the United States and the U.S. population as a whole (5%) (James et al. 2016). Most individuals with psychiatric illnesses do not die by suicide, but research has consistently shown a strong link between suicide risk and psychiatric illness (Moitra et al. 2021). In the same survey, rates of lifetime suicidal thoughts and behavior among Asian and Native Hawaiian/Pacific Islander TNG respondents were much higher than among the U.S. population. Specifically, 82% of TNG respondents reported having experienced suicidal thoughts, and 40% reported suicide attempts (James et al. 2016).

Limited literature documents adverse mental health outcomes such as anxiety and depression among TNG AAPI populations. TNG populations, generally, have reported rates of depressive and anxiety symptoms as high as 70% for trans women and 66% for trans men who are not on gender-affirming hormone therapy (Bouman et al. 2017). Among Asian and Asian American populations, the prevalence of depression and anxiety varies, with most studies reporting rates of depression among Asian Americans lower than in European Americans but higher than in Asian populations born outside the United States (Chang 2002; Kim et al. 2015). Insights from immigration studies show some differences between Asian Americans born in the United States and those born outside, with individuals born in the United States having a higher prevalence of depressive symptoms and episodes (Huang 2008; Zhu 2017). Moreover, emerging literature shows increased anxiety, depression, and posttraumatic stress symptoms for Asian Americans in the context of the COVID-19 pandemic (Hahm et al. 2021; Lozano et al. 2022). Specific reports on TNG AAPI mental health outcomes during the pandemic remain absent—a point for further, immediate research.

Social Contexts Surrounding Adverse Mental Health Outcomes Among TNG AAPI Adults

Given the interweaving identities of race/ethnicity and gender, most TNG AAPI people are positioned to face multiple stressors that are known to be associated with adverse mental health outcomes. These include social and structural stressors such as stigma, anti-Asian racism, transphobia, and harassment. Specifically, most TNG AAPI adults are constantly grappling with discrimination and stigmatization toward both LGBTQ+ and Asian American communities in mainstream culture, the marginalization and devaluation of TNG individuals in most LGBTQ+ spaces and communities, and the marginalization and intolerance of TNG bodies and identities in most AAPI societies with histories of European white colonization—all of which negatively affect mental health (Ching et al. 2018). Online social networking apps offer a salient example of these interwoven oppressions. Previous studies have reported intracommunity racism and transphobia from within larger LGBTQ+ populations. In particular, studies based on mobile apps have documented the overt ways in which systemic forms of oppression are aided by online social networking environments and interactions with other LGBTQ+ populations. These factors operate ubiquitously via the embodiment of statements such as "no femmes, no Asians" via chat exchanges or on users' profiles, to target, exclude, and marginalize mostly femme transgender and nonbinary AAPI app users (Elks 2018; Liu 2015).

More recently, in the wake of the COVID-19 pandemic, anti-Asian racism and hate crimes have taken the form of violent attacks faced by members of AAPI communities (Litam 2020). In particular, misinformed, misleading, and racist media coverage of COVID-19 has fueled anti-Asian racism and hate crimes toward AAPI communities, including violent attacks against individuals and destruction of AAPI businesses (Litam 2020). One study demonstrated a substantial increase in racial slurs and online harassment aimed at AAPI communities in online social media postings during the first year of COVID-19, particularly after the Trump administration's overt demonstration of xenophobic rhetoric toward Chinese and Chinese American populations (Tahmasbi et al. 2021).

We are not aware of any existing studies on TNG AAPIs' experiences of anti-Asian racism and hate crimes in the context of COVID-19, an area that warrants further investigation. Yet anecdotal reports and personal essays by TNG AAPIs on this issue have provided opportunities to understand how some members of TNG AAPI communities are grappling with anti-Asian racism and transphobia. One news story documented how queer AAPIs are "building counter-narratives" as a response to being "exhausted" about their COVID-19-related experiences, and "transgressions includ[ing] attempted stabbings, acid attacks, being spat on and pelted with eggs, assaults, and hospitalizations for concussions" (Chu 2020). This account demonstrates a mechanism through which TNG AAPIs are coping amid prevailing environmental and structural barriers to mental health counseling and telehealth (Kormendi and Brown 2021; Restar et al. 2021).

SERVICE UTILIZATION

Mental health stigma impacts all populations, but AAPIs are consistently reported as the most affected group, with the lowest utilization rate of mental health services. A national study revealed that only 8.6% of AAPIs sought mental health services, compared with 18% of the general U.S. population (McLean Hospital 2022; Nishi 2012). Although explanations for the low uptake of mental health services in TNG AAPI communities has not been fully explored, literature that describes why AAPIs more broadly do not seek mental health services often cites the pressure for most AAPIs to remain and be perceived as professionally successful—in short, the "model minority." This leads many AAPIs to pervasively deny mental health symptoms and avoid disclosing mental health issues out of shame and fear of being viewed in a negative light (McLean Hospital 2022). Paradoxically, such reasons for low uptake of mental health services among AAPIs are often centered around personal concerns, whereas the literature that characterizes and investigates challenges to improving mental health service uptake among TNG populations attributes it to social and structural barriers (Moagi et al. 2021; Shipherd et al. 2010). Social barriers include mental health provider discrimination and stigmatization and gender identity change efforts (conversion therapy). Structural barriers include the lack of (sufficient) health insurance, which translates to lack of access to in-network, culturally responsive and supportive mental health providers, high out-of-pocket costs, and lack of coverage specific to gender-affirming therapy and counseling services. Compounding these financial burdens, across the United States, dangerous state-level policies are being proposed and enacted that discourage or criminalize providers who seek to practice gender-affirming care, including gender-affirming counseling and therapy, creating an even more daunting barrier for TNG residents who seek care in those states. From their two bodies of literature, it is likely that most AAPIs who are TNG experience a heightened combination of barriers across personal, social, and structural levels. For example, the lack of access to culturally responsive mental health providers who deliver gender-affirming care while taking into consideration underlying contexts specific to TNG and AAPI health might present as a lack of mental health services utilization. As such, studies that aim to characterize and identify specific barriers to mental health service utilization among TNG AAPIs are critically needed to begin understanding how to tailor psychiatric care interventions for this important population.

CONCLUSION: THE NEED FOR GENDER-AFFIRMING PSYCHIATRIC CARE INTERVENTIONS

There is a public health imperative to address adverse mental health outcomes among TNG AAPIs. Bolstering research in this area is critically needed. To be effective, implementation should include tailored gender-affirming psychiatric care interventions with multilevel component design to address the interwoven barriers across personal, social, and structural levels. Such interventions could include addressing traumas that stem from racism and transphobia; addressing mental health stigma at both individual and social levels; screening for mental health in primary settings; referral linkages; supporting TNG AAPIs as mental health providers; training mental health providers to be culturally responsive in areas of both TNG and AAPI health; and improving insurance coverage, particularly in the context of COVID-19. Vital to designing such psychiatric care interventions is the chance to partner with community-based organizations and health centers that are intersectional in their work and are led by TNG and AAPI stakeholders and leaders who organize and advocate for mental health services for TNG AAPIs. Examples in the United States include Apicha Community Health Center in New York; the Asian Pacific Islander Queer Women and Transgender Community (https://apiqwtc.org/); Lavender Phoenix in San Francisco; Community Health for Asian Americans in Alameda, California;

and API Forward Movement in Los Angeles. Finally, an intersectional and disaggregated approach to intervention design will be critical to understanding how to best tailor psychiatric care interventions across such diverse communities of TNG AAPIs.

REFERENCES

Bith-Melander P, Sheoran B, Sheth L, et al: Understanding sociocultural and psychological factors affecting transgender people of color in San Francisco. J Assoc Nurses AIDS Care 21(3):207–220, 2010 20416495

Bouman WP, Claes L, Brewin N, et al: Transgender and anxiety: a comparative study between transgender people and the general population. Int J Transgend 18(1):16–26, 2017

Chang DF: Understanding the rates and distribution of mental disorders, in Asian American Mental Health: Assessment Theories and Methods. Boston, MA, Springer, 2002, pp 9–27

Ching THW, Lee SY, Chen J, et al: A model of intersectional stress and trauma in Asian American sexual and gender minorities. Psychol Violence 8(6):657–668, 2018

Chu KC: "I'm building counter-narratives": LGBTQ+ Asian Americans on how they're processing racism during coronavirus. Them, May 14, 2020. Available at: https://www.them.us/story/lgbtq-asian-americans-on-how-theyre-processing-racism-during-coronavirus. Accessed June 25, 2023.

Elks S: Gay dating app announces "zero tolerance" of racism, transphobia. Reuters, September 18, 2018. Available at: https://www.reuters.com/article/us-global-lgbt-dating/gay-dating-app-announces-zero-tolerance-of-racism-transphobia-idUSKCN1LY2TO. Accessed June 25, 2023.

Hahm HC, Ha Y, Scott JC, et al: Perceived COVID-19-related anti-Asian discrimination predicts post traumatic stress disorder symptoms among Asian and Asian American young adults. Psychiatry Res 303:114084, 2021 34242971

Huang J: Immigrant Health Status, Health Behavior and Health Assimilation in the United States. Doctoral dissertation, Chicago, IL, University of Illinois, 2008

James SE, Herman JL, Rankin S, et al: The Report of the 2015 U.S. Transgender Survey. Washington, DC, National Center for Transgender Equality, 2016. Available at: https://transequality.org/sites/default/files/docs/usts/USTS-Full-Report-Dec17.pdf. Accessed June 25, 2023.

Kim HJ, Park E, Storr CL, et al: Depression among Asian-American adults in the community: systematic review and meta-analysis. PLoS One 10(6):e0127760, 2015 26029911

Kormendi NM, Brown AD: Asian American mental health during COVID-19: a call for task-sharing interventions. SSM Ment Health 1:100006, 2021 34494013

Litam SDA: "Take your kung-flu back to Wuhan": counseling Asians, Asian Americans, and Pacific Islanders with race-based trauma related to COVID-19. Prof Couns 10(2):144–156, 2020

Liu X: "No fats, femmes, or Asians": the utility of critical race theory in examining the role of gay stock stories in the marginalization of gay Asian men. Contemp Justice Rev 2(2):255–276, 2015

Lozano P, Rueger SY, Lam H, et al: Prevalence of depression symptoms before and during the COVID-19 pandemic among two Asian American ethnic groups. J Immigr Minor Health 24(4):909–917, 2022 34643848

McLean Hospital: Why Asian Americans don't seek help for mental illness. Putting People First in Mental Health, May 1, 2022. Available at: https://www.mclean hospital.org/essential/why-asian-americans-dont-seek-help-mental-illness. Accessed June 25, 2023.

Moagi MM, van Der Wath AE, Jiyane PM, Rikhotso RS: Mental health challenges of lesbian, gay, bisexual and transgender people: An integrated literature review. Health SA 26:1487, 2021 33604059

Moitra M, Santomauro D, Degenhardt L, et al: Estimating the risk of suicide associated with mental disorders: a systematic review and meta-regression analysis. J Psychiatr Res 137:242–249, 2021 33714076

Nishi K: Mental Health Among Asian-Americans. Washington, DC, American Psychological Association, 2012. Available at: https://www.apa.org/pi/oema/resources/ethnicity-health/asian-american/article-mental-health. Accessed June 25, 2023.

Restar AJ, Jin H, Jarrett B, et al: Characterising the impact of COVID-19 environment on mental health, gender affirming services and socioeconomic loss in a global sample of transgender and non-binary people: a structural equation modelling. BMJ Glob Health 6(3):e004424, 2021 33753401

Shipherd JC, Green KE, Abramovitz S: Transgender clients: identifying and minimizing barriers to mental health treatment. J Gay Lesbian Ment Health 14(2):94–108, 2010

Substance Abuse and Mental Health Services Administration: Key substance use and mental health indicators in the United States: results from the 2019 National Survey on Drug Use and Health. U.S. Department of Health and Human Services, 2020. HHS publ. no. PEP20-07-01-001, NSDUH ser. H-55. Available at: https://www.samhsa.gov/data/sites/default/files/reports/rpt29393/2019NS DUHFFRPDFWHTML/2019NSDUHFFR090120.htm. Accessed July 17, 2023.

Tahmasbi F, Schild L, Ling C, et al: "Go eat a bat, Chang!": on the emergence of sinophobic behavior on web communities in the face of COVID-19, in WWW '21: Proceedings of the Web Conference 2021. New York, ACM, 2021. Available at: https://doi.org/10.1145/3442381.3450024. Accessed June 25, 2023.

Zhu L: Depression risks and correlates among different generations of Chinese Americans: the effects of relationships with friends and relatives. Soc Sci 6(2):56, 2017

CHAPTER 8

DoubleQueer

Being Neurodiverse and Gender Diverse

Noah Adams, M.S.W., Ph.D.
Teddy G. Goetz, M.D., M.S.
Reubs J. Walsh, B.A., M.Sc., Ph.D.
Zackary Derrick, B.A., M.P.H.

IN this chapter, we explore neurodiversity among transgender, non-binary, and/or gender-diverse (TNG) people in clinical and community settings. The authors of this chapter are experts in this area as academics and researchers, and are also members of the neurodiverse community. Neurodiversity is broad—we focus here on autism and ADHD (see Chapter 9, "Disability Justice and Access Needs for Disabled TNG People"; and Chapter 18, "Affirming Gender Identity in the Setting of Serious Mental Illness," for additional facets). We begin by outlining the literature and the importance of concepts such as neurodiversity. We then explore diagnosis and clinical practice, research equity, accessibility, criminalization and the law, and the work of neurodiverse clinicians. This chapter will be useful to a broad audience of clinicians, community health workers, scholars, and researchers. We discuss these issues separately for ADHD and autism, but readers will likely find information in both sections useful.

BACKGROUND

Autism

A growing body of literature reports on a greater incidence of autism among TNG (vs. non-TNG) people and vice versa. The cause is unclear (Turban and van Schalkwyk 2018), but posited theories often contain anti-TNG bias, such as attributing the gender dysphoria itself to OCD, social or cognitive challenges, deficits in theory of mind, or cognitive rigidity (Hillier et al. 2019; Jackson-Perry 2020). Those rationales align with professional and societal practices that view disabled people as compulsorily heterosexual and cisgender (Atkinson 2021; Barnett 2014; Kimball et al. 2018). Some clinicians have noted cases in which autistic traits in children disappear after gender affirmation (Fortunato et al. 2022).

The most compelling reason for the autism/TNG overlap may be that autistic people are simply less susceptible to the narrowing effects that prescriptive gender norms have on self-perception of gender and thus more likely to become conscious of the subtle, internal experiences that can lead a person to identify as TNG (Walsh 2021; Walsh et al. 2018). The same argument posits, conversely, that allistic (non-autistic) people are less likely to be aware of or motivated to address incongruity between others' and their own perception of their gender. This is supported by research demonstrating that autistic people are also more likely to be gay, lesbian, and bisexual (George and Stokes 2018). Clinicians should be careful not to characterize an inability to navigate the rigid social mores required to hide one's gender or sexual identity as a psychological disorder.

ADHD

The literature exploring ADHD in TNG people is less developed than that of autism. Only 17 relevant publications exist at the time of this writing, and all were published in or after 2014 (Goetz and Adams 2022). Gender-affirming care specialists wrote 65% of these articles, and 71% used medical records to report the prevalence of ADHD in a TNG sample. Only four (case reports) discussed potential personal or clinical implications of the TNG-ADHD nexus and focused on holistic diagnosis and treatment. None of the 17 articles proposed an explanation for the reported increased prevalence of TNG + ADHD experience. None of the articles, with the exception of Goetz and Adams (2022), avoided deficit-framing or included explicit authorship by TNG-ADHD individuals.

Neurodiversity

The term *neurodiversity* has a contested origin. The oldest known term in common use by the neurodiverse community is *neurotypical*, which appears to have originated with Autistic Network International (ANI) in the 1990s (Silberman 2015). *Neurodiversity* itself first appeared in print in *The Atlantic* (Blume 1998) and is credited to Judy Singer, an autistic sociologist who used it in a mailing list (Kapp 2020) and in her thesis (Singer 1998). It was almost exclusively used to describe people with autism; people with "dyslexia, ADHD, dyscalculia, and a myriad of other conditions [were] christened 'cousins.'" (Silberman 2015, p. 454).

Kassiane Asasumasu coined *neurodivergent* circa 2015 (Chapman 2021). Asasumasu hoped that the term would encompass all those with "a brain that diverges [including] Autistic people. ADHD people. People with learning disabilities. Epileptic people. People with mental illnesses. People with MS or Parkinson's or apraxia or cerebral palsy or dyspraxia" (Asasumasu 2015). Neurodiversity has subsequently widened to encompass all people with "variations…in cognitive, affectual, and sensory functioning" (Rosqvist et al. 2020, p. 1) and is defined, most broadly, as "the uniqueness of all brains" (Gillespie-Lynch et al. 2020). The neurodiversity model confronts a disease-based or medical model of health care that "views physical or cognitive differences as disabilities…to be corrected" and is "partly responsible for the creation of systemic barriers and negative stigmas the neurodivergent regularly face" (Jurgens 2020, p. 73).

AUTISM: DIAGNOSIS AND CLINICAL PRACTICE

Incidence

According to the CDC (2020), "about 1 in 44 8-year-old children have been identified with ASD (or 23.0 per 1,000 8-year-olds)." Recent research also found a similar rate (2.21%) of adults in the United States with autism (Dietz et al. 2020). These rates are notably higher than earlier prevalence estimates, which may be due to improved reporting practices, increased testing (particularly among lower-income people and people of color) (Winter et al. 2020), and multiple diagnoses being collapsed into "autism spectrum disorder" (American Psychiatric Association 2013; Hansen et al. 2015). A recent meta-synthesis by Warrier et al. (2020) found TNG individuals to have a 3.03–6.36 times greater rate of autism than cisgender individuals, in addition to elevated rates of autistic traits and ADHD.

Diagnosis

Within the United States, DSM-5-TR (American Psychiatric Association 2022) is used for diagnosis of autism. Although ADHD can occur in tandem with autism, their criteria overlap, so they need to be carefully differentiated during diagnosis. An autism diagnosis is not a neutral act, however; it may interfere with access to TNG health care by causing clinicians to be more cautious than they otherwise would be (Adams and Liang 2020; MacKinnon et al. 2020).

Diagnosis is also not universally accessible. Autism is more commonly diagnosed in children, and until recently, adult diagnosis was rare. Insurance plays a large role in the financial coverage of diagnostic costs, which often reach several thousand U.S. dollars, and may be more available to parents seeking diagnosis for children than to independent adults seeking their own diagnosis. Some people may secure financial coverage through secondary education insurance if referred for a psychoeducational assessment.

The utility of diagnosis varies. Children will often be able to access autism services only with a diagnosis; there are few services available in the United States for autistic adults. An autism diagnosis may give access to psycho-educational resources in university and workplace accommodations. Many autistic individuals also find it reassuring to put a name to their experiences and struggles. The clinician's role is to help the patient explore the pros and cons of diagnosis for them. Clinicians may find it helpful to self-reflect on their internalized notions around autism. Regardless, the autistic community is quite welcoming of people who are self diagnosed or "community diagnosed" (see Bennie 2020; Shekhar 2020).

Comorbid Conditions

Many conditions are more prevalent in autistic people than in non-autistic peers. A recent review reported higher rates of OCD, ADHD, suicidal behavior, and disorders of anxiety, mood, psychosis, sleep, impulse control, eating, and substance use (Hossain et al. 2020). Another found increased risk of sleep problems, epilepsy, self-inflicted oral soft tissue injury, peripheral hearing loss, allergies and autoimmune disease (including diabetes), gastrointestinal issues, and (among those assigned male at birth) hypospadia (Rydzewska et al. 2021, p. 12). The generalizability of these findings may be limited by the setting of individual studies (e.g., clinical vs.community) and whether the sampling strategy was reported.

Autism is a notably heterogeneous condition (see Geurts et al. 2014), and clinicians should guard against the danger of mistaking "treating a comorbidity [for] treating autism itself" (Chown 2020, p. 34). Likewise, we should resist the temptation to cleave autistic people into categories of "low" and "high" functioning, as all people function at different levels throughout their lives; for example, a person may have poor cooking skills but be highly skilled artistically. Moreover, "autistic people can be extremely cognitively able and yet have major difficulties in other domains," and their experience of being disabled can be highly "contingent upon social conditions such as stigma, rather than inherent disadvantage" (Bovell 2020, p. 50). Ultimately, cognitive ability (or perceived ability) is not synonymous with capacity to contribute to society and is not sufficient to deny gender-affirming care.

Treatment and Clinical Care

Clinical guidelines exist for autistic and TNG children and adolescents (Strang et al. 2018a) but not for adults. Emerging evidence suggests that many clinicians who serve TNG communities are reluctant to treat autistic people and are overly cautious in doing so (Adams and Liang 2020; Shumer et al. 2016; van der Miesen et al. 2018), perhaps because of differences in the ways that autistic and neurotypical TNG patients present. As has been noted, autistic people may not perceive the need to present in a stereotypically gendered manner (Walsh 2021; Walsh et al. 2018). Jacobs et al. (2014), for instance, observed that TNG autistic people may express discomfort with changing their clothing to "match" the gendered expectations of their felt gender. Although care should be taken to explain possible safety concerns related to not meeting societal gender expectations (e.g., violence and discrimination), clinicians must not make treatment conditional on physical appearance or conformity to a norm. Clinicians are advised to approach the care and treatment of TNG and autistic patients with the same openness with which they approach neurotypical patients.

A related issue is the tendency of anti-trans organizations and activists to use TNG autistic people as a "cautionary tale" against gender-affirming care broadly. This conflation is almost always undertaken without the participation of autistic individuals. A notable exception is the Cain and Velasco (2020) case report of an autistic TNG individual who discusses detransitioning because of anti-trans stigma.

Autism alone is insufficient reason to infer incapacity and deny or delay gender-affirming care. Nevertheless, it is often a factor in decisions to do just that (e.g., Zupanič et al. 2021). Lemaire et al. (2014) go so far as to direct that "if [autism] is diagnosed, rehabilitation centered on social interactions and communication should be proposed before sex reassignment surgery" (p. 397). This recommendation presumes that an autistic person can and should become "not TNG" through rehabilitation, which has never been documented to occur successfully.

Clinicians working with all TNG people should tailor "information and gender-affirming care...to allow for different learning styles [and communication challenges] specific to the individual" (Cheung et al. 2018, p. 236). These concerns do not take precedence over TNG health care, but patients "struggling with social aspects of gender transition [may benefit from]...interventions to develop interpersonal skills, increase self-esteem, and improve social and peer support" (Cheung et al. 2018, p. 236).

Applied Behavioral Analysis

Applied behavioral analysis (ABA), considered by many to be the gold standard treatment for autistic children, uses discrete operant conditioning to alter autistic behaviors to those more akin to neurotypical children. Several scholars have pointed out striking similarities between ABA and gay/trans conversion therapies (Gibson and Douglas 2018; Pyne 2020), and that the emphasis on compliance from children in ABA fosters increased vulnerability to sexual assault (Sandoval-Norton et al. 2019). Others have noted that ABA inhibits behaviors used by people with autism to self-regulate, and that it causes PTSD (Kupferstein 2018). Autistic children and adults should be supported with information about medical options and risks; however, they should never be compelled to change or hide fundamental aspects of themselves to access health care or for any other reason.

ADHD: DIAGNOSIS AND CLINICAL PRACTICE

Incidence

In a 2016 survey of parents, 6.1 million children in the United States (9.4%) had ever been diagnosed with ADHD (Centers for Disease Control and Prevention 2022). The lifetime prevalence of ADHD was found to be 8.7% among adolescents and 4.4% among adults 18–44 years old (National Institute of Mental Health n.d.). Recent systematic literature reviews (Goetz and Adams 2022; Thrower et al. 2020) found ADHD rates of 4%–20% among TNG children and adolescents (2–13 times greater than cis peers) and 4%–11% among TNG adults (3–11 times greater than cis peers). These findings are limited by "self-reported diagnoses, a bias [toward] young internet users, and, as birth-assigned sex was not [always] asked,…unlikely to be representative of transgender cohorts" (Thrower et al. 2020, p. 703). Furthermore, hyperactivity and impulsivity in TNG youth are often labeled as "externalizing behaviors" (a broad category encompassing aggression and delinquency), impeding proper diagnosis of gender dysphoria (Coleman et al. 2012; Dawson et al. 2017). There is also little research on the overlap of TNG identity and ADHD, although the literature on TNG identity and autism sometimes comments on a higher incidence of co-occurring ADHD, potentially from stress and inherent vulnerability (Warrier et al. 2020).

Diagnosis

ADHD diagnostic criteria for adults and children differ only by the number of symptoms that must be present (5+ if ≥17 years old vs. 6+ if <17). Neuropsychological testing or an intensive psychiatric interview may establish diagnosis, although it may be difficult to obtain insurance coverage for the former. As with autism, ADHD is not a neutral diagnosis and may bring with it a host of other socio-logistical problems associated with discrimination. TNG individuals are at particular risk of clinicians invalidating TNG identities, inappropriately assigning mental health diagnoses, and overmedication (Dawson et al. 2017).

Generally speaking, clinicians and researchers appear to express fewer concerns about coincident TNG and ADHD than autism. The specter of autism seems to provoke a fundamental conceptual challenge to the idea of providing gender-affirming care, perhaps because of deficit-based research that stereotypes autistic people as dependent and incapable. In contrast with autism (e.g., Lewis 2016a, 2016b), adult ADHD supports (e.g., medication, psychotherapy) are more widely available, although an official diagnosis is usually required to access them. These supports can make the difference between succeeding in one's education and employment or not (Gupta 2021).

Adult ADHD diagnosis appears to be increasingly common and socially acceptable (Jaynes 2021). However, TNG people may be less likely to obtain a diagnosis in childhood because they fail to match stereotypically gendered assumptions regarding ADHD presentation (Call 2018; Christian-Brandt et al. 2021; Janssen and Leibowitz 2018; Kuvalanka et al. 2018). Diagnosis of ADHD has historically been much less available for Black and Latinx children than white peers (Coker et al. 2016; Joho 2021), and racial and socioeconomic barriers persist (Chung et al. 2019). Among children with diagnoses, white people are most likely to receive treatment, and Asian people least (Shi et al. 2021; see also Chapter 7, "Gender-Affirming Care in Asian American and Pacific Islander Communities"). Clinicians should be well versed in cultural sensitivity regarding different experiences and presentations of ADHD and autism. The Color of Autism Foundation (n.d.) offers excellent resources that may be helpful here. Nevertheless, the cost of an ADHD diagnosis can run into the thousands of dollars, and insurance coverage may be limited. Clinicians should be prepared to advise patients regarding the pros and cons of ADHD diagnosis and to help problem-solve specific issues of access regarding diagnosis, medication, and treatment.

Comorbid Conditions

ADHD is associated with "mood and anxiety disorders, substance use disorders, and personality disorders" (Katzman et al. 2017, p. 1); physical comorbidities include allergies, neurological problems (e.g., seizures, migraines), and immunological problems (Pan and Bölte 2020). Although ADHD is not a true "condition," young people with both autism/ADHD and TNG report notably "high levels of bullying, harassment, and abuse" (Holt et al. 2016, p. 115).

Treatment and Clinical Care

Health Care Provision

Clinical guidance for working with TNG/neurodiverse patients is extremely limited, particularly for adults (as opposed to children) initiating care. Accessing any form of gender-affirming medical care can be an extremely slow process that requires a lot of waiting and uncertainty. A person looking to start hormone replacement therapy might need to wait ≥6 months for a first appointment, a week or even several months between requesting and starting it, then an even longer period before noticing changes. Likewise, going through legal processes to change one's name and gender marker can be long and arduous, consisting of dozens of logistical steps across a variety of systems. Those with ADHD may struggle with the process if they have difficulties with organizational skills, task completion, and other aspects of executive dysfunction. Yet there is no evidence that ADHD cannot be managed optimally during gender affirmation. Many neurodiverse individuals are also sensitive to stimuli and unable to wear transitional garments (e.g., binders). This does not discount their degree of gender dysphoria, but rather highlights the negotiation of multiple important, contradictory needs.

Clinicians caring for those with ADHD may need "a range of different tools and approaches to account for factors such as inattention [and] lack of organization" (Cheung et al. 2018, p. 236). This can include psychoeducation; mindfulness, behavioral, and impulse control techniques; and strategies to deal with depression triggers and stress management. Evidence supports several psychotherapeutic skills-based programs and multimodal approaches (Hesslinger et al. 2002; Philipsen et al. 2007; Solanto et al. 2008; Young and Amarasinghe 2010; Zylowska et al. 2008). An individual's experience with ADHD should not be used to invalidate their gender identity or deny access to gender-affirming health care.

Medication

For ADHD symptom management, stimulants such as methylphenidate (e.g., Concerta, Ritalin), dextroamphetamine and amphetamine mixed salts (Adderall), and lisdexamfetamine (e.g., Vyvanse) have been shown to be highly effective and safe with appropriate medical oversight (Groom and Cortese 2022). Nonstimulants such as atomoxetine (Strattera), nortriptyline (Pamelor), and bupropion (Wellbutrin) remain second-line for symptoms management but may be preferred for a specific patient for a variety of reasons (e.g., history of substance use disorder, unable to tolerate side effects of stimulant, cardiac condition) (Groom and Cortese 2022). For information about potential stimulant side effects and interactions with GAHT, see Chapter 4, "Psychopharmacological Considerations for TNG People."

ACCESSIBILITY

Physical

Clinicians may need to adapt their practices to be accessible to neurodiverse individuals. Such adaptations may be physical: for example, offering appointments with lowered lights, no scents, and a less busy environment (Lynch 2019). Clinicians should also consider alternative means of holding appointments, such as telehealth or secure messaging service.

Patients with ADHD may have difficulty keeping appointments or arriving on time. Clinicians should not draw conclusions regarding patients' potential desire for or capacity to undergo gender-affirmative care based on such factors alone. Autistic patients, on the other hand, often need appointment times to be precisely observed. Building a time buffer into appointments can help with this. Given that many autistic patients are periodically or completely nonverbal, care should be given to allow for them to respond via text or methods such as sign language (Pezzuoli et al. 2020).

Communication

Clinicians should be aware of differences between autistic and neurotypical communication styles to adequately provide services and not mistake miscommunication for incapacity. For instance, fidgeting, stimming, and lack of eye contact are normal among those with autism and not a sign of disrespect or disengagement. The disconnect between autistic and neurotypical communication has been termed the "double empathy problem," in which "the misperceptions…of the neurotypical majority influence the perceptions and behavior of autistic people such that they become increasingly separate and indeed isolated from mainstream society" (Milton 2012; Mitchell et al. 2021).

Autistic patients may be better able to respond to closed questions asked in a direct and concrete way, and clinicians should not be surprised by overly literal answers. From the autistic perspective, a question such as "How was your day?" can be too broad to answer—it might not be obvious what part of the day the question refers to, or whether it hides other social expectations. Better to "match conversation styles to those of the client, and to use more concrete starters such as 'How was the traffic?'" (Jacobs et al. 2014, p. 281). Requests and requirements should be explained and have clear rationale. An understanding of the reason for a policy will help an autistic patient to follow it. (Thus clinicians are encouraged to consider the rationale for conditions and requirements.)

This communication approach should be kept in mind when asking questions about gender, which is inherently intertwined with socialization and societal expectations. Questions regarding experience of gender identity and desire for gender-affirming care should be concrete and direct, with clinicians prepared to navigate miscommunications. Strang et al. (2018b) offer the following examples: "When did you first notice that you might be [affirmed gender]? What did you notice? …What is it like to be transgender and autistic?" (p. 40–42). The Autistic Women and Nonbinary Network has a resource to assist TNG autistic people in preparing for and obtaining TNG health care (daVanport et al. 2020).

RESEARCH EQUITY

Autism

Since 1996, >600 articles have been published that touch on people who are both TNG and autistic, with >170 in 2020 alone (N. Adams, personal communication, June 2023). Little of this originates from or accounts for their perspective and instead focuses on the supposed etiology of this overlap, with the implicit goal of reducing or eliminating it. TNG autistic people, on the other hand, frequently cite the need for research that addresses their access to health care and sexuality education (see Adams and Liang 2020).

Another oft-noted concern is the impact of *masking* (not to be confused with physically wearing masks in the pandemic), in which autistic people are encouraged or required to subvert and hide their autistic traits to appear neurotypical (Pearson and Rose 2021). Masking may exert psychiatric stressors similar to those experienced by TNG people, and the effects of hiding one's autism and minoritized gender identity can be mutually reinforcing (George and Stokes 2018; Murphy et al. 2020). Research exploring the causes and costs of masking, as well as efforts to promote awareness and understanding and ultimately decrease the degree to which it is required, would be welcome.

ADHD

The literature on the TNG-ADHD intersection is particularly young and sparse, and it focuses almost entirely on the etiology of and possible problems caused by this overlap (Goetz and Adams 2022). The lack of explicit TNG and ADHD community involvement in existing research is particularly striking. Future work is needed that moves beyond incidence, etiology, and prevention to explore this group's health care needs.

LAW, POLICE, AND CRIMINALIZATION

Research exploring the risk posed to autistic people by police violence would be useful. Police often respond to calls for mental wellness checks with disproportionate force. Combined with a frequent inability to understand an autistic person's communication and a propensity to misinterpret autistic behavior as evasive or indicative of illicit drug use, police interaction with autistic people is lethal all too frequently. A recent study found that people with autism were more likely to have an interaction with the police, and that these interactions were frequently negative and resulted in escalating the crisis (Tint et al. 2017).

Police interactions are even more frequently violent when the autistic individual is a person of color and, in particular, Black (Ball and Jeffrey-Wilensky 2020).

Autistic people may be more likely to experience institutionalization and comparatively harsh legal consequences or even indeterminate sentences owing to their presentation (e.g., the autistic and TNG woman discussed in Baker and Shweikh 2016). Again, autistic people of color are more likely than whites to experience racialized health disparities, such as delayed diagnosis, and to receive diagnoses that carry greater stigma and blame, such as conduct disorder or oppositional defiant disorder (Bishop-Fitzpatrick and Kind 2017; Mandell et al. 2007).

Research on people who are TNG and neurodivergent should involve and be led by people who are themselves at this intersection. Some leading journals in this field, such as *Autism*, now require community involvement statements (Community Involvement Reporting FAQ n.d.). It is critical, however, that participation be meaningful and not perfunctory.

NEURODIVERSE PROFESSIONALS IN TNG HEALTH CARE

Many established professionals are also members of autistic, ADHD, and TNG communities. There are distinct advantages to having a knowledgeable researcher or clinician who is a member of the community being investigated (Cabral and Smith 2011; Zane et al. 2005). For instance, communication between autistic and neurotypical people has been shown to be less effective than between two autistic people (Crompton et al. 2020).

CONCLUSION

We highlight the need for community-driven research and leadership in neuroqueer scholarship and the paucity of literature on the intersection of ADHD and TNG identities (in contrast to that on autism and TNG identities). This disparity may stem from pathologizing distinct neurodivergent experiences or a perception that they interfere in TNG health care.

Ultimately, gender-affirming care should be available to everyone, regardless of diagnoses. This may require more learning on the part of clinicians, but that is only just. Neurodiverse people are not inherently less capable, and any requirement to be cured or "managed" before care fails to understand the inherent basis of both neurodiversity and TNG identities.

REFERENCES

Adams N, Liang B: Trans and Autistic: Stories From Life at the Intersection. Philadelphia, PA, Jessica Kingsley Publishers, 2020

American Psychiatric Association: Diagnostic and Statistical Manual of Mental Disorders, 5th Edition. Arlington, VA, American Psychiatric Association, 2013

American Psychiatric Association: Diagnostic and Statistical Manual of Mental Disorders, 5th Edition, Text Revision. Washington, DC, American Psychiatric Association, 2022

Asasumasu K: PSA from the actual coiner of "neurodivergent." Lost in My Mind TARDIS (blog), 2015. Available at: https://sherlocksflataffect.tumblr.com/post/121295972384/psa-from-the-actual-coiner-of-neurodivergent. Accessed June 3, 2023.

Atkinson T: Autism Entangled: Controversies Over Disability, Sexuality, and Gender in Contemporary Culture. Ph.D. thesis, Lancaster, UK, Lancaster University, 2021. Available at: https://eprints.lancs.ac.uk/id/eprint/152153/1/2021atkinsonphd.pdf. Accessed June 3, 2023.

Baker P, Shweikh E: Autistic spectrum disorders, personality disorder and offending in a transgender patient: clinical considerations, diagnostic challenges and treatment responses. Advances in Autism 2(3):140–146, 2016

Ball E, Jeffrey-Wilensky J: Why autism training for police isn't enough. Spectrum News, 2020. Available at: https://www.spectrumnews.org/news/why-autism-training-for-police-isnt-enough/. Accessed June 3, 2023.

Barnett JP: Sexual Citizenship on the Autism Spectrum. Ph.D. thesis, Windsor, ON, University of Windsor, 2014. Available at: https://scholar.uwindsor.ca/cgi?article=6100=etd. Accessed June 3, 2023.

Bennie M: Am I Autistic? A Guide to Diagnosis for Adults. Calgary, ON, Autism Awareness Centre, Inc, 2020. Available at: https://autismawarenesscentre.com/am-i-autistic-a-guide-to-diagnosis-for-adults/. Accessed June 3, 2023.

Bishop-Fitzpatrick L, Kind AJH: A scoping review of health disparities in autism spectrum disorder. J Autism Dev Disord 47(11):3380–3391, 2017 28756549

Blume H: Neurodiversity. The Atlantic, September 1998. Available at: https://www.theatlantic.com/magazine/archive/1998/09/neurodiversity/305909/. Accessed June 3, 2023.

Bovell V: Is there an ethical case for the prevention and/or cure of autism?, in Neurodiversity Studies: A New Critical Paradigm. Edited by Rosqvist HB, Chown N, Sterling A. Abingdon, UK, Routledge, 2020, pp 39–54

Cabral RR, Smith TB: Racial/ethnic matching of clients and therapists in mental health services: a meta-analytic review of preferences, perceptions, and outcomes. J Couns Psychol 58(4):537–554, 2011 21875181

Cain LK, Velasco JC: Stranded at the intersection of gender, sexuality, and autism: Gray's story. Disabil Soc 36(3):358–375, 2020

Call D: Prepubertal children with gender dysphoria: a case to illustrate the management of co-occurring attention deficit hyperactivity disorder and disruptive behavior disorders, in Affirmative Mental Health Care for Transgender and Gender Diverse Youth. Edited by Janssen A, Leibowitz S. New York, Springer, 2018, pp 105–119

Centers for Disease Control and Prevention: Autism and Developmental Disabilities Monitoring (ADDM) Network. Atlanta, GA, Centers for Disease Control and Prevention, 2020. Available at: https://www.cdc.gov/ncbddd/autism/addm.html. Accessed June 3, 2023.

Centers for Disease Control and Prevention: Data and Statistics About ADHD. Atlanta, GA, Centers for Disease Control and Prevention, 2022. Available at: http://www.cdc.gov/ncbddd/adhd/data.html. Accessed June 3, 2023.

Chapman R: Negotiating the neurodiversity concept: towards epistemic justice in conceptualising health. Psychology Today, August 18, 2021. Available at: https://www.psychologytoday.com/ca/blog/neurodiverse-age/202108/negotiating-the-neurodiversity-concept. Accessed June 3, 2023.

Cheung AS, Ooi O, Leemaqz S, et al: Sociodemographic and clinical characteristics of transgender adults in Australia. Transgend Health 3(1):229–238, 2018 30596151

Chown N: Language games used to construct autism as pathology, in Neurodiversity Studies: A New Critical Paradigm. Edited by Rosqvist HB, Chown N, Sterling A. Abingdon, UK, Routledge, 2020, pp 27–38

Christian-Brandt AS, Philpott J, Edwards-Leeper L: "Quiero soy un niño!": family-based treatment of a Mexican American child with gender dysphoria and disruptive behaviors. Clin Pract Pediatr Psychol 9(2):203–208, 2021

Chung W, Jiang SF, Paksarian D, et al: Trends in the prevalence and incidence of attention-deficit/hyperactivity disorder among adults and children of different racial and ethnic groups. JAMA Netw Open 2(11):e1914344, 2019 31675080

Coker TR, Elliott MN, Toomey SL, et al: Racial and ethnic disparities in ADHD diagnosis and treatment. Pediatrics 138(3):e20160407, 2016 27553219

Coleman E, Bockting W, Botzer M, et al: Standards of care for the health of transsexual, transgender, and gender-nonconforming people, version 7. Int J Transgend 13(4):165–232, 2012

Community Involvement Reporting FAQ: Autism, n.d. Available at: https://journals.sagepub.com/pb-assets/cmscontent/AUT/Community-Involvement-Reporting-FAQ-1626698718.pdf. Accessed June 3, 2023.

Crompton CJ, Ropar D, Evans-Williams CVM, et al: Autistic peer-to-peer information transfer is highly effective. Autism 24(7):1704–1712, 2020 32431157

Dawson AE, Wymbs BT, Gidycz CA, et al: Exploring rates of transgender individuals and mental health concerns in an online sample. Int J Transgend 18(3):295–304, 2017

daVanport S, Rodríguez-Roldán VM, Brown LXZ: Before You Go: Know Your Rights & What to Expect at the Doctor and in the Hospital. Lincoln, NE, Autistic Women and Nonbinary Network, 2020. Available at: https://awnnetwork.org/wp-content/uploads/2020/10/Final-Version-Before-You-Go-Know-Your-Rights-Booklet.pdf. Accessed June 3, 2023.

Dietz PM, Rose CE, McArthur D, Maenner M: National and state estimates of adults with autism spectrum disorder. J Autism Dev Disord 50(12):4258–4266, 2020 32390121

Fortunato A, Giovanardi G, Innocenzi E, et al: Is it autism? A critical commentary on the co-occurrence of gender dysphoria and autism spectrum disorder. J Homosex 69(7):1204–1221, 2022 33852376

George R, Stokes MA: Sexual orientation in autism spectrum disorder. Autism Res 11(1):133–141, 2018 29159906

Geurts H, Sinzig J, Booth R, Happé F: Neuropsychological heterogeneity in executive functioning in autism spectrum disorders. Int J Dev Disabil 60(3):155–162, 2014

Gibson MF, Douglas P: Disturbing behaviors: Ole Ivar Lovaas and the queer history of autism science. Catalyst 4(2):1–28, 2018

Gillespie-Lynch K, Dwyer P, Constantino C, et al: Can we broaden the neurodiversity movement without weakening it? Participatory approaches as a framework for cross-disability alliance building, in Disability Alliances and Allies: Opportunities and Challenges. Edited by Carey AC, Ostrove JM, Fannon T. Bingley, UK, Emerald Publishing, 2020, pp 189–223

Goetz TG, Adams N: The transgender and gender diverse and attention deficit hyperactivity disorder nexus: a systematic review. J Gay Lesbian Ment Health 1–18, 2022

Groom MJ, Cortese S: Current pharmacological treatments for ADHD. Curr Top Behav Neurosci 57:19–50, 2022 35507282

Gupta D: Why an ADHD diagnosis is often out of reach for Canadian university students. Maclean's, October 7, 2021. Available at: https://www.macleans.ca/society/health/why-an-adhd-diagnosis-is-often-out-of-reach-for-canadian-university-students/. Accessed June 3, 2023.

Hansen SN, Schendel DE, Parner ET: Explaining the increase in the prevalence of autism spectrum disorders: the proportion attributable to changes in reporting practices. JAMA Pediatr 169(1):56–62, 2015 25365033

Hesslinger B, Tebartz van Elst L, Nyberg E, et al: Psychotherapy of attention deficit hyperactivity disorder in adults—a pilot study using a structured skills training program. Eur Arch Psychiatry Clin Neurosci 252(4):177–184, 2002 12242579

Hillier A, Gallop N, Mendes E, et al: LGBTQ+ and autism spectrum disorder: experiences and challenges. Int J Transgender Health 21(1):98–110, 2019 33005905

Holt V, Skagerberg E, Dunsford M: Young people with features of gender dysphoria: demographics and associated difficulties. Clin Child Psychol Psychiatry 21(1):108–118, 2016 25431051

Hossain MM, Khan N, Sultana A, et al: Prevalence of comorbid psychiatric disorders among people with autism spectrum disorder: an umbrella review of systematic reviews and meta-analyses. Psychiatry Res 287:112922, 2020 32203749

Jackson-Perry D. The autistic art of failure? Unknowing imperfect systems of sexuality and gender. Scand J Disability Res 22(1):221–229, 2020

Jacobs LA, Rachlin K, Erickson-Schroth L, Janssen A: Gender dysphoria and co-occurring autism spectrum disorders: review, case examples, and treatment considerations. LGBT Health 1(4):277–282, 2014 26789856

Janssen A, Leibowitz S (eds): Affirmative Mental Health Care for Transgender and Gender Diverse Youth: A Clinical Guide. New York, Springer, 2018

Jaynes A: I was diagnosed with ADHD as an adult. Now I realize how misunderstood this condition is. CBC Radio, April 9, 2021. Available at: https://www.cbc.ca/radio/docproject/i-was-diagnosed-with-adhd-as-an-adult-now-i-realize-how-misunderstood-this-condition-is-1.5978042. Accessed June 3, 2023.

Joho J: Privilege plays a huge role in getting an ADHD diagnosis. Mashable, June 24, 2021. Available at: https://mashable.com/article/how-to-get-adhd-diagnosis. Accessed June 3, 2023.

Jurgens A: Neurodiversity in a neurotypical world: an enactive framework for investigating autism and social institutions, in Neurodiversity Studies: A New Critical Paradigm. Edited by Rosqvist HB, Chown N, Sterling A. Abingdon, UK, Routledge, 2020, pp 73–88

Kapp SK: Autistic Community and the Neurodiversity Movement: Stories From the Frontline. London, Palgrave Macmillan, 2020

Katzman MA, Bilkey TS, Chokka PR, et al: Adult ADHD and comorbid disorders: clinical implications of a dimensional approach. BMC Psychiatry 17(1):302, 2017 28830387

Kimball E, Vaccaro A, Tissi-Gassoway N, Bobot SD: Gender, sexuality, and (dis)ability: queer perspectives on the experiences of students with disabilities. Disabil Stud Q 38(2), 2018

Kupferstein H: Evidence of increased PTSD symptoms in autistics exposed to applied behavior analysis. Adv Autism 4(1), 2018

Kuvalanka KA, Mahan DJ, McGuire JK, Hoffman TK: Perspectives of mothers of transgender and gender-nonconforming children with autism spectrum disorder. J Homosex 65(9):1167–1189, 2018 29161222

Lemaire M, Thomazeau B, Bonnet-Brilhault F: Gender identity disorder and autism spectrum disorder in a 23-year-old female. Arch Sex Behav 43(2):395–398, 2014 23835847

Lewis LF: Exploring the experience of self-diagnosis of autism spectrum disorder in adults. Arch Psychiatr Nurs 30(5):575–580, 2016a 27654240

Lewis LF: Realizing a diagnosis of autism spectrum disorder as an adult. Int J Ment Health Nurs 25(4):346–354, 2016b 26940281

Lynch C: Medical visits and autism: a better way. Psychology Today, April 6, 2019. Available at: https://www.psychologytoday.com/ca/blog/autism-and-anxiety/201904/medical-visits-and-autism-better-way. Accessed June 3, 2023.

MacKinnon KR, Grace S, Ng SL, et al: "I don't think they thought I was ready": how pre-transition assessments create care inequities for trans people with complex mental health in Canada. Int J Ment Health 49:1–25, 2020

Mandell DS, Ittenbach RF, Levy SE, Pinto-Martin JA: Disparities in diagnoses received prior to a diagnosis of autism spectrum disorder. J Autism Dev Disord 37(9):1795–1802, 2007 17160456

Milton DEM: On the ontological status of autism: the "double empathy problem." Disability Soc 27(6):883–887, 2012

Mitchell P, Sheppard E, Cassidy S: Autism and the double empathy problem: implications for development and mental health. Br J Dev Psychol 39(1):1–18, 2021 33393101

Murphy J, Prentice F, Walsh R, et al: Autism and transgender identity: implications for depression and anxiety. Res Autism Spectr Disord 69:101466, 2020

National Institute of Mental Health: Attention-Deficit/Hyperactivity Disorder (ADHD). Bethesda, MD, National Institute of Mental Health, n.d. Available at: https://www.nimh.nih.gov/health/statistics/attention-deficit-hyperactivity-disorder-adhd. Accessed June 3, 2023.

Pan P-Y, Bölte S: The association between ADHD and physical health: a co-twin control study. Sci Rep 10(1):22388, 2020 33372183

Pearson A, Rose K: A conceptual analysis of autistic masking: understanding the narrative of stigma and the illusion of choice. Autism Adulthood 3(1):52–60, 2021 36601266

Pezzuoli F, Tafaro D, Pane M, et al: Development of a new sign language translation system for people with autism spectrum disorder. Adv Neurodev Disord 4(7), 439–446, 2020

Philipsen A, Richter H, Peters J, et al: Structured group psychotherapy in adults with attention deficit hyperactivity disorder: results of an open multicentre study. J Nerv Ment Dis 195(12):1013–1019, 2007 18091195

Pyne J: "Building a person": legal and clinical personhood for autistic and trans children in Ontario. Can J Law Soc 35(2):341–365, 2020

Rosqvist HB, Stenning A, Chown N: Introduction, in Neurodiversity Studies: A New Critical Paradigm. Edited by Rosqvist HB, Chown N, Sterling A. Abingdon, UK, Routledge, 2020, pp 1–11

Rydzewska E, Dunn K, Cooper S-A: Umbrella systematic review of systematic reviews and meta-analyses on comorbid physical conditions in people with autism spectrum disorder. Br J Psychiatry 218(1):10–19, 2021 33161922

Sandoval-Norton AH, Shkedy G, Shkedy D: How much compliance is too much compliance: is long-term ABA therapy abuse? Cogent Psychol 6(1):1641258, 2019

Shekhar R: I self-diagnosed my autism because nobody else would. Here's why that needs to change. The Swaddle, May 23, 2020. Available at: https://theswaddle.com/i-self-diagnosed-my-autism-because-nobody-else-would-heres-why-that-needs-to-change/. Accessed June 3, 2023.

Shi Y, Hunter Guevara LR, Dykhoff HJ, et al: Racial disparities in diagnosis of attention-deficit/hyperactivity disorder in a US national birth cohort. JAMA Netw Open 4(3):e210321, 2021 33646315

Shumer DE, Reisner SL, Edwards-Leeper L, Tishelman A: Evaluation of Asperger syndrome in youth presenting to a gender dysphoria clinic. LGBT Health 3(5):387–390, 2016 26651183

Silberman S: Neurotribes: The Legacy of Autism and the Future of Neurodiversity. Garden City, New York, Avery, 2015

Singer J: Odd People In: The Birth of Community Amongst People on the "Autistic Spectrum." Bachelor's thesis, Sydney, Australia, University of Technology, 1998. Available at: https://www.academia.edu/27033194/Odd_People_In_The_Birth_of_Community_amongst_people_on_the_Autistic_Spectrum_A_personal_exploration_based_on_neurological_diversity. Accessed June 3, 2023.

Solanto MV, Marks DJ, Mitchell KJ, et al: Development of a new psychosocial treatment for adult ADHD. J Atten Disord 11(6):728–736, 2008 17712167

Strang JF, Meagher H, Kenworthy L, et al: Initial clinical guidelines for co-occurring autism spectrum disorder and gender dysphoria or incongruence in adolescents. J Clin Child Adolesc Psychol 47(1):105–115, 2018a 27775428

Strang JF, Powers MD, Knauss M, et al: "They thought it was an obsession": trajectories and perspectives of autistic transgender and gender-diverse adolescents. J Autism Dev Disord 48(12):4039–4055, 2018b 30140984

The Color of Autism Foundation: n.d. Available at: https://thecolorofautism.org/. Accessed June 3, 2023.

Thrower E, Bretherton I, Pang KC, et al: Prevalence of autism spectrum disorder and attention-deficit hyperactivity disorder amongst individuals with gender dysphoria: a systematic review. J Autism Dev Disord 50(3):695–706, 2020 31732891

Tint A, Palucka AM, Bradley E, et al: Correlates of police involvement among adolescents and adults with autism spectrum disorder. J Autism Dev Disord 47(9):2639–2647, 2017 28612245

Turban JL, van Schalkwyk GI: "Gender dysphoria" and autism spectrum disorder: is the link real? J Am Acad Child Adolesc Psychiatry 57(1):8–9.e2, 2018 29301673 van der Miesen AIR, de Vries ALC, Steensma TD, Hartman CA: Autistic symptoms in children and adolescents with gender dysphoria. J Autism Dev Disord 48(5):1537–1548, 2018 29189919

Walsh RJ: "Masculine" describes gender expressions, not neurobiologies: response to Dutton and Madison (2020). Sex Res Soc Policy 18(3):805–807, 2021 34721712

Walsh RJ, Krabbendam L, Dewinter J, Begeer S: Brief report: Gender identity differences in autistic adults: associations with perceptual and socio-cognitive profiles. J Autism Dev Disord 48(12):4070–4078, 2018 30062396

Wanta JW, Niforatos JD, Durbak E, et al: Mental health diagnoses among transgender patients in the clinical setting: an all-payer electronic health record study. Transgend Health 4(1):313–315, 2019 31701012

Warrier V, Greenberg DM, Weir E, et al: Elevated rates of autism, other neurodevelopmental and psychiatric diagnoses, and autistic traits in transgender and gender-diverse individuals. Nat Commun 11(1):3959, 2020 32770077

Winter AS, Fountain C, Cheslack-Postava K, Bearman PS: The social patterning of autism diagnoses reversed in California between 1992 and 2018. Proc Natl Acad Sci USA 117(48):30295–30302, 2020

World Health Organization: International Statistical Classification of Diseases and Related Health Problems, 10th Revision. Geneva, World Health Organization, 2016

Young S, Amarasinghe JM: Practitioner review: non-pharmacological treatments for ADHD: a lifespan approach. J Child Psychol Psychiatry 51(2):116–133, 2010 19891745

Zane N, Sue S, Chang J, et al: Beyond ethnic match: effects of client-therapist cognitive match in problem perception, coping orientation, and therapy goals on treatment outcomes. J Community Psychol 33(5):569–585, 2005

Zupanič S, Kruljac I, Šoštarič Zvonar M, Drobnič Radobuljac M: Case report: adolescent with autism and gender dysphoria. Front Psychiatry 12:671448, 2021 34122187

Zylowska L, Ackerman DL, Yang MH, et al: Mindfulness meditation training in adults and adolescents with ADHD: a feasibility study. J Atten Disord 11(6):737–746, 2008 18025249

CHAPTER 9

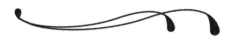

Disability Justice and Access Needs for Disabled Transgender, Nonbinary, and/or Gender-Expansive (TNG) People

Evelyn Callahan, Ph.D., M.Sc.
Brendon Holloway, M.S.W.
Vern Harner, Ph.D., M.S.W.
Shanna K. Kattari, Ph.D., M.Ed., C.S.E., A.C.S.

IN this chapter, we highlight the interconnectedness of transness and disability so that clinicians will become better able to work with people who are both disabled and TNG. We begin by defining and giving background on disability and chronic illness in general and within TNG communities, noting the high incidence of disability within TNG communities. We look at some of the key challenges that disabled and chronically ill TNG people face (specifically, gatekeeping of health care services and frequent negative medical encounters), and then we conclude with recommendations for making mental health services more accessible. Our discussion here is informed by a disability justice framework, which we discuss in more detail next.

We do not shy away from using the term *disabled*, and neither should you. There is nothing wrong with being disabled: it is simply another way of experiencing the world. Also, using the word makes it possible to organize around a disability justice framework (Andrews et al. 2019). In this chapter, disability is an extensive and inclusive umbrella term, although we recognize that individual people may not self-identify as disabled for various reasons, including stigma (Bogart et al. 2017). We also use *identity-first language* (disabled person, chronically ill person, trans person, etc.) rather than *person-first language* (e.g., person with a disability, person with a chronic illness, person who is trans). Although some organizations and individuals still use person-first language, many find it stigmatizing and clunky (Collier 2012; Gernsbacher 2017). Identity-first language is the standard within communities, and it is what we use throughout this chapter. If an individual prefers to use person-first language for themselves, then that is what you should use for them. We also use the terms *apparent* and *non-apparent* disabilities rather than *visible* or *invisible*. This usage emphasizes that although someone's disability might not be apparent to certain people or in certain circumstances, visibility or its lack is not an inherent feature of the disability. For example, a person's chronic fatigue may become apparent only when they use a cane or are on bed rest. Additionally, that person's chronic fatigue might not be apparent to nondisabled people, but to someone else who also has chronic fatigue or a similar disability, it might be extremely apparent, as they recognize the subtle signs of their own experience in others.

BACKGROUND

For this chapter, we define *disability* flexibly and acknowledge that disability is not solely an intellectual, developmental, or physical impairment of a person's body or mind: it is all of these experiences intersecting with the experiences of the environment in which an individual lives. This also encompasses society's expectations in terms of ability status (Ustün et al. 2003). In how we define disability, we include those with non-apparent disabilities (e.g., chronic pain, chronic illness, mental illness) and those whose disability or impairment varies day to day. We also include neurodivergent people, although individual neurodivergent people may or may not self-identify as disabled or chronically ill. (You can read more about the specific needs of neurodivergent TNG people in Chapter 8, "DoubleQueer.")

Disability

About 15%–20% of individuals ages 15+ have a disability (U.S. Census Bureau 2015). Disability can be chronic or acute, and an individual can be born with a disability or become disabled at any time of life (Smart 2011). Disabled individuals experience increased rates of discrimination in society (Krahn et al. 2015); disabled people are often desexualized, hypersexualized, or inscribed with heteronormativity (Abbott 2015). Because society views disabled people through a heteronormative lens, disabled individuals often find it difficult to outwardly explore gender or to resist the gender binary (Slater and Liddiard 2018).

Models of Disability

Two primary models conceptualize disability: the medical model and the social model. The *medical model* views disability as an individual deficit that needs to be cured, placing the burden on disabled people to overcome their disability or impairment (Gerben Dejong 1979; Kattari et al. 2017). Under this model, disabled people are viewed through the lens that they need to be cured or treated. This places the burden on disabled individuals to seek treatment and further reinforces that disabled people need to be cured to exist in mainstream society.

The *social model* of disability focuses on society's—or the system's—role in disability (Abberley 1987). This model places the blame on society and systems for not creating a world that is accommodating to disabled individuals. The social model accounts for the lack of accessible spaces for disabled individuals, such as doorways too narrow for wheelchairs or buildings without ramps. The social model upholds the belief that an individual's limitations are not the problem, but rather the problem is "society's failure to provide appropriate services and adequately ensure the needs of disabled people are fully taken into account" (Inclusion London 2015; Oliver 1990).

Intersection of Disability and TNG Identities

Similar to the range of disability identities, there are a wide range of gender identities under the TNG umbrella, including binary-oriented identities (e.g., trans man, trans woman), nonbinary-oriented identities (e.g., genderqueer, gender fluid), multiple gender identities, or no gender identity. An individual can be TNG and disabled regardless of other identities, such as race/ethnicity, citizenship status, and class status. In 2015, the largest survey of TNG people to date ($N=27,715$; U.S. Transgender Survey [James et al. 2016]) found that ~39% of TNG people had at least one disability. Additionally, the 2010 National Trans Discrimination Survey (Kattari et al. 2017) found that disabled TNG respondents reported significantly elevated rates of discrimination when accessing crisis centers, drug treatment programs, mental health centers, and intimate partner violence shelters. Disabled TNG people of color who participated in the survey experienced even higher rates of discrimination than white disabled TNG people.

Disability Justice

The *disability justice framework* has 10 guiding principles (Berne et al: 2018):

1. *Intersectionality:* The experience and systemic oppression of disabled people is interconnected with race, gender, class, relationship to colonization, etc.
2. *Leadership of those most impacted:* We allow those who are the most impacted and who have the most systemic knowledge to lead us.
3. *Anti-capitalist politic:* Human worth is not dependent on what and how much a person produces or does.
4. *Cross-movement solidarity:* We incorporate how other social justice movements understand disability.
5. *Recognizing wholeness:* We value people for who they are, as they are, and we view all individuals as having inherent worth outside of the capitalistic notions of productivity.
6. *Sustainability:* We pace ourselves as individuals and as a collective.
7. *Commitment to cross-disability solidarity:* We value and acknowledge the insights of all community members.
8. *Interdependence:* We attempt to meet one another's needs as we move toward liberation.
9. *Collective access:* We strive to ensure that all marginalized communities have equal access.
10. *Collective liberation:* We move together, ensuring that nobody is left behind.

The disability justice framework can be adapted for other marginalized communities. The root description of this framework is that community members support one another to ensure individual and collective needs are being met within or outside of formal systems.

Why Are Rates of Disability High in TNG Communities?

Samples of TNG people regularly report higher rates of disability and chronic illness than their cisgender peers. This includes 39% of the total sample of 27,715 in the U.S. Transgender Survey (James et al. 2016) and 55% of the 2,873 respondents in the Trans PULSE Canada study (Pyne et al. 2012). In contrast, as stated earlier, ~15%–20% of the general U.S. population are disabled (Okoro et al. 2018; U.S. Census Bureau 2015), and ~40% have a chronic disease (lasting ≥ 3 months) (Centers for Disease Control and Prevention 2009; National Center for Health Statistics 2013). It is not clear whether TNG individuals are more likely to be disabled (or vice versa) or whether disabled individuals are at times oversampled or overrepresented in TNG research.

When it comes to considering co-occurrence of transness and disability, there is a danger of falling into traps of bioessentialism—believing that TNG people have a biological predisposition to physical or mental impairment—when there is no evidence to support this. However, TNG individuals are medicalized, pathologized, and traumatized in oppressive societies, which may contribute to mental health struggles such as anxiety, depression, and PTSD. Research studies comparing the experiences of TNG individuals with and without familial/social support are exploring potential connections between these mental health struggles, behavioral "disorders" resulting from survival behaviors, and impacts of the immediate and larger environments. For example, Olson et al. (2016) saw no increased rate of depression and only slightly elevated levels of anxiety in a sample of socially transitioned trans youth (ages 3–12) with supportive families (N=73), compared with the general population of youth in that age range. In a sample of 64 genderqueer adults, Budge et al. (2014) found level of social support to be inversely associated with depression and anxiety. Rates of autism and ADHD have been reported as higher among TNG people than cisgender peers (see Chapter 8, "DoubleQueer"). Higher rates of diagnosis could reflect higher rates of autism, neurodivergence, or mental health conditions generally, or they may reflect higher rates of mental health care utilization or surveillance. Studies regarding linkages between the environment and physical disability, illness, or impairment in TNG communities have yet to be conducted.

Being TNG, or otherwise "non-normative" when it comes to one's experience of gender, has in and of itself been conceptualized as a disability. Notably, DSM included gender nonconformity as part of a diagnosable condition starting with its first edition in 1952 (American Psychiatric Association 1952; Drescher 2010). In 1994, DSM-IV shifted the diagnostic name from *gender identity disorder* (GID) to *gender dysphoria*, aiming to shift from viewing gender dysphoria or transness as inherently disordered, to instead focusing on the distress experienced due to dysphoria (American Psychiatric Association 1994; Riggs et al. 2019). A diagnostic code may be needed to obtain insurance coverage and therefore to access mental health care for gender affirmation–related care, and many TNG individuals experience these diagnoses as pathologizing. What is more, the very requirement for a diagnostic code reflects systemic barriers to access of care for TNG individuals, who are obligated to depend on a diagnostic code for their psychiatric or physical health services.

GATEKEEPING OF SERVICES

TNG individuals face numerous barriers when accessing health care. These barriers include past discriminatory experiences in health care settings

(Roberts and Fantz 2014), the need to educate medical providers and staff (Poteat et al. 2013; Roller et al. 2015), having to travel long distances to access affirming care (Kattari et al. 2020), and gatekeeping of health services. *Gatekeeping* in health care is defined as limiting an individual's or community's access to general care, specialty care, or in the case of some TNG individuals, transition-related care.

Gatekeeping of transition-related care runs rampant in health care settings, as many medical providers require letters from mental health professionals for TNG individuals to access hormones (e.g., testosterone, estrogen) and gender-affirming procedures and surgeries (e.g., facial feminization surgery, double incision top surgery).

Disabled individuals also experience extreme gatekeeping in health care settings. These barriers include services and spaces that are inaccessible, the need for accessible transportation to reach in-person services, and health care staff who are ableist. *Ableism* is the act of prejudice, victimization, or discrimination against disabled people (Hehir 2002) and coincides with able-bodied—or nondisabled—privilege. Ableism places value on physical, emotional, and mental capital and upholds socially constructed expectations of ability status (Loja et al. 2013). Ableist health care staff can actively harm disabled individuals who are seeking health care, by refusing to give a disabled person a needed diagnosis, minimizing or disbelieving their symptoms, and refusing care. Other examples of how health care staff and offices may harm disabled people: not providing an American Sign Language (ASL) interpreter when requested, maintaining physical office spaces that are not accessible, and viewing disabled people as unable to understand their own health.

Additionally, some health care staff view all health care issues as stemming from disability or the individual's TNG identity. For example, if a TNG person goes to the emergency room for a broken bone, they are asked about their gender identity and, even more inappropriately, about what's in their pants. This is known as *trans broken arm syndrome*. At its core, trans broken arm syndrome means refusing to see TNG people as people, viewing them exclusively as TNG (Knutson et al. 2016), even if they need immediate attention for an issue unrelated to their gender identity, such as a broken bone.

The intersection of disability and gender identity is not well represented in the literature, but plentiful research and shared community expertise show that disabled TNG individuals experience gatekeeping that is unique to their identities. In a common example of gatekeeping toward this community, disabled TNG people are often denied transition-related services because they are "too medically complex" or "too high risk" to treat. Because of this ableism from providers, disabled TNG individuals have to interact with multiple health care offices and staff to find a clinician who will prescribe hormones or make referrals for gender-affirming surgeries and procedures, creating more labor for the patient and more barriers to care (Goetz 2021).

Impact of Negative Medical Encounters

Previous experiences with health care providers may discourage disabled or chronically ill TNG people from fully engaging in treatment or from seeking out treatment in the first place. One factor here is the medicalization of transness. Many health systems involve primary care providers, endocrinologists, psychiatrists, surgeons, and other health care staff in essential gender-affirming care services, necessitating that TNG people interact with a higher number of health care staff and have more medical encounters than otherwise. Further, this group may have to try out different clinicians to find those who are willing to adequately support all of their identities. For example, a trans wheelchair user might go to one psychiatrist who misgenders them, then try another whose practice has stair access, before finally finding one who can provide them with appropriate care. Thus what should have been one health care interaction has become three.

These numerous medical interactions provide more opportunities to experience medical ableism and medical transphobia. Shane Neilson defines *ableism* as "practices or policies that treat people with disabilities as if they were invisible, disposable and less than human, while taking for granted able-bodiedness as humanity's default state" (Neilson 2020, p. E411). *Medical ableism* is ableism within a medical context, including within psychiatry, psychology, counseling, and any other mental health care context. Similarly, *medical transphobia* is "negative attitudes (hate, contempt, disapproval) directed toward trans people because of their being trans" that occurs in any medical context (Bettcher 2014, p. 249). These experiences are particularly relevant to mental health care: in many health care systems around the globe, people need a diagnosis from a psychiatrist to access hormones, surgeries, and other essential gender-affirming care. This is an example of gatekeeping, a step that many see as unnecessary and pathologizing; thus having to go through that process can create distrust.

In addition to the negative experiences described here, many disabled or chronically ill TNG people have experienced medical trauma. *Medical trauma* arises from "injury, acute medical illness, and medical treatment" (Marsac et al. 2014, p. 399), and it can overlap with other trauma, including trauma resulting from being trans in a transphobic society (Mizock and Lewis 2008). Medical trauma is not unique to the disabled TNG population, but again an increased number of medical interactions in turn increases the risk of medical trauma. Therefore, it is likely that clinicians working with this population will encounter people presenting with PTSD or complex PTSD (Richmond et al. 2012).

To provide disabled or chronically ill TNG people with the best possible care, it is crucial for clinicians to understand the barriers to care that they face. Experiences of medical ableism, medical transphobia, and medical trauma may dissuade people from seeking out any medical interventions. Individuals also have to make difficult choices as they try to limit their exposure to additional medical interactions. For example, a person may require gender affirmation–related health care and mental health care, in addition to their primary care clinician and specialists for their disabilities/chronic illnesses. In this example, they may choose not to seek mental health care in favor of seeking out gender affirmation–related health care, or vice versa. Clinicians should be prepared to serve individuals within this population who are reluctant to seek mental health care, or who are struggling to do so. To best address these needs, clinicians should employ a trauma-informed approach, as detailed in Chapter 11, "Trauma-Informed Mental Health Care."

Implications for Practice

It is essential to connect research and frameworks of disability justice to clinical practice, informing how clinicians show up for and support their disabled TNG clients. Inclusion happens at the micro level (interpersonal), the meso level (family systems, groups, organizations), and the macro level (institutions, policies, systems); practitioners should be prepared to do work at each level to advocate for and offer inclusive practice to their TNG disabled clients.

Ensure your practice (and that of other professionals to whom you may refer your clients) is both accessible and gender affirming. Anything less forces TNG disabled people to choose between their identities, essentially forcing them to decide between a space that they can physically (mentally, sensorily) access and a space that respects and affirms their gender and cor-related experiences. In this vein, gender-inclusive, screen reader–compatible intake forms and Americans With Disabilities Act–compliant, gender-inclusive restrooms are the absolute baseline for inclusion. Culturally responsive clinicians should also

- Follow current policies and potential bills that could impact disabled TNG people; consider writing letters and testifying for or against such policies in support of clients' needs.
- Understand some of the challenges chronically ill TNG people face that affect their gender experiences (e.g., transfeminine individuals with breast cancer who may lose access to gender-affirming hormone therapy; transmasculine or nonbinary people assigned female sex at birth

who cannot wear binders because of issues with nerve pain or adverse responses to compression).

- Have resources that affirm both gender and disability identities and experiences, including local and national groups (online and in person), books, websites, podcasts, education resources, other media, and fellow therapists.
- Be knowledgeable about local clinicians who are also inclusive across these identities (e.g., gender-inclusive and disability-aware primary care physicians, accessible gender-affirming care specialists).
- Adopt a trauma-informed lens to meet the needs of the many clients who have experienced trauma relative to their TNG identities and their disabled identities (and any other identities).
- Create offices (virtual or in person) that are physically accessible (and include this access information on the website); use HIPAA-compliant platforms that also allow for autocaptions and for people to change their display name and pronouns; encourage the use of sensory-friendly stimming items; and ensure low-scent, or even chemical-free, spaces. Office signs should include braille. Furniture should be supportive of all body types, and displayed imagery should include TNG people, disabled people, and TNG disabled people, ideally created by TNG disabled artists.
- Practice asking for everyone's *access needs* (and then work to meet them!), share your own access needs, and remind people that we all have access needs—for instance, say "my access needs are met," rather than "I don't have access needs." Access needs include general accessibility issues, concerns around being outed to other people in the same health system, transportation or technology needs, the ability to change into gender-affirming clothing, and space to take medications, eat meals, and hydrate. Any given person knows their own needs better than anyone else, and so creating a space where people are asked, and feel safe sharing, their access needs—and see that the clinician is also thinking about their needs—is an excellent way to model this.

CONCLUSION

This chapter serves as a starting point for treating TNG disabled or chronically ill people and orienting clinical practice toward disability justice. We suggest that you continue to learn and improve on the care that you provide to this population; we urge you to seek out expertise not only from other clinicians, but most importantly, from TNG disabled or chronically ill people with lived experience of accessing mental health care; of course those individuals may be clinicians as well. Finally, pass on this learning to your colleagues and lead by example as you implement these recommendations.

REFERENCES

Abberley P: The concept of oppression and the development of a social theory of disability. Disabil Handicap Soc 2(1):5–19, 1987

Abbott D: Love in a cold climate: changes in the fortunes of LGBT men and women with learning disabilities. Br J Learn Disabilities 43(2):100–105, 2015

American Psychiatric Association: Diagnostic and Statistical Manual: Mental Disorders. Washington, DC, American Psychiatric Association, 1952

American Psychiatric Association: Diagnostic and Statistical Manual of Mental Disorders, 4th Edition. Washington, DC, 1994

Andrews EE, Forber-Pratt AJ, Mona LR, et al: #SaytheWord: a disability culture commentary on the erasure of "disability." Rehabil Psychol 64(2):111–118, 2019 30762412

Berne P, Morales AL, Langstaff D, et al: Ten principles of disability justic. Women Stud Q 46(1):227–230, 2018

Bettcher TM: Transphobia. Transgend Stud Q 1(1–2):249–251, 2014

Bogart KR, Rottenstein A, Lund EM, Bouchard L: Who self-identifies as disabled? An examination of impairment and contextual predictors. Rehabil Psychol 62(4):553–562, 2017 28581320

Budge SL, Rossman HK, Howard KAS: Coping and psychological distress among genderqueer individuals: the moderating effect of social support. J LGBT Issues Couns 8(1):95–117, 2014

Centers for Disease Control and Prevention: The Power of Prevention. Atlanta, GA, Centers for Disease Control and Prevention, 2009. Available at: https://www.cdc.gov/chronicdisease/programs-impact/pop/pdfs/oral-disease-H.pdf. Accessed June 25, 2023.

Collier R: Person-first language: noble intent but to what effect? CMAJ 184(18):1977–1978, 2012 23128280

Drescher J: Queer diagnoses: parallels and contrasts in the history of homosexuality, gender variance, and the diagnostic and statistical manual. Arch Sex Behav 39(2):427–460, 2010 19838785

Gerben Dejong MPA: Independent living: from social movement to analytic paradigm. Arch Phys Med Rehabil 60(10):435–436, 1979

Gernsbacher MA: Editorial perspective: the use of person-first language in scholarly writing may accentuate stigma. J Child Psychol Psychiatry 58(7):859–861, 2017 28621486

Goetz TG: Terminal transition: an ethnographic exploration of (in)finite gender journeys. Presented at the U.S. Professional Association for Transgender Health Conference, Virtual, May 2021

Hehir T: Eliminating ableism in education. Harv Educ Rev 72(1):1–33, 2002

Inclusion London: The Social Model of Disability. London, Inclusion London, 2015. Available at: https://www.inclusionlondon.org.uk/about-us/disability-in-london/social-model/the-social-model-of-disability-and-the-cultural-model-of-deafness/. Accessed October 13, 2022.

James SE, Herman JL, Rankin S, et al: The Report of the 2015 U.S. Transgender Survey. Washington, DC, National Center for Transgender Equality, 2016. Available at: https://transequality.org/sites/default/files/docs/usts/USTS-Full-Report-Dec17.pdf. Accessed June 25, 2023.

Kattari SK, Walls NE, Speer SR: Differences in experiences of discrimination in accessing social services among transgender/gender nonconforming individuals by (dis)ability. J Soc Work Disabil Rehabil 16(2):116–140, 2017 28447917

Kattari SK, Grange J, Seelman KL, et al: Distance traveled to access knowledgeable trans-related healthcare providers. Ann LGBTQ Pub Popul Health 1(2), 2020

Knutson D, Koch JM, Arthur T, et al: "Trans broken arm": health care stories from transgender people in rural areas. J Res Women Gend 7(1):30–46, 2016

Krahn GL, Walker DK, Correa-De-Araujo R: Persons with disabilities as an unrecognized health disparity population. Am J Public Health 105(2 Suppl 2):S198–S206, 2015 25689212

Loja E, Costa ME, Hughes B, Menezes I: Disability, embodiment, and ableism: stores of resistance. Disabil Soc 28(2):190–203, 2013

Marsac ML, Kassam-Adams N, Delahanty DL, et al: Posttraumatic stress following acute medical trauma in children: a proposed model of bio-psycho-social processes during the peri-trauma period. Clin Child Fam Psychol Rev 17(4):399–411, 2014 25217001

Mizock L, Lewis TK: Trauma in transgender populations: risk, resilience, and clinical care. J Emotional Abuse 8(3):335–354, 2008

National Center for Health Statistics: Summary Health Statistics for the U.S. Population: National Health Interview Survey, 2012. Atlanta, GA, Centers for Disease Control and Prevention, 2013. Available at: http://www.cdc.gov/nchs/data/series/sr_10/sr10_259.pdf. Accessed June 25, 2023.

Neilson S: Ableism in the medical profession. CMAJ 192(15):E411–E412, 2020 32392505

Okoro CA, Hollis ND, Cyrus AC, et al: Prevalence of disabilities and health care access by disability status and type among adults — United States, 2016. MMWR Morb Mortal Weekly Rep 67(32):882–887, 2018

Oliver M: The individual and social models of disability. Paper presented at Joint Workshop of the Living Options Group and the Research Unit of the Royal College of Physicians, London, July 23, 1990. Available at: https://disability-studies.leeds.ac.uk/wp-content/uploads/sites/40/library/Oliver-in-soc-dis.pdf. Accessed June 25, 2023.

Olson KR, Durwood L, DeMeules M, McLaughlin KA: Mental health of transgender children who are supported in their identities. Pediatrics 137(3):e20153223, 2016 26921285

Poteat T, German D, Kerrigan D: Managing uncertainty: a grounded theory of stigma in transgender health care encounters. Soc Sci Med 84:22–29, 2013 23517700

Pyne J, Bauer G, Redman N, Travers R: Improving the health of trans communities: findings from the Trans PULSE Project. Conference plenary for the Trans Health Advocacy Summit, London, ON, Canada, 2012. Available at: https://transpulseproject.ca/research/improving-the-health-of-trans-communities-findings-from-the-trans-pulse-project/. Accessed June 25, 2023.

Richmond KA, Burnes T, Carroll K: Lost in trans-lation: interpreting systems of trauma for transgender clients. Traumatology 18(1):45–57, 2012

Riggs DW, Pearce R, Pfeffer CA, et al: Transnormativity in the psy disciplines: constructing pathology in the Diagnostic and Statistical Manual of Mental Disorders and standards of care. Am Psychol 74(8):912–924, 2019 31697127

Roberts TK, Fantz CR: Barriers to quality health care for the transgender population. Clin Biochem 47(10-11):983–987, 2014

Roller CG, Sedlak C, Draucker CB: Navigating the system: how transgender individuals engage in health care services. J Nursing Scholarsh 47(5):417–424, 2015

Slater J, Liddiard K: Why disability studies scholars must challenge transmisogyny and transphobia. Can J Disability Stud 7(2):83–93, 2018

Smart J: Disability Across the Developmental Life Span: For the Rehabilitation Counselor. New York, Springer, 2011

Spade D: Solidarity not charity. Soc Text 38(1):131–151, 2020

U.S. Census Bureau: 2015 American Community Survey 1-Year Estimates: Disability Characteristics. Washington, DC, U.S. Census Bureau, 2015. Available at: https://www2.census.gov/programs-surveys/acs/tech_docs/table_shells/2015/S1810.xlsx. Accessed [date].

Ustün TB, Chatterji S, Bickenbach J, et al: The International Classification of Functioning, Disability and Health: a new tool for understanding disability and health. Disabil Rehabil 25(11-12):565–571, 2003 12959329

CHAPTER 10

Caring for Displaced People

Mental Health Concerns for TNG Individuals

Hannah Janeway, M.D.
Valeria Karina Anaya, M.D.

TRANSGENDER, non-binary, and/or gender-expansive (TNG) migrants face persecution and are marginalized by intersecting oppressive forces in their communities of origin, during their forced migration, and at their destination. Structural and infrastructural violence, perpetuated by capitalism, neoliberalism, imperialism, racism, cisgenderism, and heterocentrism, create their international displacement and migration. In this chapter, we provide background for health professionals about the specific mental health needs of displaced TNG individuals.

Case Example: Genesis

Genesis (she/her) is a 38-year-old transgender woman from El Salvador. She presents in your clinic seeking treatment for insomnia. She was recently granted humanitarian parole to seek treatment in the United States for her psychological issues while she awaits her asylum hearing. She reports that she comes from a small town in El Salvador, which she left at 14 years old after witnessing her father physically abuse her mother. Her family is ashamed of her and wants her to marry a woman to "try it out."

Ever since Genesis was little, people would try to humiliate her for being gay. "But I did not care," she says. "I am what I am—why pretend to be anything else?" She became a sex worker. She states proudly that she was able to earn enough money to start her own small store. Eventually she was able to purchase a home in El Salvador. Although she was discriminated against constantly, it was not until gang members started to extort her business that her life was threatened. Neighbors and an ex-boyfriend warned her that gang members were lying in wait and helped her to escape. In Mexico, she was no safer. The police would stop her when she dressed in alignment with her gender identity. Genesis was kicked out of her apartment when her landlord saw her dressed "like I am," she says. "He took my rent money and threw my clothes on the street. I was raped by a gang of men that night on the street. It was the lowest I ever felt in my life."

Genesis says she knows that trans women don't usually reach even 35 years old, so she is very concerned about maintaining her health. Since arriving in the United States, she has not been able to sleep because of nightmares. She struggles to trust people and experiences intense mood swings, from anger to profound sadness for what she has gained and lost. She is frustrated by intrusive memories of past experiences and reports shortness of breath, heart racing, chest pressure, and feeling paralyzed when these memories come up.

STRUCTURAL FORCES OF DISPLACEMENT

According to the United Nations High Commissioner for Refugees (2022), 89.3 million individuals were forcibly displaced worldwide in 2020, an increase of 6.9 million people over 2019.

Individuals are displaced and then migrate for a variety of different reasons, including persecution related to gender or sexuality, racism, xenophobia, political affiliation, economic devastation, climate changes, civil war, and cartel violence. International literature on migration has generally divided displaced individuals into groups based roughly on the 1951 Geneva Convention (United Nations High Commissioner for Refugees 1951). These groups include asylum seekers, refugees, stateless individuals, internally displaced individuals, and economic migrants. These designations, however, are dangerous to displaced individuals and to the health care providers who treat them, as they erase the complex political, economic, and social histories that intersect to create forced migration. They instead divide migrants from one another, perilously deeming some individuals as "worthy" of migration while ignoring the upstream intersectional forces of oppression that cause all individuals to migrate. For instance, Genesis in the case example was displaced for a number of reasons, including economic pressure, gender and sexuality discrimination, and cartel-based violence. Behind each of these structural forces are economic and political histories that intersect and feed off one another.

A nuanced understanding of the structural and infrastructural violence that produces migration is essential, as it changes the ways in which clinicians see patients and their journeys. Borders are manifestations of the power of citizenship, and they uphold the inequities that create structural and infrastructural determinants of health. From a human rights perspective, clinicians must see borders for what they are: artificial lines drawn through, by, and in support of those in power. As noted by Dubal et al. (2021, p. 4): "whereas many current approaches to border health tend to individualize and depoliticize illness through a humanitarian approach to the suffering of poor people of color, it is only by paying careful attention to the underlying and ongoing histories beyond the surface that we can begin to properly construct effective treatment."

As clinicians, we must approach displaced peoples, including TNG migrants, as individuals deserving of the freedom to move, the freedom to stay, and the freedom to return. In fact, individuals in the world's global north have inequitably been bestowed with these freedoms through citizenship, borders, and militarization. Mental health professionals should see advocacy for these essential freedoms as part of their work to decrease the structural and infrastructural determinants of mental health that oppress patients and create poor health outcomes.

As evidenced in Genesis's story, the web of structural forces that create oppression and migration are frequently intersectional for TNG communities. For instance, although it is easy to place blame for Genesis's trauma and migration on the Salvadoran patriarchy or cisgenderism in Latin America, neither of these forces appeared on their own. Rather, the clinician must remember that systemic oppression arises in the context of "intersecting forms of violence—including racism, capitalism, and colonialism"—while still acknowledging the effects of sexism and cisgenderism on daily life (Dubal et al. 2021, p. 4). This approach allows the practitioner to provide mental health services through a non-oppressive lens that does not "other" the societies from which migrants come. It also highlights the reality that underlying forms of violence are still at play in the final destination of the displaced individual, whether that be the United States, Europe, or elsewhere. These forces follow individuals and continue to oppress them, determining their access to care and their ability to heal from trauma once they arrive at their destination (Dubal et al. 2021).

TNG MIGRANTS AND IMMIGRANTS

Forced migration is a risk factor for poor mental health outcomes. Migrants experience trauma pre-flight, in transit, and upon arrival at their destination, and they lack access to basic needs for survival, including housing and health care services. They face frequent detention and must live with great uncertainty about the asylum process and their future (Hynie 2018; Ryan et al. 2009; von Werthern et al. 2018). Migrants who are lesbian, gay, bisexual, transgender, queer, intersex, asexual, and more (LGBTQIA+) have even higher rates of mental distress than their non-LGBTQIA+ counterparts. A systematic review by Hermaszewska et al. (2022, p. 8) illustrates how the intersection of pervasive violence, discrimination, exclusion, and unmet needs creates "extreme deprivation and suffering, with serious consequences for mental health pre-migration and post-migration" (Alessi et al. 2016, 2021).

Pre-flight Trauma

bell hooks, the late intersectional feminist, wrote: "in an ideal world, we would all learn in childhood to love ourselves. We would grow, being secure in our worth and value, spreading love wherever we went, letting our light shine" (hooks 2000, p. 67–68). Instead, adverse childhood experiences interrupt the trajectory of self-worth and value development, especially for those living TNG experiences. TNG individuals are at increased risk for abuse and rejection from their family of origin and peers, and they often experience neglect, abuse, and household dysfunction (Schnarrs et al. 2019). These factors have an additive detrimental effect on adult physical and mental health, leading to increased levels of depression, anxiety, and suicidality compared with LGB or cisgender populations (Felitti et al. 1998; Schnarrs et al. 2019).

Beyond childhood, multiple studies of TNG people have documented pervasive and persistent violence and persecution by family members, community members, and government officials, as well as systematic social and economic exclusion—including exclusion from health care services (Alessi et al. 2021; Hermaszewska et al. 2022; Kattari et al. 2017). At the time of writing, 66 countries still criminalize LGBT people (Human Dignity Trust 2023). Many discriminatory laws that originated during early colonial times continue to endanger TNG individuals, whose sexual orientation is automatically classified as homosexual by cisheteronormative patriarchal standards. In 2021, at least 375 TNG people worldwide were murdered, 70% in Central and South America, the majority of whom were Black (Alessi et al. 2021). A meta-analysis of qualitative research of LGBTQIA+ forced migrants' experiences with violence and abuse highlighted experiences of sexual violence, conversion therapy, forced marriage, and "corrective rape" (Alessi et al. 2016; Cheney et al. 2017). People were more likely to experience abuse at a younger age if they exhibited traits of gender nonconformity (Cheney et al. 2017; Gowin et al. 2017). Given these data, the lack of legal protections for TNG individuals compounds any other reasons for flight.

Dangers and Trauma During Transit

All migrants are vulnerable during transit from the country of origin to their destination. Migrants experience abuse, extortion, imprisonment, kidnapping, sexual assault, and torture after leaving their homes. Many travel in caravans as a way to reduce these risks, but TNG individuals may be excluded from the basic protections these caravans generally provide, owing to persisting cisnormativity in the caravans themselves. TNG individuals have a harder time concealing their identity than LGB individuals and thus are more exposed to physical and sexual violence (Alessi et al. 2021). Several studies have shown that TNG Latinx migrants are more likely than their cisgender counterparts to experience sexual and psychological violence and to participate in sex work (Leyva-Flores et al. 2016, 2019).

TNG individuals are often excluded from services offered to cisgender asylum seekers and refugees at different points along the journey and at borders. Most medical services provided to these individuals along their journey do not include gender-affirming medical or psychiatric services (even though those benefits can be lifesaving). In addition, "emergency response tools such as camps, temporary shelters, sanitation facilities and supplies, centralized aid distribution areas, information points, and health centers may not be sensitive to their particular needs," which include gender-inclusive bathrooms and security (Roeder et al. 2014, p. 33). Lastly, TNG individuals are further socially marginalized and placed at risk by the lack of organizations to help navigate the complicated journey and asylum process. Broken promises of safety and inadequate training for providers create alienation from government and nongovernment organizations that can have "noted lasting effects on the patient's ability to form relationships and seek help," notes Messih (2016, p. 6). "This is especially troubling given that patients who access community resources and group activity have better outcomes than patients in isolation." In addition, at least one study has shown that TNG asylum seekers who entered the United States without legal status had deep distrust and fear of people in authority and thus did not seek help from organizations that could provide resources to help apply for asylum (Cheney et al. 2017; Hopkinson et al. 2017). These experiences also can be humiliating and harmful for the individual, increasing the sense of physical insecurity and psychological distress (Rumbach and Knight 2014). TNG migrants evaluated before entering their destination country reported very high scores for PTSD and active suicidal ideation, with as many as 72.1% reporting past or current suicidal ideation (Mollica et al. 1993).

Around the world, many TNG migrants end up in detention facilities while their asylum claims are being adjudicated (Hopkinson et al. 2017). Incarceration is inherently traumatic and contradictory to principles of mental health for all, and it can be particularly detrimental to TNG individuals. Within immigration detention facilities, TNG individuals become marginalized, are forced to endure gender-based abuses, and are subject to increased discrimination and violence by detention center personnel and fellow detainees. According to the American Civil Liberties Union, 20% of confirmed sexual abuse cases in the custody of U.S. Immigration and Customs Enforcement involve a transgender detainee (Nakamura and Skinta 2020). Known TNG asylum seekers in the

United States also face an average of 99 days in custody before being released, which is more than double the average time for cisgender individuals (Oztaskin 2019; Smoley 2020). In the absence of sound policies surrounding TNG detainees, many are placed into gender-segregated facilities based on their sex assigned at birth or into "administrative segregation," which amounts to long periods of isolation. Both scenarios increase physical and psychological harm and worsen underlying mental health issues including depression, anxiety, and PTSD. The mental health consequences of detention are augmented by lack of appropriate medical care or gender-affirmation services (McCauley and Brinkley-Rubinstein 2017). Suggestions by immigrant rights advocates for alternatives to incarceration have been largely ignored.

TNG Asylum and Refugee Claims Process

Although overlapping and intersecting structural forces drive migration, current international laws have guidelines for who should be legally recognized as an asylum seeker or refugee. Clinicians are often asked to categorize individuals for forensic evaluation or to define conditions for the purpose of granting refugee or asylum status. We believe strongly that these distinctions are fundamentally flawed, as noted earlier, but the definitions are still useful to know and understand for patient advocacy purposes.

Per Amnesty International and other large organizations that look to the 1951 Geneva Convention, a refugee is a person "who has fled their own country because they are at risk of serious human rights violations and persecution there" and whose "own government cannot or will not protect them from those dangers" (Amnesty International 2022). Specifically, the persecution must be secondary to race, religion, nationality, membership in a particular social group, or political orientation (United Nations High Commissioner for Refugees 2022). An asylum seeker is similar to a refugee but has not yet been legally recognized as such. Individuals who are outside of the United States can apply for refugee status, usually through the U.N. High Commission for Refugees.

International guidelines and individual case law, including the Yogyakarta Principles and the updated Istanbul Protocol, have established TNG identities as meeting the criteria for asylum. Canada became the first Western country to grant asylum to LGBTQIA+ individuals in 1992; 2 years later, the United States recognized LGBTQIA+ individuals as part of a particular "social group" and therefore meeting one of the crucial criteria for asylum. Despite these advances, the assessment used to explore TNG claims for asylum is often problematic. In the United Kingdom, for instance, the interviewers are asked to "explore what the applicant is claiming to be their current gender identity and establish the range of behavior and activities of life that inform or affect the individual's gender identity, or how they are perceived" (Bach

2013, p. 35). In this way, a standard has been set to define what it means to be and behave in a way that is "legitimately transgender." This promotes the idea that to be transgender, the individual must be in some phase of "transition" as perceived by society. In contrast, transgender theory establishes gender identity as internal to the individual and not reliant on any particular changes to the body itself (Vogler 2019). For this reason, those identifying as non-binary or genderqueer also face difficulties in the asylum process.

TNG migrants are in a particularly difficult situation in relation to the asylum process. Many may not feel comfortable disclosing their identity early in their claims process because of safety concerns during interrogation or confinement; others may not even identify as TNG owing to internalized shame or cultural understandings of their own gender identity or sexuality.

Unfortunately, hiding gender identity during part of the asylum process can later be used against TNG people in court, as a way to deny asylum claims (Eckstrand and Potter 2017). "In transgender individuals, proof of identity is problematic [citation removed], as some may have transitioned and/or no longer identify as the gender listed on accepted forms of identification" (Messih 2016, p. 6).

Most importantly, many individuals who have fled persecution secondary to their gender identity have had little to no assistance in their own process of gender affirmation. Organizations that serve displaced individuals at points of border entry or in refugee camps should provide gender-affirmation services as part of their emergency medical care, as has been modeled by Refugee Health Alliance. Many TNG individuals who enter the United States without legal status are unaware that they can apply for asylum or that they have 1 year to do so after entering (longer if they can prove extenuating circumstances) (Cheney et al. 2017). Organizations such as the Transgender Law Center, Immigration Equality, Immigrant Legal Resource Center, The Queer Detainee Empowerment Project, and Rainbow Railroad assist TNG migrants with immigration law and resettlement resources. Clinicians can refer patients to these or other local LGBTQIA+ organizations for legal assistance.

Cultural Bereavement and Acculturation

Cultural bereavement was described by Eisenbruch (1991) as an experience resulting from loss of social roles, social networks, identity, and values when migrants are obligated to acculturate or assimilate in their host country. Of note, Eisenbruch sought to distinguish these experiences from Western interpretation of traumatic distress or PTSD. From his work with Cambodian refugees, Eisenbruch identified a culturally bereaved person as living in the past, being visited by supernatural forces when asleep or awake, and experiencing feelings of guilt or anger. Of note, cultural bereavement will differ based on geographical and cultural context.

Not mentioned by Eisenbruch, however, is how loss of homeland is experienced alongside the psychological trauma of witnessing or experiencing violence during forced migration and relocation (Tippens et al. 2021). There is a dearth of research documenting the experiences of TNG migrants as they acculturate and their particular experiences of cultural bereavement. We can extrapolate that the loss of social roles may have already taken place during any period of family rejection; conversely, migrants may be able to gain access to a more expansive LGBTQIA+ community on the journey.

The trajectory through cultural bereavement may be affected by the receiving country's levels of xenophobia, racism, ageism, homophobia, and cisgenderism. Bhugra et al. (2011) described how cultural bereavement may also be minimized if a migrant is able to maintain ties to the culture of origin through increased ethnic density, improved social support, or maintenance of religious beliefs and practices. Particularly for TNG migrants, the social networks of their homeland were more likely to be a chosen family (as birth families are often perpetrators of abuse), and their ability to retain exposure to cultural norms through ethnic communities in the host country is not a given (Shidlo and Ahola 2013). It is not uncommon for LGBTQIA+ migrants to meet and find each other, forming their own enclave during travel or in a new host community. These bonds are delicate, however, and can trigger additional psychological distress when challenged by within-group cultural and language differences, fluctuating economic situations, changing asylum status, and racism.

Acculturation is the "process through which immigrants acquire the beliefs, values, and behaviors of a host country, while either preserving or modifying those of their host country of origin" (Fuks et al. 2018, p. 298). In the United States, the attitude toward immigrants often obliges assimilation or replacement of cultural values with those of the host country (Jeter 2007). But the reality is, avoiding acculturation may have economic consequences (Fuks et al. 2018). For TNG migrants, their cultural identity, sexual orientation, or gender identity dynamically intersect and inform each other during the acculturation process. For example, strongly identifying culturally with one's homeland may result in a struggle to recognize or accept one's sexual orientation or gender identity (internally); before migration, this is likely reinforced through stigmatization and state-sanctioned violence or discrimination. Once in a new host country, TNG migrants may gravitate toward the validation of their sexual orientation or gender identity, which in turn means distancing themselves from their cultural identity. The TNG migrant may continue to examine and discard any internalized stigma, and continue to distance themselves culturally from their country of origin, until they feel secure in their identity and, ideally, reintegrate the positive aspects of their culture into it.

Many TNG migrants face significant social barriers to care and overall wellness during their journey and upon arrival at their destination. Studies have shown that social determinants of health are a determining factor in mental health outcomes in the forced migrant population (Hynie 2018). TNG migrants often lack familial or social support from communities of origin that other migrants may have on arrival, increasing their material and social exclusion. For instance, in the case example, Genesis frequently found herself unhoused during her journey and upon arrival to the United States. Shelter provides relative safety and helps reinforce a sense of self, belonging, and community. Daily struggles to eat, bathe, and use the toilet become all-consuming, further affecting the person's ability to thrive. When housing is insecure, patients still seek routine, certainty, and space for belonging. However, the difficulty of maintaining that belonging exacerbates underlying mental illness or precipitates new episodes of mental illness.

MENTAL HEALTH RECOMMENDATIONS

As mental health providers, we have a significant amount of power and privilege that can be used or even sacrificed to promote the well-being of our patients. The work of practicing empathy requires rigorous self-interrogation of the differences in power and privilege between ourselves and our TNG forced migrant patients. A radical interrogation is required of Western conceptualizations of PTSD and sexual orientation and gender identities, as well as the disempowerment that these may represent to those who must conform. Ultimately, we can embody safety and acceptance for our patients, take note of avoidance and self-preservation patterns, interpret mental health symptoms, and advocate for our patients by learning how to write asylum evaluations or humanitarian parole letters and advocating against policies that reinforce borders and barriers to movement.

As providers, we can take note that TNG forced migrants take on risk every day and use strategies to protect themselves. These strategies might prevent them from connecting with others, hindering their own social integration and well-being in their new host country.

Resettlement may be especially difficult for TNG forced migrants as they struggle with socioeconomic loss, limited knowledge of language and customs, or lack of work skills. Of particular relevance to TNG asylum seekers, *minority stress theory* (Abreu et al. 2021; Frost and Meyer 2023) specifies the challenges of identity concealment and the protective function of LGBTQIA+ community connectedness (Frost and Meyer 2012) and social support (Hatzenbuehler 2009) related to sexual and gender minority mental health. The World Health Organization (20192019) states that gender is one of the core social determinants of inequalities in health and recognizes that "transphobia and discrimination are major barriers to healthcare access.... Legal gender recognition, represented through documents reflecting a person's gender identity, is important for protection, dignity and health" (WHO 2019, p. 2–3). Mental health providers can facilitate a sense of safety if they practice empathy and self-interrogate their own power and privilege. As trained clinicians, we can provide psychiatric services but also recognize that connecting our TNG forced migrant patients with access to legal assistance, housing, food, and gender-affirming care has just as much of an impact on their health as traditional health services.

Long-term experiences with rejection and invalidation can lead TNG forced migrants to expect rejection. Mental health providers may note that TNG forced migrants avoid their own ethnic community, as perpetrators of violence and abuse were often family, community members, and government officials. TNG forced migrant patients may also avoid religion and faith-based communities (Kahn et al. 2017). Although reactions vary geographically, religious contexts may magnify feelings of internalized homophobia or cisgenderism that can trigger internalizing mental health symptoms such as depression and anxiety. The patient's level of connection to their faith-based community may depend on whether they hide their gender identity or sexual identity (Kahn et al. 2017). If patients have been forced to hide their TNG identities, they may still have significant social connection and support but also may seek additional support from LGBTQIA+ communities. Mental health providers may wish to use creative outreach strategies to promote a sense of connection and community. For example, a mainstream health care organization may consider offering group therapy for migrants who might not feel safe to affiliate with LGBTQIA+ community organizations. Efforts to provide group experiences tend to ease the resettlement stressors for TNG forced migrants, giving them opportunities to network, socially integrate, and form alternative surrogate kinship structures (Hwahng et al. 2019). Online community support or experiences may also be beneficial. Community-led intervention and peer support from other TNG forced migrants can broaden coping capacity, knowledge, and access to vital resources such as hormones (Hermaszewska et al. 2022). Evidence supports the efficacy of peer support in protecting against poor mental health outcomes for transgender people (Bockting et al. 2013).

As mental health clinicians, we can learn how to perform forensic asylum evaluations, which are interviews that differ little from our normally extensive and thorough medical history-taking (Janeway et al. 2022). Forensic evaluations have been found to almost double the chance that someone will be granted asylum (Atkinson et al. 2021), and as previously discussed, obtaining asylum status is associated with decreased mental distress. Adjudicators do expect sequential accounts of persecution, however. This is complicated: trauma is often cumulative and may not present neatly as defined by traditional Western conceptual frameworks. The early traumatic events of TNG forced migrants have the potential to influence core aspects of themselves, their ability to make sense of the world, and their ability to regulate emotion, cope with stress, and seek safety. There is a policy expectation for the TNG migrant to "prove themselves" as having gender incongruence, but the nuanced realities of TNG individuals' identities may not be what adjudicators expect (Eckstrand and Potter 2017). It may be helpful to document shifts over time in broader aspects of gender identity, such as internal processes of self-discovery (e.g., hiding gender nonconforming behaviors, navigating fears of disappointing families of origin). It is important to educate others that the coming out process may have been slowed or altered in the migrant's country of origin, as they may have had limited relationships with gender-expansive people or may have been in a marriage with children. TNG individuals may experience significant shifts in identity even before they begin the asylum application process, and such shifts in identity can be considered normative in this context (e.g., believing they are lesbian or gay but later expressing that they are transgender) (Shidlo and Ahola 2013).

CONCLUSION

Many forced migrant TNG individuals suffer from significant mental health consequences as a result of a lifetime of cumulative trauma. Common diagnoses include recurrent depression, dissociative disorders, panic disorder, generalized anxiety disorder, social anxiety, traumatic brain injury, and substance use disorders. It is important to note that these are interpretations of mental health symptom clusters that are viewed through a lens rooted in ableism and white supremacy. The concepts of gender identity that we clinicians seek in the narratives of TNG forced migrants are also rooted in white supremacy, which seeks to define nontraditional gender identities as "other" and as requiring a coming-out process of disclosure and announcement that has repeatedly proven dangerous to psychological and physical existence. Furthermore, the claims process has the potential to worsen psychological symptoms and negatively impact well-being, as TNG migrants are repeatedly asked to develop a consistent persecution narrative and "perform" their gender identity through the lens of white supremacist ideologies. Through critical self-reflection and understanding the structural and infrastructural violence that creates migration, mental health providers have an opportunity to act in solidarity with their patients. This includes (but goes beyond) simple patient treatment and advocacy confined to healing the downstream effects of structural violence.

This knowledge should move mental health providers to actively engage in work that takes aim at the upstream causes of health inequity, including capitalism, colonialism, imperialism, white supremacy, and cisgenderism, which created borders and continue to reinforce their existence.

REFERENCES

Abreu RL, Gonzalez KA, Capielo Rosario C, et al: "What American dream is this?": the effect of Trump's presidency on immigrant Latinx transgender people. J Couns Psychol 68(6):657–669, 2021 34180690

Alessi EJ, Kahn S, Chatterji S: "The darkest times of my life": recollections of child abuse among forced migrants persecuted because of their sexual orientation and gender identity. Child Abuse Negl 51:93–105, 2016 26615778

Alessi EJ, Cheung S, Kahn S, Yu M: A scoping review of the experiences of violence and abuse among sexual and gender minority migrants across the migration trajectory. Trauma Violence Abuse 22(5):1339–1355, 2021 34812109

Amnesty International: Refugees, asylum seekers and migrants, in What We Do. London, Amnesty International, 2022. Available at: https://www.amnesty.org/en/what-we-do/refugees-asylum-seekers-and-migrants/. Accessed August 28, 2022.

Atkinson HG, Wyka K, Hampton K, et al: Impact of forensic medical evaluations on immigration relief grant rates and correlates of outcomes in the United States. J Forensic Leg Med 84:102272, 2021 34743036

Bach J: Assessing transgender asylum claims. Forced Migr Rev 42:34–35, 2013

Bhugra D, Gupta S, Bhui K, et al: WPA guidance on mental health and mental health care in migrants. World Psychiatry 10(1):2–10, 2011 21379345

Bockting WO, Miner MH, Swinburne Romine RE, et al: Stigma, mental health, and resilience in an online sample of the US transgender population. Am J Public Health 103(5):943–951, 2013 23488522

Cheney MK, Gowin MJ, Taylor EL, et al: Living outside the gender box in Mexico: testimony of transgender Mexican asylum seekers. Am J Public Health 107(10):1646–1652, 2017 28817317

Dubal SB, Samra SS, Janeway HH: Beyond border health: infrastructural violence and the health of border abolition. Soc Sci Med 279:113967, 2021

Eckstrand KL, Potter J (eds): Trauma, Resilience, and Health Promotion in LGBT Patients: What Every Healthcare Provider Should Know. Cham, Switzerland, Springer International, 2017

Eisenbruch M: From post-traumatic stress disorder to cultural bereavement: diagnosis of Southeast Asian refugees. Soc Sci Med 33(6):673–680, 1991

Felitti VJ, Anda RF, Nordenberg D, et al: Relationship of childhood abuse and household dysfunction to many of the leading causes of death in adults. The Adverse Childhood Experiences (ACE) Study. Am J Prev Med 14(4):245–258, 1998 9635069

Frost DM, Meyer IH: Measuring community connectedness among diverse sexual minority populations. J Sex Res 49(1):36–49, 2012 21512945

Frost DM, Meyer IH: Minority stress theory: application, critique, and continued relevance. Curr Opin Psychol 51:101579, 2023

Fuks N, Smith NG, Peláez S, et al: Acculturation experiences among lesbian, gay, bisexual, and transgender immigrants in Canada. Couns Psychol 46(3):296–332, 2018

Gowin M, Taylor EL, Dunnington J, et al: Needs of a silent minority: Mexican transgender asylum seekers. Health Promot Pract 18(3):332–340, 2017 28187690

Hatzenbuehler ML: How does sexual minority stigma "get under the skin"? A psychological mediation framework. Psychol Bull 135(5):707–730, 2009 19702379

Hermaszewska S, Sweeney A, Camminga B, et al: Lived experiences of transgender forced migrants and their mental health outcomes: systematic review and meta-ethnography. BJPsych Open 8(3):e91, 2022 35535515

hooks b. All About Love: New Visions. New York, William Morrow, 2000

Hopkinson RA, Keatley E, Glaeser E, et al: Persecution experiences and mental health of LGBT asylum seekers. J Homosex 64(12):1650–1666, 2017 27831853

Human Dignity Trust: Map of criminalisation. 2023. Available at: https://www.human dignitytrust.org/lgbt-the-law/map-of-criminalisation/. Accessed June 15, 2023.

Hwahng SJ, Allen B, Zadoretzky C, et al: Alternative kinship structures, resilience and social support among immigrant trans Latinas in the USA. Cult Health Sex 21(1):1–15, 2019 29658825

Hynie M: The social determinants of refugee mental health in the post-migration context: a critical review. Can J Psychiatry 63(5):297–303, 2018 29202665

Janeway H, Anaya K, Ahola J, et al: Module 9: Sexual orientation, gender identity, and asylum: Evaluating LGBTQIA+ asylum seekers. In Asylum Medicine Training Initiative: Asylum Medicine Introductory Curriculum. Edited by Emery E, DeFries T. Panopto, 2022. Available at: https://pro.panopto.com/Panopto/Pages/Viewer.aspx?tid=4c878e34-047c-4592-8215-aeda013256d5. Accessed July 17, 2023.

Jeter A: Assimilation versus acculturation. Blog entry, 2007. Available at: http://archiejeter.blogspot.com/2007/08/assimilation-versus-acculturation.html. Accessed July 17, 2023.

Kahn S, Alessi E, Woolner L, et al: Promoting the wellbeing of lesbian, gay, bisexual and transgender forced migrants in Canada: providers' perspectives. Cult Health Sex 19(10):1165–1179, 2017 28322629

Kattari SK, Walls NE, Whitfield DL, Langenderfer Magruder L: Racial and ethnic differences in experiences of discrimination in accessing social services among transgender/gender-nonconforming people. J Ethn Cult Divers Soc Work 26(3):217–235, 2017

Leyva-Flores R, Infante C, Servan-Mori E, et al: HIV prevalence among Central American migrants in transit through Mexico to the USA, 2009–2013. J Immigr Minority Health 18:1482–1488, 2016

Leyva-Flores R, Infante C, Gutierrez JP, et al: Migrants in transit through Mexico to the US: experiences with violence and related factors, 2009–2015. PLoS One 14(8):e0220775, 2019 31433820

McCauley E, Brinkley-Rubinstein L: Institutionalization and incarceration of LGBT individuals. In Trauma, Resilience, and Health Promotion in LGBT Patients: What Every Healthcare Provider Should Know. Cham, Switzerland, Springer, 2017, pp. 149–161

Messih M: Mental health in LGBT refugee populations. Am J Psychiatry Resid J 11(7):5–7, 2016

Mollica RF, Donelan K, Tor S, et al: The effect of trauma and confinement on functional health and mental health status of Cambodians living in Thailand-Cambodia border camps. JAMA 270(5):581–586, 1993

Nakamura N, Skinta M: LGBTQ Asylum Seekers: How Clinicians Can Help. Washington, DC, American Psychological Association, 2020

Oztaskin M: The harrowing, two-year detention of a transgender asylum seeker. The New Yorker, October 31, 2019. Available at: https://www.newyorker.com/news/dispatch/the-harrowing-two-year-detention-of-a-transgender-asylum-seeker. Accessed June 24, 2023.

Pega F, Veale JF: The case for the World Health Organization's Commission on Social Determinants of Health to address gender identity. Am J Public Health 105(3):e58–e62, 2015 25602894

Roeder LW, Rumbach J, Knight K: Issues of Gender and Sexual Orientation in Humanitarian Emergencies: Risks and Risk Reduction. Cham, Switzerland, Springer International, 2014

Rumbach J, Knight K: Sexual and gender minorities in humanitarian emergencies. In Issues of gender and sexual orientation in humanitarian emergencies: Risks and Risk Reduction. Cham, Switzerland, Springer International, 2014, pp. 33–74

Ryan DA, Kelly FE, Kelly BD: Mental health among persons awaiting an asylum outcome in Western countries: a literature review. Int J Ment Health 38(3):88–111, 2009

Schnarrs PW, Stone AL, Salcido R Jr, et al: Differences in adverse childhood experiences (ACEs) and quality of physical and mental health between transgender and cisgender sexual minorities. J Psychiatr Res 119:1–6, 2019 31518909

Shidlo A, Ahola J: Mental health challenges of LGBT forced migrants. Forced Migr Rev 42:9–11, 2013

Smoley M: The detention of trans asylum seekers in the U.S. InReach, September 11, 2020. Available at: https://inreach.org/detention-trans-asylum-seekers-usa/. Accessed June 24, 2023.

Tippens JA, Roselius K, Padasas I, et al: Cultural bereavement and resilience in refugee resettlement: a photovoice study with Yazidi women in the Midwest United States. Qual Health Res 31(8):1486–1503, 2021 33884945

United Nations High Commissioner for Refugees: Global Trends, 2022. Available at: https://www.unhcr.org/globaltrends.html. Accessed September 26, 2022.

United Nations High Commissioner for Refugees: Convention and Protocol Relating to the Status of Refugees, 1951. Available at: https://www.unhcr.org/3b66c2aa10.html. Accessed March 6, 2023.

Vogler S: Determining transgender: adjudicating gender identity in U.S. asylum law. Gender Soc 33(3):439–462, 2019

von Werthern M, Robjant K, Chui Z, et al: The impact of immigration detention on mental health: a systematic review. BMC Psychiatry 18(1):382, 2018 30522460

World Health Organization: Transgender health in the context of ICD-11. Regional Office for Europe, WHO, 2019. Available at: https://www.ichatten.no/WHO%20europa%20om%20IOCD%2011.pdf. Accessed November 23, 2011.

CHAPTER 11

Trauma-Informed Mental Health Care With Transgender, Non-binary, and/or Gender-Expansive (TNG) Communities

Sebastian M. Barr, Ph.D.
Gene Dockery, Ph.D.
Jaimie Cory, M.Ed.
Jae Sevelius, Ph.D.

> "I believe that healing from gendered trauma lives in the spaces
> between us…. If we can start to notice the wound
> [of gendered trauma], engage with it critically,
> start to clean it up within and between ourselves,
> we can start to plant seeds for another world of possibilities."
>
> —*Alex Iantaffi, Gender Trauma: Healing Cultural, Social,
> and Historical Gendered Trauma (Iantaffi 2020, p. 202)*

TRAUMA-INFORMED MENTAL HEALTH CARE WITH TNG COMMUNITIES

TNG people experience trauma in ways that impact their mental health and shape how they seek and engage in mental health care. Given the ubiquity of trauma and traumatic stress in TNG communities, clinicians require an affirming, trauma-informed approach to be truly competent in their work with TNG clients. Here, we first describe how trauma affects TNG communities, then discuss models of trauma-informed care and their integration into mental health care delivery. As much of the trauma TNG people face is oppression-related, we also briefly identify ways in which clinicians can and should engage in advocacy. We conclude by reflecting on the potential effects of engaging in this work for clinicians—particularly TNG clinicians—including vicarious traumatization.

TRAUMA IN TNG COMMUNITIES

Psychological Distress and Traumatic Stress

TNG people are more likely than cisgender peers to experience psychological distress (Wanta et al. 2019). Members of TNG communities have increased odds of receiving a psychiatric diagnosis, including PTSD, mood disorders, anxiety disorders, and psychotic spectrum disorders (Barr et al. 2021, 2022; Wanta et al. 2019). Although some diagnoses are attributable to clinician bias and misattribution of symptoms and experiences that stem from gender dysphoria (Barr et al. 2021), psychological suffering in TNG communities is a real concern. The gender *minority stress model* (Testa et al. 2017; see Chapter 2, "Stigma and Mental Health Inequities"), which has been supported by a robust and growing body of evidence (e.g., Valentine and Shipherd 2018), demonstrates that the risk of psychological distress faced by TNG people is explained by a convergence of oppression- and marginalization-related factors, as well as gender dysphoria (Lindley and Galupo 2020).

In addition to high prevalence rates of psychiatric diagnoses, the intersection of vulnerabilities among TNG populations (e.g., insecure attachment and high rates of suicidality, dissociation, anxiety symptoms, depressive symptoms, and hypervigilance) (Giovanardi et al. 2018; Hanna et al. 2019; Kuper et al. 2019; Surace et al. 2021) with aspects of complex PTSD presentations (Briere and Spinazzola 2005) has led numerous scholars to use a trauma framework for conceptualizing the psychological impacts of being a TNG person in today's society (Barr et al. 2022; Richmond et al. 2012). A trauma framework contextualizes these various health disparities and frames TNG mental health within the reality of gender minority stress, elucidating the relationships between oppression- and marginalization-related minority stressors and negative mental health outcomes in TNG communities (Dockery and McLuckie 2021; Levenson et al. 2023). In other words, the overall picture of mental health risk in TNG communities may be most accurately and robustly described thus: TNG people face high rates of traumatization and complex PTSD. At the time of writing, there are no known studies looking at complex PTSD as an outcome, but recent studies have documented a 44% prevalence of current clinically significant PTSD symptoms (DSM-5-TR; American Psychiatric Association 2022) in TNG-identified samples (Barr et al. 2022; Reisner et al. 2016), compared with an estimated 8% lifetime prevalence of PTSD in the general U.S. population (Kilpatrick et al. 2013).

Victimization and Trauma Exposure

TNG people face notably high rates of violence, such as physical assault and harassment, sexual assault, domestic abuse, and childhood abuse, among other traumatic events that satisfy Criterion A of the PTSD diagnosis (Barr et al. 2022; James et al. 2016; Shipherd et al. 2011). The risk is even greater for TNG people who face marginalization related to multiple identities (e.g., racism for TNG people of color and Indigenous or Two-Spirit people)—particularly TNG women of color (James et al. 2016)—and for TNG people who have more expansive gender expressions (Shipherd et al. 2011). This increased risk of victimization is due in part to anti-TNG hatred, as well as the marginalization and oppression that place TNG people at greater risk of poverty, homelessness, and dependence on work in underground economies, all of which increase the risk of victimization and other trauma (Valentine and Shipherd 2018).

Further, exposure to violence does not need to be direct and personal to have traumatic impact. Research has implicated social media exposure, specifically, in collective trauma and vicarious traumatization of marginalized communities (Pickles 2020; Zhang et al. 2021). Although social media often serves as a valuable source of support and information (Cannon et al. 2017; Selkie et al. 2020), it is often used to share stories of violence against TNG and LGBTQ+ communities (Pickles 2020). Thus, a TNG person who has not directly experienced this type of trauma may develop traumatic stress due to awareness of and exposure to community trauma.

Anti-TNG Bias and Non-affirmation as Insidious/Complex Trauma

Along with traditionally defined traumas (i.e., Criterion A–qualifying traumas), it is important to consider the trauma of encountering interpersonal and systemic bias (Richmond et al. 2012). The Substance Abuse and Mental Health Services Administration (2014) defines trauma more expansively than DSM-5-TR: "an event, series of events, or set of circumstances that is experienced by an individual as physically or emotionally harmful or life threatening and that has lasting adverse effects on the individual's functioning and mental, physical, social, emotional, or spiritual well-being" (p. 7).

By adopting a wider definition of trauma than that found in DSM, mental health clinicians and researchers have elucidated nuances of complex trauma (Cloitre 2020; Karatzias et al. 2020), unique features of racial trauma including gendered racism (Abdullah et al. 2021; Comas-Díaz et al. 2019; Helms et al. 2010), and historical and community trauma (Hartmann et al. 2019). Similarly, TNG mental health scholars have demonstrated that experiences of anti-TNG bias (harassment, discrimination, and violence) as well as non-affirmation of a person's gender identity (e.g., frequent misgendering) predict severity of posttraumatic stress, even after controlling for traditional trauma exposure (Barr et al. 2022; Reisner et al. 2016). Given that these sources of potential traumatization in TNG lives can be insidious and diffuse, trauma among TNG people may be untraceable to a singular event (Stanley 2021). As such, conceptualizations of trauma or traumatic stress that require individuals to identify singular, discrete experiences of harm fail to capture the full extent of the trauma faced by TNG people.

Medical Care and Mental Health Care as Sources of Trauma

Clinicians must recognize that medical and mental health care institutions and clinicians often inflict trauma on TNG people. TNG people have been denied life-improving or lifesaving care through outright discrimination and barriers to accessing gender-affirming care (e.g., lack of insurance coverage, mandated mental health evaluations) (James et al. 2016; MacKinnon et al. 2020). Denial of care constitutes a threat to physical and psychological safety and can be experienced as traumatic. Further, health care spaces routinely fail to affirm the identities and bodies of TNG people (Cicero et al. 2019), particularly of those multiply marginalized by medical and mental health institutions (e.g., people of color with racism, people in larger bodies with fatphobia). For example, TNG people report experiencing misgendering, negative comments about their bodies or identities, clinicians who center their sex assigned at birth in a manner that induces or heightens dysphoria, pathologization (e.g., being treated as crazy or deviant), and outright harassment (Cicero et al. 2019; Heng et al. 2018; Hines et al. 2019). This occurs interpersonally (e.g., by clinicians and staff) and systemically (e.g., in medical charts, institutional policies) (Ram et al. 2022). Non-affirmation in medical settings can cause severe harm. In a sample of TNG adults, negative interactions with health care clinicians were associated with worsened mental health (Kattari et al. 2019). In a report on TNG health care experiences, a participant described the pain of being repeatedly misgendered while in the hospital as worse than the pain of the appendicitis that sent them there (James et al. 2016).

Another aspect of health care trauma sequelae is the experience of being triggered by health care spaces, clinicians, and other memory cues and associations. Because of this, TNG people often report heightened levels of physiological distress and emotional dysregulation when having to interface with health care staff and systems (Cicero et al. 2019; Heng et al. 2018). TNG people often avoid medical and mental health care in terms of both prevention and treatment (Lerner and Robles 2017). This avoidance is an adaptive protective response (i.e., avoiding a source of dangerous harm) as well as an aspect of posttraumatic stress (i.e., generalizing the avoidance of appropriate fear-based stimuli to more diffuse avoidance). Regardless of the adaptive versus maladaptive nature of the avoidance, this reduced help-seeking contributes to health disparities in TNG communities (James et al. 2016).

DEFINING TRAUMA-INFORMED CARE

Because TNG people are likely to experience trauma, interdisciplinary affirmative care must adopt trauma-informed care to reduce harm to TNG individuals and communities (Rafferty 2021). The National Center for Trauma-Informed Care defines *trauma-informed care* as a strengths-based approach rooted in understanding and responding to the impact of trauma that emphasizes physical, psychological, and emotional safety for clinicians and survivors to create opportunities for empowerment (Marsac et al. 2016). Being trauma-informed is not merely a practice protocol, but rather a holistic way of thinking and engaging with clients that requires the clinician to comprehend the nature and neurobiology of trauma while also seeing the entire person, not just a victim (Bent-Goodley 2019).

Six Guiding Principles of Trauma-Informed Care

CDC guidance on trauma-informed care includes six principles: a) safety; b) trustworthiness and transparency; c) peer support; d) collaboration and mutuality; e) empowerment, voice, and choice; and f) cultural, historical, and gender issues (Centers for Disease Control and Prevention 2020). The first principle, *safety*, is the anchor of trauma-informed care (Bent-Goodley 2019). TNG clients report that safety includes a nonthreatening environment, gender-inclusive bathrooms, and actions from the clinician that demonstrate their commitment to addressing barriers for TNG people (Hall and DeLaney 2021). *Trustworthiness and transparency*, the second principle, involves creating predictable and nonjudgmental spaces (Bent-Goodley 2019) to remove access barriers. For TNG clients, this includes validating their identities, being well informed on TNG health, and providing consistency (Hall and DeLaney 2021). The third principle, *peer support*, builds community that furthers the process of healing (Bent-Goodley 2019); this may include facilitating therapy groups for TNG individuals.

Collaboration and mutuality, the next principle, focuses on working in partnership with the client and giving them power in the therapeutic relationship (Bent-Goodley 2019). In this vein, TNG clients noted that they felt heard when their feedback was used to shape interventions and their expertise was respected by clinicians (Hall and DeLaney 2021). This leads directly to the fifth principle, *empowerment, voice, and choice*, which means providing support, encouragement, and strategies for self-empowerment (Bent-Goodley 2019). Empowering TNG individuals in the therapeutic process includes assisting them in accessing medical gender affirmation, providing transition support, and supporting the development of self-advocacy skills (Hall and DeLaney 2021). *Cultural, historical, and gender issues*, the final principle, is about being culturally responsive by addressing systemic challenges, discrimination, community trauma, and historical trauma (Bent-Goodley 2019). This includes understanding and acknowledging the intersectional identities of TNG clients and disrupting and changing established hegemonic norms.

Four Rs of Trauma-Informed Care

The Substance Abuse and Mental Health Services Administration (2014) developed a framework for implementing components of trauma-informed care, identified as the *four Rs*, which should be established systemwide: realization of the possibility that any individual may present with a trauma history, recognition of the signs and symptoms of trauma, responding effectively to signs and symptoms of trauma by implementing trauma-informed care at all levels of care and trauma-focused care as appropriate, and resisting retraumatization of all clients and staff.

The first of the principles, *realization* of the possibility of trauma, includes an awareness of the diversity of experiences that can be traumatizing, as well as understanding that clients' behavior and presenting concerns can be related to ongoing or historical trauma. In many instances, identified mental health disorders or other forms of emotional distress may be exacerbated or even caused by events that are identified by the client as traumatizing (Substance Abuse and Mental Health Services Administration 2014). This is true even if clients do not meet full diagnostic criteria for PTSD; for marginalized clients, many sources of insidious trauma may be involved. The second principle, *recognition* of the signs and symptoms of trauma, requires knowledge of the variety of clinical presentations clients may have in response to traumatic events. Some common responses include reexperiencing (which includes intrusive memories and trauma responses to trigger cues), avoiding internal and external reminders of the trauma, and altering arousal (e.g., hypervigilance, dissociation), as well as affect dysregulation, negative self-concept, and disturbances in interpersonal relationships (World Health Organization 2018). The third principle, *responding* to signs and symptoms of trauma, is most effective if used by all staff who have been trained in methods of anticipating potential sources of perceived threat and methods of fostering an environment of physical and emotional safety. The fourth principle, *resisting retraumatization*, involves attentiveness to the ways in which clients with trauma histories are likely to encounter triggers of their traumatic histories by the very nature of engaging in mental health care (Substance Abuse and Mental Health Services Administration 2014). To prevent retraumatization, systems must avoid any unnecessary circumstances that nontherapeutically contribute to trauma responses and help clients prepare for those triggers and mitigate the impact.

APPLYING A TRAUMA-INFORMED LENS TO TNG MENTAL HEALTH CARE

In addition to in-depth understanding of the principles of trauma-informed care generally, we recommend clinicians seek thorough training in the unique experiences and needs of TNG communities, with special attention paid to multiply marginalized TNG people (e.g., Black and Indigenous TNG people and all TNG people of color; disabled, neurodivergent, and older TNG people), whose stories and needs are often decentered in psychiatric and psychological literature and who are likely to face diverse sources of trauma (Cyrus 2017; Singh 2017) (see Chapters 5, 11, and 14).

Importance of Affirmation to Reduce Retraumatization and Establish Safety

In psychiatric settings, retraumatization and lack of safety often manifest for TNG clients as repeated non-affirmation and bias (White and Fontenot 2019). Clinicians often perpetuate overt cisgenderism, invalidation and non-affirmation, pathologization of identity, and insensitivity to intersectionality (Snow et al. 2019). Being a trauma-informed system means clinical spaces (including digital spaces such as websites and client portals) need to be free of bias, inclusive of diversity, and affirming of clients' genders and intersecting identities. Efforts to reduce bias and cultivate affirmation must be intentional and holistic, inclusive of all staff and spaces that potential clients will encounter (Hall and DeLaney 2021). See Chapter 24, "Gender-Affirming Health Care Environments," for a thorough review of best practices for creating inclusive and affirming mental health care spaces.

Some aspects of psychiatric assessment and treatment, although necessary, still function as triggers and require a harm reduction approach. For example, electronic health record (EHR) systems overemphasize assigned sex and legal name, and hospital systems and insurance companies often require psychiatric diagnoses that include outdated language (e.g., gender identity disorder) for billing purposes or access to gender-affirming care (Ram et al. 2022). Clinicians can incorporate the principles of transparency, collaboration, and empowerment to reduce the impact of triggers and sources of retraumatization. Importantly, clinicians should engage in advocacy efforts to make treatment settings and processes safer and less likely to retraumatize clients (see later section Advocacy and Community Engagement). In particular, readiness and referral letters for gender-affirming medical care can be sources of retraumatization. To offset the non-affirmation inherent in the letter-writing arrangement, clinicians should be explicit in their affirmation of the client's gender and self-understanding of gender affirmation needs (see Chapter 21, "Psychiatric Evaluations in Support of Gender-Affirming Surgery," on letter writing). In taking a trauma-informed approach to letter writing, clinicians should strive to collaborate and document, rather than assess or evaluate. Clients should review the letter, and the clinician should make any requested changes in a timely manner. We support the pledge of the Gender Affirming Letter Access Project (2023) and join their call for clinicians to offer letter writing in a minimal number of sessions (as few as one, with telehealth options) at no cost.

Treatment Relationship Considerations

People who have experienced interpersonal trauma often develop interpersonal styles that protect them from future harm (Muller 2009; Van Nieuwenhove and Meganck 2020). This may be particularly true for TNG clients in health care contexts, given the medical or psychiatric trauma TNG people experience and the cissexism of medical institutions (Ansara 2012; Puckett et al. 2021). Individuals who face intersecting forces of oppression in health care (e.g., TNG people of color; TNG people with larger bodies) may be particularly likely to use protective interaction styles in client-clinician relationships, even more so when clinicians are cisgender.

When entering therapeutic or clinical relationships, TNG clients are likely to be guarded (withholding of information they experience as vulnerable) or vigilant (watchful for errors; sensitive to potential bias/non-affirmation). They may disengage from treatment relationships (dissociate or become less emotionally present; be late or absent for sessions; withdraw from treatment entirely) more readily than others following a misstep or failure of empathy by the clinician. Alternatively, clients may adopt an overly accommodating or "people-pleasing" interpersonal style and avoid transparency and conflict. It is important to recognize that these patterned behaviors may be adaptive trauma responses and to understand that they may or may not be conscious or intentional on the client's part. Understanding these nuances can help clinicians avoid acting on challenging countertransference reactions to the client, such as feeling frustrated, hopeless, or even hostile (Dalenberg 2004; Wilson and Lindy 1994) (see Chapter 12, "How Cis?").

By providing a relational experience that is consistent, warm, striving toward understanding, free of retaliation, and validating, clinicians provide the necessary foundation of relational safety (Briere and Scott 2015). The therapeutic relationship can also be a source of healing, trauma recovery, and growth (Herman 2015). For example, clients with relational trauma histories (including non-affirmation and bias) who engage defensively do so out of self-protective instincts based on beliefs that others (or health care staff specifically) are unsafe. Allowing them to experience this fear while simultaneously perceiving the clinician as trustworthy, steady, and affirming can be corrective through what Briere and Scott (2015) describe as counterconditioning. The safety experienced in a treatment relationship can, over time, modify a patient's belief that all people (or all clinicians) are unsafe. Thus individuals with relational traumatic stress may be able to engage in future interpersonal encounters with more openness and flexibility and increase their capacity for meaningful relationships with others.

Diagnostic Considerations

Misdiagnosis is a serious concern when working with TNG clients, as gender dysphoria and traumatization may present in a way similar to symptoms of unrelated diagnoses (Barr et al. 2022; Goldhammer et al. 2019). Although research on psychiatric practice demonstrates that psychotherapy and psychopharmacologic treatment planning should be dictated by transdiagnostic factors (e.g., reactance/resistance, culture, preference, spirituality) (see Norcross and Wampold 2011 for review), there are some differential diagnoses that significantly affect treatment approach, particularly when trauma or oppression-related factors are understood to be a source of the presenting symptomatology (e.g., Brown 2004; Comas-Díaz 2016). Additionally, diagnostic or formulation accuracy is critically important for TNG clients, because psychiatric diagnoses and perceived distress or dysfunction can be used as a barrier for needed gender affirmation and gender-affirming medical care (MacKinnon et al. 2020).

Assessment/Identification of Trauma History

Fundamental to the task of accurately conceptualizing the sources of a client's presenting distress/symptomology is assessment and identification of past sources of trauma. Clinical guidance for gender-affirming care has repeatedly called for thorough evaluation of trauma, including systemic violence and other forms of bias and non-affirmation in addition to the more traditionally assessed traumas (e.g., American Psychological Association 2015; Richmond et al. 2012). As noted earlier, insidious trauma may not be internalized by clients as discrete events. Additionally, TNG clients may enter into health care relationships defended against vulnerability or with a heightened level of physiological arousal and emotional dysregulation. Therefore, it may be ineffective or harmful to directly inquire about trauma histories and other experiences of oppression and non-affirmation, particularly in early sessions. Assessment and history-gathering should be considered an ongoing process that involves a combination of attunement to what the client brings in and direct inquiry from the clinician over time. Additionally, the task of trauma history-gathering (explicit or implicit) should include attention to experiences of invalidation, non-affirmation, bias, and other interpersonal and systemic sources of oppression-based trauma.

When exploration of trauma history is tolerable to the client, it may be validating to have a mental health clinician recognizing the potential impact of the client's past and present challenges as a TNG person, and it can be empowering to help the client give voice to what they have survived and continue to survive (Pantalone et al. 2017; Singh and McKleroy 2011).

Treatment Planning Considerations

Psychoeducation about trauma and gender minority stress can be transformative for TNG people seeking mental health care (Austin and Craig 2015; Budge et al. 2021). Clinicians should be knowledgeable enough to explain (in lay terms) trauma and traumatic stress, the gender minority stress model (see Chapter 2, "Stigma and Mental Health Inequities"), and the ways in which anti-TNG bias, non-affirmation, and intersecting oppression-based stress (e.g., racial trauma) can cause or exacerbate traumatic stress for clients. Helping clients conceptualize their experiences through a trauma or gender minority stress framework may be grounding and can help introduce clients to the tasks of therapeutic work.

Although this chapter discusses trauma-informed care and not trauma-focused care (which explicitly addresses traumatic experiences and targets trauma-related symptoms), clinicians can borrow from principles of trauma-focused care in planning treatment for clients who are carrying a high trauma burden. The *tripartite* or *triphasic* model of trauma therapy proposed by Dr. Judith Herman (2015) offers a helpful transtheoretical approach to therapeutic work with traumatized individuals. The three phases are broadly categorized as stabilization and the establishment of a sense of safety; remembrance or processing; and reconnection or reintegration, although progression through the phases is not necessarily linear. We recommend that clinicians consider adapting treatments to fit this model (see discussion in Barr et al. 2022 for expanded application of the tripartite model in work with members of TNG communities).

Advocacy and Community Engagement

Mental health clinician advocacy is a critical component of trauma-informed care and should address power asymmetry; protect and enforce human rights; and foster social justice through empowerment (Newbigging and Ridley 2018). Indeed, without advocacy, clinicians are endorsing the silence, violence, and injustice that have contributed to clients' traumatic stress (Marshall-Lee et al. 2019). Effective advocacy requires working with those receiving or needing care and integrating their input into the design and implementation of these efforts (Elliott et al. 2005). Failure to do so can result in advocacy that is unethical and paternalistic (American Counseling Association 2018; Newbigging and Ridley 2018), reinforces existing power structures, and harms clients and communities (Stylianos and Kehyayan 2012).

Many of the experiences that traumatize TNG people are structural, continued, and persistent, so trauma-informed advocacy is needed to ensure TNG communities' well-being. *Trauma-informed advocacy* works to reduce experiences of trauma and retraumatization and can occur on multiple levels. On an individual level, it can include connecting the individual with medical providers who will not misgender, deadname, or dehumanize them. Examples of community-level advocacy are public awareness campaigns in schools or community events to reduce stigma around TNG identities. Policy-level advocacy includes providers taking an active role in drafting public policy, advocating, and decision-making (Marshall-Lee et al. 2019).

Impact on Clinician: Secondary Traumatization and Triggered Responses

Finally, clinicians and systems working to implement effective trauma-informed care also must consider how such work may impact clinicians themselves. Clinicians who work with clients with a history of trauma may develop secondary traumatic stress: emotional duress resulting from vicarious exposure to trauma. Mental health clinicians are at increased risk of secondary traumatic stress because of the prolonged and often intimate and emotionally intense exposure to clients' stories of trauma (Chrestman 1995). TNG clinicians, especially those with shared or similar experiences of trauma, may be particularly affected (Cory 2021), but no one is immune to being greatly impacted by this work.

Signs of *secondary traumatization* include symptoms of posttraumatic stress (hypervigilance, avoidance, reexperiencing or intrusive thoughts and memories, and change in mood). Survivor's guilt, anger, and some relational or countertransference emotions are also signs of secondary traumatization, as are cognitive impairment, exhaustion, and compassion fatigue—difficulty holding empathy and warmth for others (Figley 1995, 2002; Pryce et al. 2007). Thus, in addition to being distressing for the clinician, secondary traumatic stress can reduce the ability to be an effective and caring provider. Secondary trauma has also been linked to experiences of burnout, but research suggests that systemic and organizational factors, such as workload, perceived institutional support, work-life balance, and lack of bias, are most important in burnout prevention (Bell and Kulkarni 2003).

To prevent and manage secondary traumatic stress at the individual level, clinicians should cultivate awareness of their reactions to clients and their stories, as well as early signs of secondary traumatization (Marsac and Ragsdale 2020). Professional supervision can be effective in preventing and reducing secondary trauma (Joubert et al. 2013). For TNG clinicians, we recommend seeking out TNG-identified supervisors or group supervision spaces with other TNG providers when possible. Additionally, clinicians should resist the urge to avoid the thoughts and feelings they are having (Osofsky et al. 2008). Two non-avoidant ways of sitting with secondary trauma and related feelings are mindfulness practices and constructive reflection (Harrison and Westwood 2009), which can happen in supervision or through the clinician's own therapy; also helpful are expressive formats such as writing and art (Cory 2021).

Mental health care organizations and systems are ultimately responsible for preventing secondary traumatization. In addition to creating space for clinicians to engage in the individual strategies above (such as by providing effective professional supervision, allowing protected time for peer supervision, and accommodating employees' regular psychotherapy), work should be dedicated to minimizing the following well-established organizational contributors to secondary traumatization: large caseloads, caseloads with majority traumatized clients (particularly those with a history of interpersonal violence), lack of trauma training, and unsupportive work environments and cultures (Sutton et al. 2022).

REFERENCES

Abdullah T, Graham-LoPresti JR, Tahirkheli NN, et al: Microaggressions and post-traumatic stress disorder symptom scores among Black Americans: exploring the link. Traumatology 20:1–10, 2021

American Counseling Association: American Counseling Association Advocacy Competencies. Alexandria, VA, American Counseling Association, 2018. Available at: https://www.counseling.org/docs/default-source/competencies/aca-advocacy-competencies-updated-may-2020.pdf?sfvrsn=f410212c_4. Accessed October 25, 2021.

American Psychiatric Association: Diagnostic and Statistical Manual of Mental Disorders, 5th Edition, Text Revision. Washington, DC, American Psychiatric Association, 2022

American Psychological Association: Guidelines for psychological practice with transgender and gender nonconforming people. Am Psychol 70(9):832–864, 2015 26653312

Ansara YG: Cisgenderism in medical settings: challenging structural violence through collaborative partnerships, in Out of the Ordinary: Representations of LGBT Lives. Edited by Rivers I, Ward R. Newcastle Upon Tyne, UK, Cambridge Scholars Publishing, 2012, pp 93–111

Austin A, Craig SL: Transgender affirmative cognitive behavioral therapy: clinical considerations and applications. Prof Psychol Res Pr 46(1):21, 2015

Barr SM, Roberts D, Thakkar LN: Psychosis in transgender individuals: a review of the literature and a call for more research. Psychiatry Res 306:114272, 2021 34808496

Barr SM, Snyder KE, Adelson J, Budge SL: Posttraumatic stress in the trans community: the roles of anti-transgender bias, non-affirmation, and internalized transphobia. Psychol Sex Orientat Gend Divers 9(4):410–421, 2022

Bell H, Kulkarni S, Dalton L: Organizational prevention of vicarious trauma. Fam Soc 84:463–470, 2003

Bent-Goodley TB: The necessity of trauma-informed practice in contemporary social work. Soc Work 64(1):5–8, 2019 30428068

Briere J, Scott C: Complex trauma in adolescents and adults: effects and treatment. Psychiatr Clin 38(3):515–527, 2015

Briere J, Spinazzola J: Phenomenology and psychological assessment of complex posttraumatic states. J Trauma Stress 18(5):401–412, 2005 16281238

Brown LS: Feminist paradigms of trauma treatment. Psychotherapy (Chic) 41(4):464–471, 2004

Budge SL, Sinnard MT, Hoyt WT: Longitudinal effects of psychotherapy with transgender and nonbinary clients: a randomized controlled pilot trial. Psychotherapy (Chic) 58(1):1–11, 2021 32567869

Cannon Y, Speedlin S, Avera J, et al: Transition, connection, disconnection, and social media: examining the digital lived experiences of transgender individuals. J LGBT Issues Couns 11(2):68–87, 2017

Centers for Disease Control and Prevention: Infographic: 6 guiding principles to a trauma-informed approach, in Center for Preparedness and Response: Communication Resources. Atlanta, GA, Centers for Disease Control and Prevention, 2020

Chrestman KR: Secondary exposure to trauma and self reported distress among therapists, in Secondary Traumatic Stress: Self-Care Issues for Clinicians, Researchers, and Educators. Edited by Stamm BH. Derwood, MD, The Sidran Press, 1995, pp 29–36

Cicero EC, Reisner SL, Silva SG, et al: Health care experiences of transgender adults: an integrated mixed research literature review. ANS Adv Nurs Sci 42(2):123–138, 2019 30839332

Cloitre M: ICD-11 complex post-traumatic stress disorder: simplifying diagnosis in trauma populations. Br J Psychiatry 216(3):129–131, 2020 32345416

Comas-Díaz L: Racial trauma recovery: a race-informed therapeutic approach to racial wounds, in The Cost of Racism for People of Color: Contextualizing Experiences of Discrimination. Edited by Alvarez AN, Liang C, Neville HA. Washington, DC, American Psychological Association, 2016, pp 249–272

Comas-Díaz L, Hall GN, Neville HA: Racial trauma: theory, research, and healing: introduction to the special issue. Am Psychol 74(1):1–5, 2019 30652895

Cory JS: Living trans trauma/treating trans trauma. Paper presented at Transgender Professional Association for Transgender Health, "Converging Crises: Transgender Health, Rights, and Activism (virtual, July 31 and August 1, 2021)

Cyrus K: Multiple minorities as multiply marginalized: applying the minority stress theory to LGBTQ people of color. J Gay Lesbian Ment Health 21(3):194–202, 2017

Dalenberg CJ: Maintaining the safe and effective therapeutic relationship in the context of distrust and anger: countertransference and complex trauma. Psychotherapy (Chic) 41(4):438, 2004

Dockery G, McLuckie A: From living in fear towards living queer: a workshop on trauma-informed queer space-making. Presented at the Kenyon Queer and Trans Studies Conference, virtual from Gambier, OH, April 9–11, 2021

Elliott DE, Bjelajac P, Fallot RD, et al: Trauma-informed or trauma-denied: principles and implementation of trauma-informed services for women. J Community Psychol 33(4):461–477, 2005

Figley C: Compassion Fatigue: Coping With Secondary Traumatic Stress Disorder in Those Who Treat the Traumatized. New York, Brunner-Routledge, 1995

Figley CR: Compassion fatigue: psychotherapists' chronic lack of self care. J Clin Psychol 58(11):1433–1441, 2002 12412153

Gender Affirming Letter Access Project. Sign the Pledge. Available at: https://thegalap.org/sign-the-pledge. Accessed July 17, 2023.

Giovanardi G, Vitelli R, Maggiora Vergano C, et al: Attachment patterns and complex trauma in a sample of adults diagnosed with gender dysphoria. Front Psychol 9:60, 2018 29449822

Goldhammer H, Crall C, Keuroghlian AS: Distinguishing and addressing gender minority stress and borderline personality symptoms. Harv Rev Psychiatry 27(5):317–325, 2019 31490187

Hall SF, DeLaney MJ: A trauma-informed exploration of the mental health and community support experiences of transgender and gender-expansive adults. J Homosex 68(8):1278–1297, 2021 31799893

Hanna B, Desai R, Parekh T, et al: Psychiatric disorders in the U.S. transgender population. Ann Epidemiol 39:1–7.e1, 2019 31679894

Harrison RL, Westwood MJ: Preventing vicarious traumatization of mental health therapists: identifying protective practices. Psychotherapy (Chic) 46(2):203–219, 2009 22122619

Hartmann WE, Wendt DC, Burrage RL, et al: American Indian historical trauma: anticolonial prescriptions for healing, resilience, and survivance. Am Psychol 74(1):6–19, 2019 30652896

Helms JE, Nicolas G, Green CE: Racism and ethnoviolence as trauma: enhancing professional training. Traumatology 16(4):53–62, 2010

Heng A, Heal C, Banks J, Preston R: Transgender peoples' experiences and perspectives about general healthcare: a systematic review Int J Transgend 19(4):1–20, 2018

Herman JL: Trauma and Recovery: The Aftermath of Violence—From Domestic Abuse to Political Terror. London, Hachette UK, 2015

Hines DD, Laury ER, Habermann B: They just don't get me: a qualitative analysis of transgender women's health care experiences and clinician interactions. J Assoc Nurses AIDS Care 30(5):e82–e95, 2019 31461741

Iantaffi A: Gender Trauma: Healing Cultural, Social, and Historical Gendered Trauma. Philadelphia, Jessica Kingsley Publishers, 2020

James SE, Herman JL, Rankin S, et al: The Report of the 2015 U.S. Transgender Survey. Washington, DC, National Center for Transgender Equality, 2016

Joubert L, Hocking A, Hampson R: Social work in oncology—managing vicarious trauma—the positive impact of professional supervision. Soc Work Health Care 52(2–3):296–310, 2013

Karatzias T, Shevlin M, Hyland P, et al: The network structure of ICD-11 complex post-traumatic stress disorder across different traumatic life events. World Psychiatry 19(3):400–401, 2020 32931094

Kattari S, Bakko M, Hecht H, Kattari L: Correlations between healthcare provider interactions and mental health among transgender and nonbinary adults. SSM Popul Health, 201931872041

Kilpatrick DG, Resnick HS, Milanak ME, et al: National estimates of exposure to traumatic events and PTSD prevalence using DSM-IV and DSM-5 criteria. J Trauma Stress 26(5):537–547, 2013 24151000

Kuper LE, Mathews S, Lau M: Baseline mental health and psychosocial functioning of transgender adolescents seeking gender-affirming hormone therapy. J Dev Behav Pediatr 40(8):589–596, 2019

Lerner J, Robles G: Perceived barriers and facilitators to health care utilization in the United States for transgender people: a review of recent literature. J Health Care Poor Underserved 28:127–152, 2017

Levenson JS, Craig SL, Austin A: Trauma-informed and affirmative mental health practices with LGBTQ+ clients. Psychol Serv 20(Suppl 1):134–144, 2023 33856846

Lindley L, Galupo MP: Gender dysphoria and minority stress: support for inclusion of gender dysphoria as a proximal stressor. Psychol Sex Orientat Gend Divers 7:265–275, 2020

MacKinnon KR, Grace D, Ng SL, et al: "I don't think they thought I was ready": how pre-transition assessments create care inequities for trans people with complex mental health in Canada. Int J Ment Health 49(1):56–80, 2020

Marsac M, Ragsdale L: Tips for recognizing, managing secondary traumatic stress in yourself. AAP News, May 21, 2020. Available at: https://publications.aap.org/aapnews/news/14395. Accessed October 14, 2021.

Marsac ML, Kassam-Adams N, Hildenbrand AK, et al: Implementing a trauma-informed approach in pediatric health care networks. JAMA Pediatr 170(1):70–77, 2016 26571032

Marshall-Lee ED, Hinger C, Popovic R, et al: Social justice advocacy in mental health services: consumer, community, training, and policy perspectives. Psychol Serv 17(Suppl 1):12–21, 2019 30998032

Muller RT: Trauma and dismissing (avoidant) attachment: intervention strategies in individual psychotherapy. Psychotherapy (Chic) 46(1):68–81, 2009 22122571

Newbigging K, Ridley J: Epistemic struggles: the role of advocacy in promoting epistemic justice and rights in mental health. Soc Sci Med 219:36–44, 2018 30359905

Norcross JC, Wampold BE: What works for whom: tailoring psychotherapy to the person. J Clin Psychol 67(2):127–132, 2011 21108312

Osofsky JD, Putnam FW, Lederman C: How to maintain emotional health when working with trauma. Juv Fam Court J 59(4):91–102, 2008

Pantalone DW, Valentine SE, Shipherd JC: Working with survivors of trauma in the sexual minority and transgender and gender nonconforming populations, in Handbook of Sexual Orientation and Gender Diversity in Counseling and Psychotherapy. Edited by DeBord KA, Fischer AR, Bieschke KJ, Perez RM. Washington, DC, American Psychological Association, 2017, pp 183–211

Pickles J: Sociality of hate: the transmission of victimization of LGBT+ people through social media. Int Rev Victimol 27(3):311–327, 2020

Pryce J, Shackelford K, Pryce D: Secondary Traumatic Stress and the Child Welfare Professional. Chicago, IL, Lyceum Books, 2007

Puckett JA, Aboussouan AB, Ralston AL, et al: Systems of cissexism and the daily production of stress for transgender and gender diverse people. Int J Transgend Health 24(1):113–126, 2021 36713141

Rafferty J: Childhood abuse among transgender youth: a trauma-informed approach. Pediatrics 148(2):e2021050216, 2021 34226248

Ram A, Kronk CA, Eleazer JR, et al: Transphobia, encoded: an examination of trans-specific terminology in SNOMED CT and ICD-10-CM. J Am Med Inform Assoc 29(2):404–410, 2022 34569604

Reisner SL, White Hughto JM, Gamarel KE, et al: Discriminatory experiences associated with posttraumatic stress disorder symptoms among transgender adults. J Couns Psychol 63(5):509–519, 2016 26866637

Richmond KA, Burnes T, Carroll K: Lost in trans-lation: interpreting systems of trauma for transgender clients. Traumatology 18(1):45–57, 2012

Selkie E, Adkins V, Masters E, et al: Transgender adolescents' uses of social media for social support. J Adolesc Health 66(3):275–280, 2020 31690534

Shipherd JC, Maguen S, Skidmore WC, Abramovitz SM: Potentially traumatic events in a transgender sample: frequency and associated symptoms. Traumatology 17(2):56–67, 2011

Singh AA: Understanding trauma and supporting resilience with LGBT people of color, in Trauma, Resilience, and Health Promotion in LGBT Patients. Edited by Eckstrand KL, Potter J. Cham, Switzerland, Springer, 2017, pp 113–119

Singh AA, McKleroy VS: "Just getting out of bed is a revolutionary act": the resilience of transgender people of color who have survived traumatic life events. Traumatology 17(2):34–44, 2011

Snow A, Cerel J, Loeffler DN, Flaherty C: Barriers to mental health care for transgender and gender-nonconforming adults: a systematic literature review. Health Soc Work 44(3):149–155, 2019 31359065

Stanley EA: Atmospheres of Violence: Structuring Antagonism and the Trans/Queer Ungovernable. Raleigh, NC, Duke University Press, 2021

Stylianos S, Kehyayan V: Advocacy: critical component in a comprehensive mental health system. Am J Orthopsychiatry 82(1):115–120, 2012 22239401

Substance Abuse and Mental Health Services Administration: SAMHSA's Concept of Trauma and Guidance for a Trauma-Informed Approach. Rockville, MD, Substance Abuse and Mental Health Services Administration, 2014. Available at: https://ncsacw.samhsa.gov/userfiles/files/SAMHSA_Trauma.pdf. Accessed October 14, 2021.

Surace T, Fusar-Poli L, Vozza L, et al: Lifetime prevalence of suicidal ideation and suicidal behaviors in gender non-conforming youths: a meta-analysis. Eur Child Adolesc Psychiatry 30(8):1147–1161, 2021 32170434

Sutton L, Rowe S, Hammerton G, Billings J: The contribution of organisational factors to vicarious trauma in mental health professionals: a systematic review and narrative synthesis. Eur J Psychotraumatol 13(1):2022278, 2022 35140879

Testa RJ, Michaels MS, Bliss W, et al: Suicidal ideation in transgender people: gender minority stress and interpersonal theory factors. J Abnorm Psychol 126(1):125–136, 2017 27831708

Valentine SE, Shipherd JC: A systematic review of social stress and mental health among transgender and gender non-conforming people in the United States. Clin Psychol Rev 66:24–38, 2018 29627104

Van Nieuwenhove K, Meganck R: Core interpersonal patterns in complex trauma and the process of change in psychodynamic therapy: a case comparison study. Front Psychol 11:122, 2020 32116927

Wanta JW, Niforatos JD, Durbak E, et al: Mental health diagnoses among transgender patients in the clinical setting: an all-payer electronic health record study. Transgend Health 4(1):313–315, 2019 31701012

White BP, Fontenot HB: Transgender and non-conforming persons' mental healthcare experiences: an integrative review. Arch Psychiatr Nurs 33(2):203–210, 2019

Wilson JP, Lindy JD: Empathic strain and countertransference, in Countertransference in the Treatment of PTSD. Edited by Wilson JP, Lindy JD. New York, Guilford, 1994, pp. 1–30

World Health Organization: International Classification of Diseases, 11th Revision. Geneva, World Health Organization, 2018

Zhang YT, Li RT, Sun XJ, et al: Social media exposure, psychological distress, emotion regulation, and depression during the COVID-19 outbreak in community samples in China. Front Psychiatry 12:644899, 2021 34054602

CHAPTER 12

How Cis?

Recognizing and Managing Transphobic Countertransference in Psychotherapy

Tobias Wiggins, Ph.D.

IN the past 10 years, we have witnessed dramatic shifts in the previously sanctioned pathologization of gender nonconformance in Western medicine. In turn, many Two-Spirit, transgender, non-binary, and gender expansive (2TNG)[1] people are newly seeking out the mental health care that they may have previously avoided to circumvent medical discrimination. Affirming scholars and clinicians have responded by developing clinical guides to help bolster inclusive, well-informed practices for psychotherapy.[2] These innovative educational efforts focus on establishing supportive environments, advancing culturally responsive care, dismantling long-standing systemic

---

[1] In this chapter, "trans" and "2TNG" are used as umbrella terms for all those who do not identify with the gender assigned to them at birth, such as those who are Two-Spirit, transgender, non-binary, gender fluid, agender, and genderqueer. "Gender nonconformance" is used when individuals may be perceived to be outside of societal gender norms yet may or may not identify with gender assigned at birth.

[2] In *A Clinician's Guide to Gender-Affirming Care*, Chang et al. (2018) provided a comprehensive overview of foundational knowledge for most therapeutic modalities, including dismantling cisgender normativity, respecting client self-determination, understanding trans historical contexts, honing diagnostic skills, and identifying challenges to effective treatment. Similarly, in *Counselling Skills for Working with Gender Diversity and Identity*, Beattie and Lenihan (2018) focused on counselor reflexivity and education in addressing identity, dysphoria, and self-care. Some texts have begun to address more precise issues, such as working with trans survivors of sexual violence (Rymer and Cartei 2019) and those with specific intersecting identities, such as trans and non-binary youth (Jones 2019) and autistic trans people (Gratton 2019). Others have gone beyond introductory topics, offering theories of gendered consciousness for the clinic that address issues of embodiment and trans subjectivity as natural variation (Langer 2019).

barriers, and expanding our understanding of gender's complex manifestations within psychotherapy. Yet many of these resources have overlooked the identification and management of what emerging scholarship has called *transphobic countertransference* (TCT), referring to the ways in which a clinician's unconscious prejudice can be felt, and potentially acted out, within the consulting room.

In his pivotal article "Unthinkable Anxieties: Reading Transphobic Countertransferences in a Century of Psychoanalytic Writing," trans psychoanalyst Griffin Hansbury (2017) first articulated some of the specific clinical anxieties that emerge when working with trans and gender nonconforming patients. His analysis hinged on the conviction that TCT is a form of psychotic prejudice, rooted in an earlier stage of development and thus "emanat[ing] from the analyst's primitive infantile anxieties" (Hansbury 2017, p. 387). A few clinicians have since built on Hansbury's framework, interrogating additional manifestations of TCT that do not fit neatly within the psychotic frame. For example, in "Are We Safe Analysts? Cisgender Countertransferential Fantasies in the Treatment of Transgender Patients," Porchat and Santos (2021) discerned several positive countertransferential impediments they had faced working with their 2TNG patients in psychotherapy. Rather than "experienc[ing] a transgender patient as a breakup of personal continuity, a disruption to their own experience of reality and embodiment" (Hansbury 2017, p. 388), these trans-affirming analysts found that it was their vigilant attempts to be "safe analysts"—that is, to not be transphobic—that led to premature, defensive responses that restricted a capacity for listening and space for the patient's idiosyncratic experiences.

In this chapter, I aim to synthesize and develop this burgeoning field of inquiry regarding the impacts of countertransference in clinical interactions between cisgender mental health practitioners and trans patients. Historically, the inquiring psychiatric gaze on gender nonconforming subjects was exclusively pathological: diagnosing 2TNG experience as perverse (Wiggins 2020), paraphilic, disordered, and dysphoric (Drescher 2014). With recent cultural shifts, however, trans people now participate in professional fields from which they were previously barred, a legitimization that is generating unprecedented inquiries and interventions.

The emergence of more 2TNG clinicians shifts the power dynamics of knowledge creation, providing insights far beyond the taxonomically repetitious psychiatrist's question, "Why are you trans?", to what Hansbury (2017) calls "How trans?" Put another way: "What are trans lives lived?" This query is especially pertinent considering many trans subjects, and in particular trans women of colour (Snorton and Haritaworn 2013), still encounter the realities of a necropolitical climate, which "subjugate[s]...life to the power of death" (Mbembe 2003, p. 39) through entrenched social conditions. This newly legitimized yet enduringly marginal perspective facilitates interrogation of the conditions under which such quotidian violence occurs, asking instead: "How cis?"

The question *how cis?* can be taken at face value (e.g., a consideration of what triggers common cisgender countertransferential enactments in psychotherapy). Equally, it can provide a comedic reversal meant to rattle the gate that preserves a disproportionate number of cisgender people in the mental health professions speaking for trans subjects.

Here I normalize two underdiscussed elements of clinical work with 2TNG populations: first, the undeniable presence of transphobia within the consulting room; and relatedly, the impact and uses of TCT in psychotherapy of any orientation. *Transphobia* is typically understood as any hostile, negative, and discriminatory attitude toward 2TNG people, including different types of violence and harassment (Ansara and Friedman 2016). Yet as Bettcher (2014) underscores, clear definitions of transphobia are stretched by its diverse and manifold iterations, which may be overt or covert and may be directed at gender nonconformance, but also, at trans people who do conform to binary gender norms. Like other forms of oppression, transphobia is an ever-evolving social phenomenon that is systemic, invisibilized, and a constitutive force. Therefore, the established tradition of routine yet cruel trans pathologization in psychiatry (Suess Schwend 2020), paired with clinicians' socialization in unconscious bias, will not simply dissolve if such discrimination becomes outmoded. In fact, expecting clinical approaches and views to change suddenly—with no close study of their genesis, no acknowledgment or reparation, and little to no trans-affirming education—leads to vast affective difficulties such as clinician confusion, anxiety, or shame.

Ultimately, this is a fertile ground for defenses that manifest in clinical countertransference. Theories of countertransference originated within psychoanalytic traditions (Stefana 2018) and have become common parlance within most modalities of Western psychology (American Psychological Association 2020; Fritscher 2021). Given its current household status and theoretically decontextualized usage, many of the principal tenets, controversies, and developments of clinical countertransference have been overlooked. Accordingly, here I trace the term's background to better substantiate its unique value in psychotherapy with 2TNG people. Fittingly, upon its identification, countertransference was both gendered and concealed. Since then, the utility of a clinician's feelings in reaction to a patient has been polarized, regarded by some as a therapeutic hindrance to be overcome and by others as one of the most valuable tools a therapist can employ.

Drawing from these contentions, clinical transphobia is framed here as an "unresolved issue" that gains utility only through its identification. Borrowing from Hansbury's (2017) foundation, I define *psychotic TCT* as a set of infantile affective distortions, and contribute two additional common forms of TCT to this conceptualization: *perverse TCT*, relating to the internalized law and omnipotence of diagnosis; and *neurotic TCT*, in which the clinician's previously held gendered meanings and social learning materialize. Ultimately, this investigation aims to help cisgender therapists better recognize their own distinct and heterogeneous reactions to 2TNG gender difference in the consulting room and, further, to curtail potential enactments. By normalizing otherwise disavowed transphobic affects, clinicians should be better able to creatively manage the therapeutic space to promote psychological growth and healing.

A BRIEF HISTORY OF COUNTERTRANSFERENCE

A tone of secrecy accompanied the birth of *countertransference*. Although Sigmund Freud coined the term, he did not provide much more than a cursory definition and words of caution. Its very first mention can be found in personal letters between Freud and his colleague Carl Jung in June 1909. Jung was seeking advice regarding a clandestine erotic transference with his then-patient Sabina Spielrein, who later became a pioneering woman psychoanalyst. In a sympathetic response, Freud stressed that "such experiences, though painful, are necessary and hard to avoid" and that "they help us to develop the thick skin we need and to dominate 'counter-transference,' which is after all a permanent problem for us" (McGuire 1974, pp. 230–231). It was almost a full year after this initial mention that the term *counter-transference* appeared publicly in Freud's address at the second International Psychoanalytic Congress in March 1910. His paper, which aimed to advance and expand the budding field, peripherally declares, "we have become aware of the 'counter-transference,' which arises in [the physician] as a result of the patient's influence on his[3] unconscious feelings." Freud emphasized the importance of a therapist's own self-analysis, because an analyst's countertransference neuroses and resistances would limit a successful clinical practice.

Despite its clear significance, a full article or lecture on countertransference never emerged from the founder of psychoanalysis. This absence is perhaps due to the professional risk presented by fully acknowledging what was considered a barrier to effective treatment (especially within the already-controversial occupation of listening to free-associations as remedy). Freud later wrote to Jung: "I believe an article on 'counter-transference' is sorely

---

[3] The use of he/him gender pronouns as default in original psychoanalytic texts reveals an entrenched legacy of sexism and binarism in psychoanalysis and psychiatry. They have been left intact so as not to obfuscate that heritage.

needed; of course, we could not publish it, we should have to circulate copies among ourselves" (McGuire 1974, p. 476).

Countertransference was conceived in close relationship to *transference love*, that is, a patient's feelings about a person in their past, most prominently a parent, being unconsciously directed toward the therapist (Freud 1910). For most psychoanalytic modalities, transference became a cornerstone of treatment, illuminating hidden parts of a patient's psychic life otherwise inaccessible to interpretation. From the so-called narrow perspective (Gabbard 2001), countertransference was accordingly conceptualized as the analyst's own transference to the patient, a result of the therapist's unmanaged neurosis. The sometimes sexual nature of the transference further cloaked therapists' countertransferential feelings in the taboo of unethical erotic attachment to a patient. Freud strictly maintained that countertransference must be mastered and overcome, which led succeeding clinicians to see it as an obstacle or hindrance to treatment (Stefana 2018).

Notably, in its initial iteration, countertransference was gendered through sexist enactments, which could also be considered countertransferential. During Freud's time, most patients were upper-class white women diagnosed with "hysteria," cast by patriarchal norms as dangerous "instinctual creatures who threatened the spiritual, orderly world of men" (Stefana 2018, p.11). Such concerns clearly biased male physicians' ethical boundaries and views of their women patients. The "domination" of a clinician's feelings for the patient reflected not only naturalized male power and the sexualization of women, but further, a gendered splitting between unruly women patients who were saturated in transference and the rational analytical men who could "displace affects" by developing a "thick skin" (McGuire 1974, pp. 230–231). In this way, clinicians unconsciously acted out some of their unresolved gendered issues—internalized sexist power structures and stereotypes—even within the coining of the term. The vulnerability of countertransference lay in what it exposed without sanction, potentially overthrowing the guarded veil of medical authority.

Most scholars consider the article by Paula Heimann (1950), "On Counter-transference," to be the primary turning point away from a classic view that saw countertransference as exclusively a source of trouble.[4] Heimann contended that the therapist's avoidance of all emotional reaction is actually a misreading of Freud; instead, the feelings that a patient stirs in the other "represent one of the most important tools for his work" (p. 81). Al-

---

[4] Although Heinmann's paper was able to shift therapeutic convention in the 1950s, other analysts had preempted her approach but had much less success in spreading their perspectives. Freud's contemporary, Sandor Ferenczi, for example, controversially favored relationality in treatment and the inevitability of countertransference—views that ultimately fractured his close relationship with Freud (McGuire 1974).

though unorthodox in this regard, Heimann stayed faithful to psychoanalytic tradition, maintaining that analysts should be fully analyzed to prevent their own issues from entering the clinic. While parts of the analyst's felt experience were no longer labeled an obstacle, those feelings should not belong to the "real person" of the therapist. Instead, the countertransference feelings must be analyzed as the patient's creation and therefore a potent window into the patient's unconscious. Heimann emphasized relationality but stressed that separation must be upheld given the therapist's function as a container for patients' affects. Their task should be to "*sustain* the feelings which are stirred... to *subordinate* them to the analytic task in which he functions as the patient's mirror reflection" (Heimann 1950, p. 82, emphasis in original).

This shift to considering the clinician's reactions as potentially generative sparked an elaboration of two opposing countertransference types: one that originates from the therapist's own unresolved issues and one that purely belongs to the patient as provoked in the therapist (Tarnopolsky 1995). Building on Heimann's relational interventions, a third cluster of perspectives then emerged that began to acknowledge the jointly created nature of countertransference (Aron 2009; Bion 1962; Ogden 1994). This intersubjective frame specified that the patient's influence on the therapist's feelings could not occur in isolation, as the analyst must also contribute their own internal world. Although the patient may incite a particular response, the specifics of that response would always be colored by the therapist's identity, experience, and personality (Gabbard 2001). This viewpoint moved the therapist further away from an objective stance, closer to subjectivity and an interaction between two psychic lives. Odgen (1994), for example, underscored that working with countertransference includes forming an *analytic third*, the intersubjective cocreation of shared feelings, thoughts, and fantasies.

To maintain an ethical stance, intersubjective approaches underscore mutuality while preserving asymmetry, meaning that the therapist and patient are connected but exist in different clinical locations (Zachrisson 2009). It is essential that the therapist, while remaining aware of their inner world, does not unthinkingly enact their own needs or unconscious conflicts, coopting the space meant for the patient's exploration and healing. The elements of heightened vulnerability in a relational psychotherapeutic context include entanglement of the dyad and true exposure of the "real person" of the therapist. The prospect that a clinician unintentionally confuses their own feelings for those of their patient is an ever-present risk and must be monitored (Gabbard 2001).

From Freud's classic view to diverse relational perspectives, disagreements in theories of countertransference have mostly surrounded questions of the therapist's and patient's affective contributions, as well as their subsequent utility. In sum, early models saw countertransference as a hindrance, made up completely of the analyst's neurosis; interventions in the 1950s acknowledged the force and benefit of the patient's affects; and interpersonal views have since provided mediation on various possibilities for the hybridity of therapeutic space. While seemingly disparate, all perspectives do agree that the countertransferential response will become problematic only if unconsciously acted out—wherein the therapist cannot successfully manage or account for their own personal issues and the provocations of their patient. The risk of enactment increases in a contemporary context that inadequately attends to the ubiquity of prejudice in psychotherapy and its assorted transferences and countertransferences. Unmanaged TCT is consequently more likely to emerge in such therapeutic settings, in which the clinician often has no more than a cursory understanding of trans life or legacies of medical gender pathologization, and perhaps more importantly, has not themselves undertaken a deep exploration of their own gendered history and its investments.

THREE TRANSPHOBIC COUNTERTRANSFERENCES

The normalization of a mental health professional's psychotic countertransference may seem like a groundless endeavor. Yet a psychoanalytic frame can dismantle diagnostic conventions that have supplied a narrow view of symptomatology as reserved for people with mental illness. *Psychotic TCT*, as proposed by Hansbury (2017), refers not to psychosis proper, but rather a set of affective experiences distorting reality that any clinician may have in the face of gender difference. Freud (1926) wrote extensively about *neurotic anxieties*, which, unlike realistic anxieties, arise from maladaptive trepidations evoked by the dangers of unconscious conflicts. For example, a neurotic anxiety might redundantly anticipate a trauma that occurred in the past. Hansbury argued that *psychotic anxiety* hearkens back to an even earlier, preverbal stage of development. He drew primarily from Winnicott's concept (1965) of "unthinkable anxieties" in childhood when the infant is in an absolute state of dependence on the caregiver. During this primordial and vulnerable time in development, the subject has not established agency of the body, a clear differentiation between self and other, or the capacity to use language. The result is a threatening sense that, without appropriate protection, they risk "going to pieces, falling for ever, having no relationship to the body... [or] orientation" (Winnicott 1965, p. 58). This everyday psychosis of natal aliveness follows us into adulthood and can be aroused with the appropriate disruptions; "given the right circumstances, we all can lose ourselves, however momentarily, in the swirl of infantile psychotic anxieties" (Hansbury 2017, pp. 387–388).

Analyzing a century of psychoanalytic writing, Hansbury showcased the recurrent portrayal of 2TNG people as rupturing reality and causing a fracture in the psychoanalyst's personal continuity. While clinicians easefully accorded psychosis to any patient presenting with unconventional gendered or sexed desires, they also inadvertently recorded their own symptoms of psychotic anxiety. Within published case studies, therapists recounted "a vague but constant distress sensation of uncomfortableness, incomprehension, and distress" (Torres 1996, p. 19) and "a nameless terror...feel[ing] the ground under me giving way" (Shapiro 1993, p. 372). One therapist wrote, "I was likely to get close to my own 'madness'" (Quinodoz 1998, p. 97). The fear of "going crazy" was amplified when conceding to believe or support 2TNG identities, even with minor acts such as correct pronoun use (Hansbury 2017, p. 391). In this way, clinicians behaved as if another's nonconformance threatened their own gender and bodily cohesion, an anxiety that was primarily contained through a fixation on etiology.

In contemporary psychotherapeutic settings, psychotic TCT can present as a persistent emotional dysregulation, a fixation on the cause of trans identity, the ascription of gender nonconformance to monstrosity, panic about gender-affirming surgery, the association of surgery with "mutilation," or an experience of the patient's gendered explorations as overly problematic and demanding. Although the focus of Hansbury's article is the clinician's unresolved issues, one could mindfully note—with a critical eye to the historical collapsing of transness with psychosis—that such breaks in continuity can also be cocreated. For example, a patient could internalize, project, and act out transphobic discourses about their own "madness"; transitioning or questioning gender can leave a trans person feeling undone, struggling with language, and corporeally disoriented. It is essential that therapists account for their contributions to psychotic TCT, as such disquieting intersubjective episodes are likely to be defensively assigned to patients.

Perversion is another symbolically loaded appellation; used diagnostically in early psychiatry practice, it has since been revoked as a professional anachronism (Downing 2015). Psychoanalysis certainly contributed to pejorative associations, but it also offered insights into the psychical function of perversion when freed from any stereotypical sexual behaviors and identities, such as homosexuality. For Freud (1938), *perverse defense* is a mechanism in which a subject uses a special object to help ignore an upsetting reality. The chosen object acts as a kind of screen, so that a difficult truth can be acknowledged but also overlooked. In this way, through disavowal, the perverse function allows one to say: "I know very well, but all the same" (Mannoni 1969). The mechanism can be effectively used by any subject in need of psychical protections and allows for certainty in the face of affective disruption. The repeatedly invoked object provides the comfort of sameness and a feeling of omnipotent knowledge when experiencing doubt.

Elsewhere, I have argued that DSM acts as such an object for clinicians who feel unsettled when treating gender nonconforming patients (Wiggins 2020). Precise and detailed criteria for gender disorders have been laid out since DSM-III (American Psychiatric Association 2008), where they were used to dictate the thresholds of 2TNG identity that, in turn, delineated access to hormones and surgeries (Lev 2006). Gender difference can be unfamiliar and disruptive of binary ideologies, and rigid diagnostic criteria can act as a legitimized salve, bringing order and structure to gender uncertainty.

Some clinicians recognize the limitations of medical models and seek only an instrumental approach to diagnosis. Meanwhile, 2TNG people have learned to ambivalently adhere to clinical expectations to receive unrestricted care. Judith Butler (2004) called this process a "series of individuals not quite believing what they say" (p. 91), but further noted that some identification with the procedure may be inevitable. Perverse defenses therefore allow the therapist to observe the diversity of 2TNG experiences and the restrictive nature of diagnosis, but still protectively authorize the dominance of such objects of classification.

As a form of TCT, perversion manifests in unconscious overidentification with diagnostic criteria in the consulting room. A therapist may struggle to listen to or attempt genuine understanding with a patient whose gender exceeds the available categorizations, which have been built on extremely narrow, Eurocentric medical conceptions and "wrong body" narratives (Engdahl 2014). Not easily traceable within these partitions are those who identify as non-binary, gender fluid, or Two Spirit; those do not have corporeal distress yet still want to change their body; and those who have not known they were trans since childhood, for example. Care has repeatedly been denied to 2TNG subjects who fall outside taxonomic recognition, but care is also refused benevolently on the grounds of clinical inexperience (Puckett et al. 2018). *Perverse TCT* can take the form of passive failures to educate oneself, thus casting trans people into an area of "specialization" out of reach. Clinicians may also carry unconscious guilt about the historical violence of their vocations or DSM nosology—a guilt that, if acted out, could compound their avoidance or amplify fetishistic use of the newest, most politically sound manual. 2TNG patients may contribute to perverse TCT by repressing experiences that do not fit into a classificatory mold, marking them as shameful, fallacious, or even dangerous. Given our social backdrop, they might also struggle to trust mental health professionals (Mizock and Lewis 2008), either consciously or unconsciously, completely disavowing practitioners' competency and protectively casting all psychotherapy as a barrier to 2TNG affirmation.

Finally, *neurotic TCT* appears in the clinic as one of the most multifaceted and (if accounted for) potentially useful aspects of treatment. The diagnosis of pathological neurosis has been applied to a wide scope of cognitive disorders throughout psychiatric history (Køppe 2009). Overarchingly, any mental health problem that lacked an organic cause yet produced behavioral or somatic symptoms could be considered neurotic. For Freud (1917), neurosis was a creative expression of an unresolved psychological conflict, or a part of the subject's past that had become stuck, gone unarticulated, and subsequently found an unconscious iteration. Although he differentiated between neurosis and normality—categorizing his neurotic patients as obsessional, hysteric, or phobic—Freud (1970) also argued that "ostensible healthy life is interspersed with a great number of trivial and in practice unimportant symptoms" (p. 510). The notion that neurosis is an ordinary part of psychic life was developed further by Jacques Lacan (2006), who conceptualized neurosis not as a symptom, but rather as the most common psychological structure any individual can have. Put simply, most people carry repressed and troublesome material from their previous relationships and lived experiences, and that content regularly slips out through non-debilitating yet routine actions, perceptions, and fantasies.

For cis and trans subjects alike, gender is heavily imbued with repressed meanings, as it is developmentally molded from the fabric of our most influential kinships, our identification with loved objects, and the often-restricted parameters of social convention (Butler 2004; Gozlan 2008). Nevertheless, a resolute clinical fixation on the causes of nonconformance has encouraged a trained focus on queer and trans people's gender alone, resulting in little deliberation on the psychic life of the therapist's gender within the clinical dyad. Neurotic TCT therefore encompasses the diverse, under-considered elements of gender's unique happenings, their personal significance, and subsequent ways of being and relating. By acknowledging neurotic TCT, a much-needed, habitual analysis of the imaginary life of a clinician's gender can emerge. When gender functions defensively, clinicians may struggle with a variety of TCT enactments (e.g., the bureaucratic delay of access to hormones or surgery; asking unsuitable or inappropriate questions; a loss of therapeutic attention), many of which can be easefully justified through current treatment standards that doubt trans existence and restrict affirming services.

Accounting for neurotic TCT should include a continuous process of self-reflection and self-analysis. This specific countertransference can be evoked from a variety of sources, such as the therapist's own childhood experiences, internalization of a caregiver's gendered roles and expectations, and even the transmission of their ancestors' gendered lives, including historical gender or sexual trauma. These intricate personal backgrounds are further spliced with the abundant social worlds of gender, which have been continually redefined across time, culture, and geopolitical location. The psychic life of these fluid yet forceful norms can include clinical adherence or strong aversion. A Western psychiatrist may, for example, expect a trans woman patient to adhere to norms of white femininity—donning makeup, and speaking softly; another clinician may have anxiety with that same patient, troubled by her complicity with racialized sexist stereotypes.

As 2TNG people take up more public discursive space, therapists may additionally unconsciously grapple with discourses that vacillate between trans acceptance and continued overt transphobic violence. This internal conflict includes integrating an ethical imperative to "do no harm" with the clinician's own understanding of what psychological harm entails. Such debates are particularly visible in the moral panic currently engulfing trans children, whose existence has been weaponized by conservative leaders to justify the abatement of gender-affirming care (Harper and Dey 2022). In contrast, if trans-affirming clinicians get stuck in a rigid narrative about how to create a safe space, they may struggle to listen to their patients (Porchat and Santos 2021). For example, in idealizing the affirming narrative that trans people should be able to move freely through genders, Porchat foreclosed her capacity to perceive her patient's desire for normativity: her client "did not wish to be a 'different' [fluid] kind of man" (p. 417). Ironically, seeking to minimize the harms of clinical transphobia can also generate forms of neurotic TCT that confine subjectivity.

It is not possible or desirable to completely overcome the manifold symptoms of a therapist's neurosis, as they stem from meaningful pasts and identities. Rather, practitioners can instead work to form an ethical and responsive relationship to those symptoms. If taking a relational approach, clinicians must prepare both to hold and differentiate the layers of their own gendered transference, but further, be prepared to manage challenging unmetabolized affects from their 2TNG patients. Adding to gender's inherent complexities, 2TNG patients may project material from their experiences of transphobia, such as the massive gender trauma of continual misrecognition (Saketopoulou 2014), or the residue of severe exclusion, rejection, and discrimination (Grant et al. 2011). By managing and working with the cocreated TCT, therapists will avoid acting out their own gendered fantasies and will have the capacity to discern how the patient has evoked specific reactions in them. Through mutuality, the psychotherapeutic container can hold the burdensome psychological elements that many trans people carry—elements that may not otherwise find expression.

In this chapter, I provide a short introduction to the history and theoretical trajectory of countertransference, which began as hindrance, evolved to be seen as a projection of the patient's affects, and finally, has been understood as a cocreated phenomenon. Each perspective issues its own unique technical approach, but all converge on the importance of identifying and accounting for the therapist's psychological conflicts. If we acknowledge that discrimination against 2TNG people is a vast and pressing social issue, and further, that the psychic life of a therapist's gender has largely been excluded from clinical considerations, there is no doubt that quotidian transphobia will emerge in the countertransference as an unresolved problem. I explore three types of TCT: *psychotic TCT*, in which the therapist's infantile anxieties erupt and cause significant dysregulation; *perverse TCT*, in which difference is disavowed through the comfort of systems of classification; and *neurotic TCT*, in which the clinician's own repressed gendered fantasies impact their perception and behavior. While each type maps a distinct constellation of symptomatic preoccupations, they may certainly overlap or occur simultaneously. Clinicians may choose to understand TCT as only a personal barrier to overcome, or they may understand their own transference as co-constituted. Regardless of one's therapeutic modality or theoretical orientation, sustained attentiveness to the three types of TCT, when applied alongside affirmative approaches to trans mental health care, will both alleviate unintentional harm and further clarify the profuse impacts of normalized transphobia.

REFERENCES

American Psychiatric Association: Diagnostic and Statistical Manual of Mental Disorders, 3rd Edition. Washington, DC, American Psychiatric Association, 1980

American Psychological Association: Countertransference, in APA Dictionary of Psychology. Washington, DC, American Psychological Association, 2020. Available at: https://dictionary.apa.org/countertransference. Accessed June 14, 2022.

Ansara YG, Friedman EJ: Transphobia, in The Wiley Blackwell Encyclopedia of Gender and Sexuality Studies. Edited by Wong A, Wickramasinghe M, hoogland r, Naples NA. Hoboken, NJ, John Wiley and Sons, 2016, pp. 1–3

Aron L: A Meeting of Minds: Mutuality in Psychoanalysis. New York, Routledge, 2009

Beattie M, Lenihan P: Counselling Skills for Working With Gender Diversity and Identity. London, Jessica Kingsley Publishers, 2018

Bettcher TM: Transphobia. Transgender Studies Quarterly 1(1–2):249–251, 2014

Bion W: Learning From Experience. London, Karnac Books, 1962

Butler J: Undoing Gender. New York, Routledge, 2004

Chang SC, Singh A, Dickey LM: A Clinician's Guide to Gender-Affirming Care: Working With Transgender and Gender Nonconforming Clients. Oakland, CA, New Harbinger Publications, 2018

Downing L: Heteronormativity and repronormativity in sexological "perversion theory" and the DSM-5's "paraphilic disorder" diagnoses. Arch Sex Behav 44(5):1139–1145, 2015 25894646

Drescher J: Gender identity diagnoses: History and controversies, in Gender Dysphoria and Disorders of Sex Development. Edited by Kreukels BPC, Steensma TD, de Vries ALC. Boston, MA, Springer, 2014, pp 137–150

Engdahl U: Wrong body. Transgend Stud Q 1(1–2):267–269, 2014

Freud S: The future prospects of psycho-analytic therapy (1910), in The Standard Edition of the Complete Psychological Works of Sigmund Freud. Translated and edited by Strachey J. London, Hogarth, 1957, pp 139–152

Freud S: Inhibitions, symptoms and anxiety (1926), in The Standard Edition of the Complete Psychological Works of Sigmund Freud. Translated and edited by Strachey J. London, Hogarth, 1959, pp 77–175Freud S: Splitting of the ego in the process of defence (1938), in The Standard Edition of the Complete Psychological Works of Sigmund Freud, Vol XXIII, 1937–1939: Moses and Monotheism, An Outline of Psycho-Analysis and Other Works. London, Hogarth, 1964, pp 271–278Freud S: Introductory Lectures on Psychoanalysis (1917). Translated and edited by Strachey J. New York, W.W. Norton and Company, 1966

Fritscher L: What is counter-transference? Verywell Mind, July 31, 2021. Available at: https://www.verywellmind.com/counter-transference-2671577. Accessed August 3, 2022.

Gabbard GO: A contemporary psychoanalytic model of countertransference. J Clin Psychol 57(8):983–991, 2001 11449380

Gozlan O: The accident of gender. Psychoanal Rev 95(4):541–570, 2008 18721032

Grant J, Mottet L, Tanis J: Injustice at Every Turn: A Report of the National Transgender Discrimination Survey. Washington, DC, National Center for Transgender Equality, 2011

Gratton FV: Supporting Transgender Autistic Youth and Adults: A Guide for Professionals and Families. London, Jessica Kingsley, 2019

Hansbury G: Unthinkable anxieties: reading transphobic countertransferences in a century of psychoanalytic writing. Transgend Stud Q 4(3–4):384–404, 2017

Harper KB, Dey S: Transgender Texas kids are terrified after governor orders that parents be investigated for child abuse. Texas Tribune, February 28, 2022. Available at: https://www.texastribune.org/2022/02/28/texas-transgender-child-abuse/. Accessed April 2, 2022.

Heimann P: On counter-transference. Int J Psychoanal 31:81–84, 1950

Jones T: Improving Services for Transgender and Gender Variant Youth. London, Jessica Kingsley Publishers, 2019

Køppe S: Neurosis: aspects of its conceptual development in the nineteenth century. Hist Psychiatry 20(77 Pt 1):27–46, 2009 20617639

Lacan J: Ecrits. Translated by Fink B. New York, W.W. Norton and Company, 2006

Langer SJ: Theorizing Transgender Identity for Clinical Practice: A New Model for Understanding Gender. London, Jessica Kingsley Publishers, 2019

Lev AI: Disordering gender identity: gender identity disorder in the DSM-IV-TR. J Psychol Human Sex 17(3–4):35–36, 2006

Mannoni O: "I know well, but all the same…," in Perversion and the Social Relation. Edited by Rothenberg MA, Fink B, Mannoni O, et al. Raleigh, NC, Duke University Press, 1969, pp 68–92

Mbembe A: Necropolitics. Publ Cult 15(1):11–40, 2003

McGuire W (ed): The Freud/Jung Letters: The Correspondence Between Sigmund Freud and C.G. Jung. Princeton, NJ, Princeton University Press, 1974

Mizock L, Lewis T: Trauma in transgender populations: risk, resilience, and clinical care. J Emotional Abuse 8(3):335–354, 2008

Ogden TH: The analytic third: working with intersubjective clinical facts. Int J Psychoanal 75(Pt 1):3–19, 1994 8005761

Porchat P, Santos B: "Are we safe analysts?": cisgender countertransferential fantasies in the treatment of transgender patients. Psychoanal Rev 108(4):411–431, 2021 34851704

Puckett JA, Cleary P, Rossman K, et al: Barriers to gender-affirming care for transgender and gender nonconforming individuals. Sex Res Soc Policy 15(1):48–59, 2018 29527241

Quinodoz D: A fe/male transsexual patient in psychoanalysis. Int J Psychoanal 79(Pt 1):95–111, 1998 9587811

Rymer S, Cartei V: Working With Trans Survivors of Sexual Violence: A Guide for Professionals. London, Jessica Kingsley Publishers, 2019

Saketopoulou A: Mourning the body as bedrock: developmental considerations in treating transsexual patients analytically. J Am Psychoanal Assoc 62(5):773–806, 2014 25277869

Shapiro SA: Gender-role stereotypes and clinical process: commentary on papers by Gruenthal and Hirsch. Psychoanal Dialogues 3(3):371–387, 1993

Snorton R, Haritaworn J: Trans necropolitics: a transnational reflection on violence, death, and the trans of color afterlife, in The Transgender Studies Reader Remix. Edited by Stryker S, Aizura A. New York, Routledge, 2013, pp 305–316

Stefana A: History of Countertransference: From Freud to the British Object Relations School. New York, Routledge, 2018

Suess Schwend A: Trans health care from a depathologization and human rights perspective. Public Health Rev 41(1):3, 2020 32099728

Tarnopolsky A: Understanding countertransference. Psychoanal Psychother 9(2):185–194, 1995

Torres MAG: Transsexualism: some considerations on aggression, transference and countertransference. Int Forum Psychoanal 5(1):11–21, 1996

Wiggins T: A perverse solution to misplaced distress. Transgend Stud Q 7(1):56–76, 2020

Winnicott D: The Maturational Processes and the Facilitating Environment: Studies in the Theory of Emotional Development. London, Hogarth, 1965

Zachrisson A: Countertransference and changes in the conception of the psychoanalytic relationship. Int Forum Psychoanal 18(3):177–188, 2009

Working With Transgender, Non-binary, and/or Gender-Expansive (TNG) Youth and Their Families

Néstor Noyola, Ph.D.
Hyun-Hee "Heather" Kim, M.D.
Aude Henin, Ph.D.

MANY children and adolescents in the United States identify as TNG. A recent population-based study suggested that ~3% of youth define themselves as TNG (Rider et al. 2018), and recent estimates suggest that >50% of them also identify as Black, Indigenous, and people of color (BIPOC) (Herman et al. 2017). In this chapter, we provide an overview of mental health among TNG youth and their families, with a focus on the North American context. As an interdisciplinary team of mental health clinicians with a commitment to health equity, we focus here on providing an overview of the alarming inequities experienced among TNG youth and the opportunities for using the gender minority stress and resilience model (GMSR) (see Chapter 2, "Stigma and Mental Health Inequities") and intersectionality theory to inform clinical care.

Psychology and psychiatry (and related fields) have played a significant role in creating and perpetuating oppression of TNG youth (Davy and Toze 2018). Although there have been advances in these fields, such advances are created within systems of oppression that shape the U.S. capitalist society. For example, DSM-5-TR (American Psychiatric Association 2022) continued to enforce social conformity to a rigid gender binary by pathologizing TNG people's distress as reflective of mental illness (Davy and Toze 2018). The American Psychiatric Association acknowledged a change from its historical focus on gender identity to gender dysphoria as the central clinical concern and clarified that not all TNG people experience gender dysphoria in relation to gender incongruence. Despite this shift, the inclusion of gender-related diagnoses in DSM still contributes to the stigmatization and pathologization of gender diversity (Davy and Toze 2018). This pathologizing is further reinforced by the medical-industrial complex (Relman 1980), which requires specific, billable diagnoses to be tied to medical interventions for coverage. Thus, a critical stance toward psychological and psychiatric theory, research, and practice is necessary for working with TNG youth and their families.

MENTAL HEALTH INEQUITIES AMONG TNG YOUTH

Working with TNG youth and their families requires an understanding of the mental health disparities that TNG youth face as a demographic. Because of the dearth of population-based studies that focus on mental health outcomes among TNG youth and their families, it is difficult to provide prevalence estimates. Nonetheless, the literature shows a clear trend that mental health disparities disproportionately affect TNG youth. In the following sections, we draw primarily from data reported by Johns and colleagues (Johns et al. 2019) from the 2017 Youth Risk Behavior Survey (YRBS), a national system of surveys conducted by the CDC that includes U.S. national, state, territorial, tribal government, and local school-based surveys of representative samples of students in grades 9–12. In 2017, for the first time, some survey sites asked participants about their gender identity (Johns et al. 2019). An advantage of the 2017 YRBS data is that it is population based, but a limitation is that all TNG students were grouped together, potentially obscuring intragroup differences (e.g., differences between TNG youth who identify as binary or non-binary).

TNG youth report elevated rates of mental health difficulties and suicidality compared with their cisgender peers (Johns et al. 2019). In the 2017 YRBS, >53% of TNG youth reported experiencing sadness or hopelessness more often than not for at least two consecutive weeks that led them to discontinue their usual activities in the 12 months preceding the survey (vs. cisgender boys, 21%, and cisgender girls, 39%). Similar disparities were reported in suicide-related outcomes: ~44% of TNG youth reported having thought seriously about suicide (cisgender boys, 11%; cisgender girls, 20%), and ~35% reported having attempted suicide at least once in the past 12 months (cisgender boys, 6%; cisgender girls, 9%). TNG youth also reported elevated rates of lifetime substance use, including cigarettes, alcohol, cannabis, cocaine, heroin, methamphetamines, ecstasy, and inhalants, and misuse of prescription opioids (Johns et al. 2019). Among 2017 YRBS respondents, alcohol was the most widely used substance among TNG youth, with ~70% endorsing lifetime use (cisgender boys, 53%; cisgender girls, 63%). Strikingly, 26% of TNG youth endorsed lifetime heroin use (cisgender boys, 2%; cisgender girls, <1%), and 25% of TNG youth endorsed lifetime methamphetamine use (cisgender boys, 2%; cisgender girls, 1%).

ADAPTING GMSR FOR TNG YOUTH

In this section, to make sense of some of the drivers of these disparities, we integrate GMSR with intersectionality theory. GMSR is a useful framework—albeit with some serious limitations—for understanding the drivers of mental health inequities among TNG youth (see Chapter 2, "Stigma and Mental Health Inequities"). When integrated with intersectionality theory, the model can provide mental health providers with a useful starting point for conceptualization and treatment planning, as well as for advocacy.

Intersectionality Theory

Intersectional activists have for centuries demonstrated that focusing on single axes of oppression (e.g., attending to racism as if it operates separately from sexism and classism) benefits the most socially privileged within an oppressed social group (Buchanan and Wiklund 2020). Seminal critical race theory and legal studies scholar Kimberlé Crenshaw put forth a framework for *intersectionality theory* in 1989, in which she analyzed how contemporary feminist and antiracist theorists and activists failed to consider how racism and sexism together shape BIPOC women's experiences of domestic violence and rape and, in the process, perpetuated violence against BIPOC women (Crenshaw 1989).

One of the most glaring limitations of GMSR is that it does not consider race and ethnicity (Tan et al. 2020). Most TNG youth are also BIPOC and simultaneously navigate a range of race-based and class-based minority stressors, as well as intersectional forms of stress, such as marginalization from the white TNG community (Chang and Singh 2016). Moreover, resilience factors may differ based on TNG youths' social position within our racialized, gendered, and classed society. For instance, community connectedness (a resilience factor proposed in the GMSR model) by itself (i.e., without structural change) may not be equally protective for all TNG youth. In a recent study using a representative sample of California's secondary school population, Vance et al. (2021) found that school connectedness and caring adult relationships were protective factors in the context of minority stressors for depressive symptoms and suicidal ideation for non-Latinx white TNG youth but not for Black and Latinx TNG youth. Thus, TNG youths' gender identities must be understood within the sociocultural and political context.

Intersectionality's emphasis is on changing the conditions that give rise to inequities among multiply marginalized populations. Although GMSR locates the sources of minority stress as external to people, it tends to focus on the individual's perceptions, thoughts, and behaviors of stress. For instance, the model posits that the deleterious effects of minority stress can be managed through coping and social support (Hendricks and Testa 2012). An exclusive focus on coping and social support in the context of oppression frames psychological distress as what must be changed, rather than the systems of oppression that gave rise to that distress (Phillips et al. 2015). Distress alleviation is fine, but coping and social support by themselves are unlikely to lead to changes in the oppressive systems that give rise to factors causing distress (French et al. 2020; Vance et al. 2021) or to curtail future experiences of gender minority distress.

Expanding GMSR for Younger Patients

Another significant limitation of GMSR is that it was developed for adults. Toomey (2021) recently adapted the GMSR model for TNG youth, building on the model of Hendricks and Testa (2012) by drawing focus on contexts of development, gender dysphoria as a domain of minority stress, access and use of affirmative physical and mental health care, and developmental considerations.

Regarding contexts of development, the adapted model calls for attention to the experience of distal minority stressors across different contexts of development, including family, school, peer relationships, social media, racial and ethnic communities, and Two-Spirit, lesbian, gay, bisexual, transgender, queer, intersex, asexual, and more (2SLGBTQIA+) communities (Toomey 2021). Specifically, Toomey highlights that stress may be experienced differently within and across these contexts. Indeed, data from the YRBS highlight that TNG high school students experience high levels of violence in school and peer relationships. TNG high school students were more likely than their cisgender peers to report feeling unsafe traveling to and from school (26.9%) and to have been threatened or injured with a weapon at school (23.8%). Even more reported being bullied at school (34.6%) and online (29.6%) (Johns et al. 2019). TNG high school students also experience high levels of violence in intimate relationships; 23.8% have been raped or victimized physically (26.4%) or sexually (22.9%) in dating contexts (Johns et al. 2019).

Given that gender dysphoria is correlated with mental health and well-being, Toomey (2021) proposed intra- and interpersonal gender dysphoria as key sources of minority stress that contribute to health inequities among TNG youth. In the adapted model, a distinction is made between the distress caused by the incongruence of one's gender identity, expression, and anatomy (i.e., intrapersonal gender dysphoria) and the distress caused by people and contexts that deny or refuse to acknowledge TNG youth's existence (i.e., interpersonal gender dysphoria), such as lack of access to appropriately gendered bathrooms.

Toomey (2021) highlights the critical role of access and use of gender-affirming health care. As Toomey notes, health care systems continue to pathologize TNG youth's gender identities and expressions; as such, there is a crucial need for clinicians to provide gender-affirming care. Moreover, GMSR highlights that youth, particularly younger children, are legally limited in their agency and autonomy to independently navigate resources. Parents and guardians, with the legal responsibility of caring for a child, often act as gatekeepers of affirmative resources across contexts, granting or denying permission to access affirmative health care. As such, it is important to attend to power dynamics within families as they navigate health care systems.

Finally, although Toomey does not include specific developmental considerations, the adapted model calls for considering how physical, cognitive, social, and psychosocial development shape the impact on health and well-being of minority stressors, general life stress, and access to affirmative health care. We encourage researchers and health providers to refrain from using these considerations to dismiss TNG youths' thoughts and feelings or to constrain their agency; adultism—or adults' unwarranted use of their power over youth's autonomy—is a significant source of stress among TNG youth (Singh 2013; Singh et al. 2014; Tan and Weisbart 2022).

Recent systematic reviews of risk and resilience factors related to mental health among TNG youth offer evidence for factors beyond those identified in the GMSR model (Johns et al. 2018; Tankersley et al. 2021). In one such article, Tankersley et al. (2021) found several common risk factors for mental health problems, including physical and verbal abuse, discrimination, social isolation, lower quality of peer relations, lower levels of self-esteem, weight dissatisfaction, and older age. In the other, Johns et al. (2018) used Bronfenbrenner's bioecological theory of development to review the empirical literature on protective factors for mental health among TNG youth. They found evidence for protective factors at multiple levels, such as self-esteem at the individual level; support from parents, peers, and trusted adults at the relationships level; and school policies and 2SLGBTQIA+ organizational resources at the community level. Of note, the researchers highlighted a glaring dearth of empirical work on societal-level protective factors (Johns et al. 2018).

STRESS AND RESILIENCE AMONG TNG YOUTH AND THEIR FAMILIES

Family acceptance and rejection are crucial to the mental well-being of TNG youth (Malpas et al. 2022). Acceptance and rejection are not dichotomous; different domains of acceptance and rejection may be differentially associated with mental health outcomes. For instance, in a preliminary study investigating domains of family attitude (e.g., acceptance, warmth, hostility, indifference, and undifferentiated rejection) and TNG youth's expressed feelings around their affirmed gender, Pariseau et al. (2019) found that primary caregivers' past support was significantly associated with lower levels of depression and anxiety symptoms. Moreover, they found that secondary caregivers' indifference was significantly associated with higher levels of depression and anxiety symptoms, and that sibling support was significantly and inversely associated with externalizing problems and suicidal ideation.

Families and caregivers may have a wide range of reactions and experiences as they navigate their relationships with their TNG children (Abreu et al. 2019; Matsuno et al. 2022; Pullen Sansfaçon et al. 2022). In a recent systematic literature review of research on the experiences of parents of TNG youth, Abreu et al. (2019) found that upon learning about their child's gender identity, parents experienced grief, loss, and mourning, including the perceived loss of previously held visions for their children's future based on their sex assigned at birth. Additionally, some parents experienced difficulties making sense of previously held ideologies, religious traditions, assumptions, prejudices, and beliefs around gender and sexuality. Some parents reported feeling overwhelmed by their lack of knowledge about TNG identities and communities, which contributed to their initial negative reactions and difficulties in understanding their children. Nonetheless, and importantly, some parents also reported experiencing a variety of strong, positive, and loving reactions across studies. Of note, Abreu et al. (2019) found that across studies, many parents reported undergoing a process of transformation as their relationships with their TNG children progressed. This process was characterized by the development of new parental behaviors, including actively seeking information and other resources to understand their children's TNG identities; changing previously held negative beliefs; seeking support; connecting with TNG communities; gaining a deeper awareness and understanding of discrimination; and developing empathy. Moreover, parents described several benefits to having a TNG child, including an improved parent-child relationship, affirmation of enacted values such as unconditional positive love for their children, increased involvement in activism, and new, personal narratives around their children and their role as parents.

In addition to navigating their relationships with their children, parents of TNG youth face various gender-based stressors themselves (Abreu et al. 2019; Hidalgo and Chen 2019; Katz-Wise et al. 2021; Matsuno et al. 2022). In a recent qualitative interview study, Hidalgo and Chen (2019) found that parents of TNG youth reported facing discrimination (e.g., perceived scrutiny from other parents and community members; travel-related discrimination), rejection from extended adult family members and other parents, verbal victimization (e.g., being labeled as a "bad parent"), and non-affirmation (e.g., witnessing the misgendering of their children; navigating non-affirming family interactions). Parents reported several proximal stressors, such as internalizing gender-based stigma (e.g., stigma against gender-nonconforming behaviors), anticipating experiences of minority stress for their children (e.g., fear that their child would be victimized), and navigating disclosure of their children's gender identity journeys in interactions with others. Parents noted that these stressors contribute to negative emotions and social isolation.

ADDRESSING GENDER MINORITY STRESSORS AND RESILIENCE WITH PSYCHOSOCIAL INTERVENTIONS

Increasingly, researchers and clinicians have begun to provide gender-affirming psychosocial interventions to promote well-being, guide TNG youth and their families to make sense of minority stressors they experience, and support the development of their resiliency, including living authentically in their gender identities. These interventions integrate tenets from the Gender Affirmative Model (GAM) (Hidalgo et al. 2013):

a) gender variations are not disorders;
b) gender presentations are diverse and varied across cultures, therefore requiring our cultural sensitivity;
c) to the best of our knowledge at present, gender involves an interweaving of biology; development and socialization; and culture and context, with all three bearing on any individual's gender self;
d) gender may be fluid and is not binary, both at a particular time and if and when it changes within an individual across time;
e) if there is pathology, it more often stems from cultural reactions (e.g., transphobia, homophobia, sexism) rather than from within the child.

Unfortunately, there is little research or outcome data on gender-affirming psychosocial interventions specifically designed for TNG youth and their families (Austin et al. 2018; Malpas et al. 2022). One promising intervention is AFFIRM, a gender-affirmative cognitive-behavioral coping skills group intervention for TNG youth that was designed through a community-based research approach. The aim of the intervention is "promoting positive change and healthy coping through the creation of a safe, affirming, and collaborative therapeutic experience" (Austin et al. 2018, p. 2). In their preliminary investigation, Austin et al. found that there was a statistically significant reduction in depression scores immediately after the intervention and 3 months later, compared with baseline depression scores. In contrast, there was no statistically significant change in reflective coping skills (other coping skills were not measured). Of note, TNG youth participants reported high levels of satisfaction, although they did recommend greater attention to intersectionality and the experiences of BIPOC TNG youth throughout the intervention. Overall, despite their limitations, these results suggest that AFFIRM may help address depression among TNG youth. Recently, the researchers found similar results for a telehealth version of AFFIRM (Craig et al. 2021).

Given the paucity of research on gender-affirming psychosocial interventions specifically for TNG youth, next we offer practical suggestions for using cognitive-behavioral therapy (CBT), an evidence-based intervention for a range of mental problems, from a gender-affirming approach to address the mental health impacts of minority stressors among TNG youth and their families.

Understanding Minority Stress

Gender-affirmative interventions should include explicit discussions about minority stressors experienced by TNG youth, including individual, interpersonal, community, institutional, and cultural transnegativity as it intersects with other systems of oppression such as white supremacy and racism, the impact on health, and strategies to mitigate the negative effects of these stressors on well-being. One common goal is to normalize anxiety and depression as understandable reactions to ongoing minority stressors and to help youth accurately attribute the cause of these symptoms. For example, a child's gender itself is not the cause of bullying that they experience, but rather, a peer's prejudice, which stems from transnegativity. As part of psychoeducation, TNG youth may monitor physiologic, cognitive, emotional, and behavioral reactions to minority stress and be guided to link previous and current experiences of minority stressors with specific emotional reactions and behaviors. TNG youth and their experiences are rich and varied, and thus it may be useful to help TNG youth and families explore how dimensions of their multiple and overlapping racial/ethnic, gender, and sexual social identities (among others) relate to privilege and oppression in different social contexts and how this may influence the minority stressors they experience (Golden and Oransky 2019). Accurate recognition of sociocultural and political context and minority stressors, as well as their impact, is a pillar of culturally sensitive gender-affirming care (Chang and Singh 2016).

Identifying and Restructuring Negative Cognitions About Minority Status

Cognitions are shaped by early life experiences, which for TNG youth may involve a range of experiences with discrimination, violence, abuse, rejection, and invalidation. Cognitive strategies, a core aspect of most CBT interventions, focus on the mediating impact of automatic thoughts and beliefs on emotions and behaviors. The goal is to identify unhelpful or maladaptive self-talk and foster more adaptive, helpful, or realistic thought patterns. Gender-affirming interventions may offer explicit discussion of negative self-talk about gender identity as shaped by minority stressors, as well as strategies to challenge this self-talk. In addition, cognitive strategies may be used to address proximal gender minority stressors such as internalized transphobia, expectations of rejection, and rumination on past experiences of minority stress.

Given that these proximal factors are suggested as mediating factors for the impact of distal stressors on mental health outcomes (Hatzenbuehler 2009), they are important targets for intervention. TNG youth and their families can be guided to better understand how previous experiences have shaped negative core beliefs about themselves, their gender, and their relationships to others; recognize automatic thoughts that arise from these core beliefs; and adopt more adaptive self-talk. Some approaches with 2SLGBTQIA+ youth also incorporate compassion-focused cognitive and experiential techniques to decrease shame and internalized stigma, foster self-compassion and empathy, and cultivate a nonjudgmental perspective toward one's experiences (Bluth et al. 2021).

Addressing Hypervigilance

One of the consequences of repeated experiences with discrimination, violence, abuse, rejection, and invalidation for many TNG youth is chronic hypervigilance to potential threats (Rood et al. 2017). This hypervigilance is associated with increased physiological arousal, unhelpful thinking patterns, avoidance behaviors, and decreased self-regulation capacity, which may be adaptive in some contexts but disadvantageous in others (Bögels and Mansell 2004; Hatzenbuehler 2009; Hatzenbuehler et al. 2009). Trauma-informed CBT, which addresses hypervigilance, can be used to help TNG youth recognize triggers for hypervigilance, implement relaxation and mindfulness strategies to reduce physiologic symptoms of stress, challenge inaccurate threat-related cognitions, and differentiate safe versus unsafe situations (Alessi and Martin 2017; Black et al. 2012).

Facilitating Emotional Regulation

Because gender identity develops early in life, repeated invalidation, denigration, or dismissal of TNG identities over childhood may teach youth to ignore their internal sense of self or instincts; ignore or suppress gender-related emotions and thoughts; and conceal gender-nonconforming behaviors to conform to cisgender societal norms and expectations. Growing up and existing in persistently invalidating environments increases risk for emotional dysregulation in several ways: decreasing awareness of internal states and emotional recognition; limiting coping tools that could help manage negative emotional states; and increasing experiential avoidance (Skerven et al. 2018). Gender dysphoria may further exacerbate these difficulties and increase risks for depression, anxiety, suicidality, and self-injury behaviors.

Emotion regulation and distress tolerance skills, drawn from dialectical behavioral therapy (DBT), teach youth to recognize and label various emotional states (including physiologic, affective, cognitive, and behavioral aspects of emotions), their triggers, and their consequences (Linehan 1993; Miller et al. 2007). To develop a range of skills to manage and tolerate intense negative emotional states in a nondestructive manner, TNG youth can learn strategies to tolerate intense negative emotions, including mindfulness, distraction, and self-soothing techniques. Strategies to enhance overall well-being (e.g., exercise, sleep hygiene, activity scheduling) may also enhance resilience and reduce vulnerability to negative mood states.

Using Exposure to Address Avoidance Behaviors

Progressive exposure is one of the best-established interventions to address anxiety-based avoidance, with demonstrated effectiveness for all anxiety disorders, trauma-related disorders, and obsessive-compulsive disorders (Barlow et al. 2016). Based on classic (extinction learning) and operant conditioning models, clients are asked to gradually confront anxiety-provoking situations without engaging in avoidance or safety-seeking behaviors. With repeated exposure practice, clients experience reduced anxiety in previously feared situations, an enhanced sense of mastery and competence, and skills to cope with anxiety symptoms. Whenever appropriate, exposure exercises should incorporate issues of relevance to TNG youth (e.g., coming out; using a bathroom that accords with their gender identity). Many interventions also include a focus on assertiveness skills, both directly (e.g., when being misgendered) and indirectly (e.g., when initiating a new relationship). These may be important in addressing difficult interpersonal relationships (Coyne et al. 2020) as well as enhancing health-related behaviors (e.g., substance refusal skills, sexual health negotiations).

Fostering Sources of Resilience

It is essential, in any discussion of behavioral health, to highlight known sources of resilience in TNG youth, both to avoid pathologizing gender diversity and to offer targets for behavioral health interventions that can enhance well-being and positive outcomes. There is evidence that social support (especially parental and familial support and affirmation) is a powerful protective factor for TNG people, especially youth (Johns et al. 2018). Several studies emphasize the mental health benefits of parental acceptance and support, with increased self-esteem and decreased substance use, suicidal thoughts, and depression (Malpas et al. 2022). Conversely, family rejection or maltreatment is associated with increased risk of depression, suicidal ideation and behaviors, substance use disorders, and homelessness (Seibel et al. 2018; Toomey 2021).

In addition, having community support improves mental health outcomes among TNG people. For example, having an effective Gay-Straight Alliance (now called Gender & Sexuality Alliances) in school enhances well-being and positive mental health outcomes in young adulthood and buffers young people against the negative effects of 2SLGBTQIA+-associated school victimization (Toomey et al. 2011). It is important to be mindful that BIPOC TNG youth may experience complex combinations of support and rejection around their gender, sexual, and racial and ethnic identities (e.g., feeling supported around their racial identities but not around their gender identities or vice versa), which may lead to simultaneous feelings of empowerment and disempowerment (Golden and Oransky 2019). Finally, focusing on the unique strengths of TNG people, including enhancing pride in diverse gender identities, further enhances resilience, as does supporting community building and social activities (Singh 2013; Singh et al. 2014). Clients may identify TNG role models and community champions and benefit from increasing positive representation of TNG people in media, literature, and education to foster self-esteem, pride, and hope for the future.

WORKING WITH FAMILIES OF TNG YOUTH

Involving parents and other family members in care is often a critical aspect of gender-affirming interventions (Malpas et al. 2022). Families may benefit from psychoeducation around gender identity and expression, developmental processes in identity formation, and gender affirmation. Providing accurate information is also an important part of informed consent for medical affirmation procedures. Parents may have misconceptions, concerns, and fears about their child's TNG identity and may benefit from specific guidance on how best to support and advocate for their child. Clinicians may offer pragmatic suggestions around additional resources, including support groups for parents or children and social affirmation procedures. Parents may benefit from separate meetings to discuss and manage their own feelings of grief, guilt, and anxiety and to identify and challenge negative or transphobic beliefs. In families experiencing significant distress or conflict around supporting a child, family therapy may be warranted to address underlying family vulnerabilities and maladaptive patterns of interaction and communication. The overarching goals of family interventions are to help families align with their TNG child and progressively address impediments to providing a supportive and affirming family culture.

CONCLUSION

TNG youth are a racially and ethnically diverse group who experience alarming mental health inequities in the context of transnegativity and its intersections with multiple systems of oppression. Researchers and clinicians have a critical role in guiding TNG youth and their families to make sense of their experiences with minority stressors and to foster their resilience in the service of authentic living. We advocate for a (continued) critical stance toward the pathologizing of gender in psychology and psychiatry, the integration of intersectionality theory and developmentally informed GMSR models, and a gender-affirmative approach to evidence-based interventions. Importantly, we encourage researchers and clinicians to actively advocate for change at the micro, meso, and macro levels of society to ensure the well-being of TNG youth.

REFERENCES

Abreu RL, Rosenkrantz DE, Ryser-Oatman JT, et al: Parental reactions to transgender and gender diverse children: a literature review. J GLBT Fam Stud 15(5):461–485, 2019

Alessi EJ, Martin JI: Intersection of trauma and identity, in Trauma, Resilience, and Health Promotion in LGBT Patients: What Every Healthcare Provider Should Know. Cham, Springer International, 2017, pp 3–14

American Psychiatric Association: Diagnostic and Statistical Manual of Mental Disorders, 5th Edition, Text Revision. Arlington, VA, American Psychiatric Association, 2022

Austin A, Craig SL, D'Souza SA: An AFFIRMative cognitive behavioral intervention for transgender youth: preliminary effectiveness. Prof Psychol Res Pr 49(1):1–8, 2018

Barlow DH, Allen LB, Choate ML: Toward a unified treatment for emotional disorders—republished article. Behav Ther 47(6):838–853, 2016 27993336

Black PJ, Woodworth M, Tremblay M, Carpenter T: A review of trauma-informed treatment for adolescents. Can Psychol 53(3):192–203, 2012

Bluth K, Lathren C, Clepper-Faith M, et al: Improving mental health among transgender adolescents: implementing mindful self-compassion for teens. J Adolesc Res 38:2, 271–302, 2021

Bögels SM, Mansell W: Attention processes in the maintenance and treatment of social phobia: hypervigilance, avoidance and self-focused attention. Clin Psychol Rev 24(7):827–856, 2004 15501558

Buchanan NCT, Wiklund LO: Why clinical science must change or die: integrating intersectionality and social justice. Women Ther 43(3–4):309–329, 2020

Chang SC, Singh AA: Affirming psychological practice with transgender and gender nonconforming people of color. Psychol Sex Orientat Gend Divers 3:140–147, 2016

Coyne CA, Poquiz JL, Janssen A, Chen D: Evidence-based psychological practice for transgender and non-binary youth: defining the need, framework for treatment adaptation, and future directions. Evid Based Pract Child Adolesc Ment Health 5(3):340–353, 2020

Craig SL, Leung VWY, Pascoe R, et al: AFFIRM online: utilising an affirmative cognitive-behavioural digital intervention to improve mental health, access, and engagement among LGBTQA+ youth and young adults. Int J Environ Res Public Health 18(4):1–18, 2021 33562876

Crenshaw K: Demarginalizing the intersection of race and sex: a black feminist critique of antidiscrimination doctrine, feminist theory and antiracist politics. Univ Chic Leg Forum 1989(1):139–167, 1989

Davy Z, Toze M: What is gender dysphoria? A critical systematic narrative review. Transgend Health 3(1):159–169, 2018 30426079

French BH, Lewis JA, Mosley DV, et al: Toward a psychological framework of radical healing in communities of color. Couns Psychol 48(1):14–46, 2020

Golden RL, Oransky M: An intersectional approach to therapy with transgender adolescents and their families. Arch Sex Behav 48(7):2011–2025, 2019 30604170

Hatzenbuehler ML: How does sexual minority stigma "get under the skin"? A psychological mediation framework. Psychol Bull 135(5):707–730, 2009 19702379

Hatzenbuehler ML, Nolen-Hoeksema S, Dovidio J: How does stigma "'get under the skin'"? The mediating role of emotion regulation. Psychol Sci 20(10):1282–1289, 2009 19765237

Hendricks ML, Testa RJ: A conceptual framework for clinical work with transgender and gender nonconforming clients: an adaptation of the minority stress model. Prof Psychol Res Pr 43(5):460–467, 2012

Herman JL, Flores AR, Brown TNT, et al: Age of Individuals Who Identify as Transgender in the United States. Los Angeles, CA, The Williams Institute, 2017. Available at: https://williamsinstitute.law.ucla.edu/wp-content/uploads/Age-Trans-Individuals-Jan-2017.pdf. Accessed December 1, 2021.

Hidalgo MA, Chen D: Experiences of gender minority stress in cisgender parents of transgender/gender-expansive prepubertal children: a qualitative study. J Fam Issues 40(7):865–886, 2019

Hidalgo MA, Ehrensaft D, Tishelman AC, et al: The gender affirmative model: what we know and what we aim to learn. Hum Development 56(5):285–290, 2013

Johns MM, Beltran O, Armstrong HL, et al: Protective factors among transgender and gender variant youth: a systematic review by socioecological level. J Prim Prev 39(3):263–301, 2018 29700674

Johns MM, Lowry R, Andrzejewski J, et al: Transgender identity and experiences of violence victimization, substance use, suicide risk, and sexual risk behaviors among high school students—19 states and large urban school districts, 2017. MMWR Morb Mortal Wkly Rep 68(3):67–71, 2019 30677012

Katz-Wise SL, Galman SC, Friedman LE, Kidd KM: Parent/caregiver narratives of challenges related to raising transgender and/or nonbinary youth. J Fam Issues 43:12, 3321–3345 2021

Linehan MM: Cognitive-behavioral treatment of borderline personality disorder. New York, Guilford, 1993

Malpas J, Pellicane MJ, Glaeser E: Family-based interventions with transgender and gender expansive youth: systematic review and best practice recommendations. Transgend Health 7(1):7–29, 2022 36644030

Matsuno E, McConnell E, Dolan CV, Israel T: "I am fortunate to have a transgender child": an investigation into the barriers and facilitators to support among parents of trans and nonbinary youth. LGBTQ+ Family: An Interdisciplinary Journal 18(1):1–19, 2022

Miller AL, Rathus JH, DuBose AP, et al: Dialectical Behavior Therapy for Adolescents. New York, Guilford, 2007

Pariseau EM, Chevalier L, Long KA, et al: The relationship between family acceptance-rejection and transgender youth psychosocial functioning. Clin Pract Pediatr Psychol 7(3):267–277, 2019

Phillips NL, Adams G, Salter PS: Beyond adaptation: decolonizing approaches to coping with oppression. J Soc Polit Psych 3(1):365–387, 2015

Pullen Sansfaçon A, Medico D, Gelly M, et al: Blossoming child, mourning parent: a qualitative study of trans children and their parents navigating transition. J Child Fam Stud 31(7):1771–1784, 2022

Relman AS: The new medical-industrial complex. N Engl J Med 303(17):963–970, 1980 7412851

Rider GN, McMorris BJ, Gower AL, et al: Health and care utilization of transgender and gender nonconforming youth: a population-based study. Pediatrics 141(3):e20171683, 2018 29437861

Rood BA, Reisner SL, Puckett JA, et al: Internalized transphobia: exploring perceptions of social messages in transgender and gender-nonconforming adults. Int J Transgend 18(4):411–426, 2017

Seibel BL, de Brito Silva B, Fontanari AMV, et al: The impact of the parental support on risk factors in the process of gender affirmation of transgender and gender diverse people. Front Psychol 9:399, 2018 29651262

Singh AA: Transgender youth of color and resilience: negotiating oppression and finding support. Sex Roles 68(11–12):690–702, 2013

Singh AA, Meng SE, Hansen AW: "I am my own gender": resilience strategies of trans youth. J Couns Dev 92(2):208–218, 2014

Skerven K, Whicker DR, Lemaire KL: Applying dialectical behaviour therapy to structural and internalized stigma with LGBTQ+ clients. Cogn Behav Therap 12:e9, 2018

Tan KKH, Treharne GJ, Ellis SJ, et al: Gender minority stress: a critical review. J Homosex 67(10):1471–1489, 2020 30912709

Tan S, Weisbart C: 'I'm me, and I'm Chinese and also transgender': coming out complexities of Asian-Canadian transgender youth. Journal of LGBT Youth 1–27, 2022

Tankersley AP, Grafsky EL, Dike J, Jones RT: Risk and resilience factors for mental health among transgender and gender nonconforming (TGNC) youth: a systematic review. Clin Child Fam Psychol Rev 24(2):183–206, 2021 33594611

Toomey RB: Advancing research on minority stress and resilience in trans children and adolescents in the 21st century. Child Dev Perspect 15(2):96–102, 2021

Toomey RB, Ryan C, Diaz RM, Russell ST: High school gay-straight alliances (GSAs) and young adult well-being: an examination of GSA presence, participation, and perceived effectiveness. Appl Dev Sci 15(4):175–185, 2011 22102782

Vance SR Jr, Boyer CB, Glidden DV, Sevelius J: Mental health and psychosocial risk and protective factors among Black and Latinx transgender youth compared with peers. JAMA Netw Open 4(3):e213256, 2021 33769506

Caring for the Mental Health Needs of Transgender, Non-binary, and/or Gender-Expansive (TNG) Older Adults

Brett Dolotina, B.S.
Gabrielle Morgan, B.S.
Lisa Krinsky, M.S.W., L.I.C.S.W.

TNG older adults (≥50 years of age) comprise ~1 million people, about 0.3% of the United States adult population (Brown 2022). With increasing acceptance of gender diversity and access to gender-affirming health care, this number is expected to rise. However, the medical field has not yet met the mental health needs of this population, who face intersecting and amplified discrimination based on both gender identity and age (Witten 2016) and have worse mental health than their cisgender peers (Fredriksen-Goldsen et al. 2014). Here, we outline the role of clinicians in providing gender-affirming psychiatric care for TNG older adults.

GENERATIONAL AND CULTURAL CONTEXT: A LIFE COURSE PERSPECTIVE

The cultural and sociohistorical contexts within which TNG older adults have lived directly impact their well-being. This may be conceptualized through *life course theory*, the notion that life events influence health trajectories (Aldwin et al. 2006, 2017; Elder 1994; Siverskog 2015). As of writing this chapter, members of this population were born between 1940 and 1973. During this time, TNG people were often called "transsexuals," a term now considered pejorative (Cook-Daniels 2016), and faced high levels of stigma, harassment, discrimination, and violence (Slagstad 2021).

Popular culture had little TNG representation until 1952, when Christine Jorgensen, a 25-year-old U.S. veteran, underwent genital reconstructive surgery (GRS) in Denmark. The U.S. media firestorm around Jorgensen's story allowed more individuals to see reflections of their own gender identity experience, claim the label of transsexuality, and seek gender-affirming surgeries themselves (Brevard 2011; Scarpella 2010).

As gender-affirming health care developed, the first GRS program in the United States opened at Johns Hopkins Hospital (Baltimore, Maryland) in 1966, followed by similar clinics at other universities across the country. Applicants needed to meet several stringent requirements to receive care, such as clear narratives of lifelong distress about being "born in the wrong body" and an attraction to people of the "opposite" sex. These requirements, on top of an already exclusionary health care system, greatly limited access to GRS; only 24 of the 2,000 people who sought GRS at Johns Hopkins received surgery in its first 2.5 years of operations (Meyerowitz 2004).

In 1979, the first professional TNG health organization was founded. Named the Harry Benjamin International Gender Dysphoria Association after one of the first U.S. physicians to care for transgender patients (Meyerowitz 2004), the organization renamed itself the World Professional Association for Transgender Health (WPATH) in 2007. Shortly after its creation, WPATH issued Standards of Care, protocols for clinicians to follow when working with TNG patients. These protocols required TNG individuals to undergo considerable psychological counseling before accessing gender-affirming procedures (World Professional Association for Transgender Health 2012). Initially, some university clinics disregarded the WPATH Standards of Care and continued with their strict university policies for gender-affirming procedures (Meyerowitz 2004). However, clinicians worldwide soon began to use the protocols as a starting point in guiding their provision of gender-affirming medical care.

In 1980, the American Psychiatric Association formalized a new diagnosis, *gender identity disorder* (American Psychiatric Association 1980), signifying that an individual identified as transgender. The APA modified this diagnosis to *gender dysphoria* in 2013 with the intention of separating objective TNG identity from the subjective distress caused by a person's gender not aligning with societal expectations for their sex assigned at birth. Critiques remain as to whether this distinction was materially beneficial for TNG people (Davy 2015).

It became much easier for TNG individuals to build community and access information on TNG experiences with expanded use of the internet in the 1990s. Individuals could now widely and privately find information on social and medical gender affirmation. Partly as a result, the number of people identifying as TNG and becoming visible markedly increased, as did the number of organizations and conferences specifically for TNG individuals. The Transgender Aging Network, for example, was founded in 1998 with the primary goal of connecting professionals interested in the betterment of older TNG people; however, it quickly became a space for older TNG adults to find each other, seek advice, and build community.

Mental Health Disparities

There are limited data on the mental health disparities experienced by TNG older adults. Reasons for this include poor data collection tools for gender identity in national epidemiological surveys (Witten 2009, 2017), as well as a deep mistrust of health researchers among TNG people owing to a long-standing history of extraction, whereby researchers draw out information from TNG communities without a commitment to meaningfully involve or invest in them (American Psychological Association 2015). Research clearly shows that TNG older adults face disproportionate mental illness as a result of the multiplicative effects of transphobia and ageism (Witten 2016). In one study, TNG older adults reported more depression, perceived stress, and poor physical health than cisgender older adults in their sample (Fredriksen-Goldsen et al. 2014). Data on suicidality among TNG older adults is scant, although a systematic review of suicidality among TNG adults estimated a lifetime prevalence of 55%, with a range of 28.9%–96.5% (Adams et al. 2017). The U.S. Transgender Survey estimated that 40% of the 27,715 TNG adult respondents reported having attempted suicide at least once in their life (Herman et al. 2019). One qualitative study noted that 14 of the 88 TNG older adults in their sample specifically discussed suicidality in detail during their interviews, accentuating the prevalence of mental health challenges among this population (Gaveras et al. 2021).

Multiple structural-, community-, and individual-level factors affect mental health and access to gender-affirming psychiatric care for TNG older adults. Societal stigma (such as ageism and transphobia) often manifest as discrimination (e.g., social stress, prejudice, physical violence) (Kcomt 2019). Indeed, in one study, most TNG older adults listed gender and age as the main reasons for the discrimination they experienced in the past year (White Hughto and Reisner 2018). Further, in that study, TNG older adults who experienced gender- or age-related discrimination were 5.68 and 2.04 times more likely, respectively, to experience depressive distress. TNG older adults also often experience financial barriers to accessing health care. Nearly half of TNG older adults live below two times the federal poverty level (Fredriksen-Goldsen et al. 2014). TNG older adults are thus likely to lack insurance, further delaying medical care and exacerbating mental health challenges (Downing and Przedworski 2018; Wilson et al. 2015).

In addition to these structural and institutional barriers, TNG older adults have lower levels of social support (Fredriksen-Goldsen et al. 2014) and experience high rates of family rejection and stress (Factor and Rothblum 2007), factors that have been shown to result in loneliness and psychological distress in this population (Fredriksen-Goldsen et al. 2014). Moreover, TNG older adults with additional marginalized identities experience amplified mental health disparities due to structural racism, ableism, classism, ageism, and other oppressions along minoritized social positionalities (Bowleg 2021). Indeed, on top of financial and transportation barriers, TNG older adults of color face barriers to accessing health care at culturally responsive queer and TNG centers, especially in majority-white neighborhoods (Linscott and Krinsky 2016). Future research should steer development of tailored clinical interventions, led by the voices of TNG older adults who face additional structural oppressions based on race, ethnicity, socioeconomic class, education, and immigration status. Clinicians must consider the multifaceted lived experiences of TNG older adults to provide comprehensive, affirming care.

Affirmative Psychiatric Care

Gender-affirming care consists of a flexible, sensitive, and responsive approach to health care that comprehensively attends to the medical and mental health needs of TNG individuals while wholeheartedly affirming their gender identities. Providing gender-affirming psychiatric care is indispensable in supporting the mental health and well-being of TNG older adults (Jarrett et al. 2021; Wernick et al. 2019). Clinicians looking to gain insight into gender-affirming care should consult Chapter 24, "Gender-Affirming Mental Health Care Environments," which provides a broad overview of considerations that should be made in clinical practice to ensure a welcoming and safe space for TNG individuals in general: respect for a patient's pronouns and chosen name, use of empirically supported protocols, support in addressing internalized shame, and an earnest commitment to self-reflection, continuing education, and cultural humility.

Self-determination (e.g., the agency a patient has in navigating their gender identity, care options, and treatment plans) is a central component of gender-affirming psychiatric care. This is especially pertinent among TNG older adults who may be experiencing a loss of agency because of others being involved in their care, as is common among aging adults. For example, an adult child who is caring for a TNG older parent may use incorrect pronouns or disregard their TNG identity entirely, which inherently influences a clinician to proceed in the same manner. Clinicians should advocate for the patient and adhere to the patient's self-identified name and pronouns, regardless of disagreement from family or others.

As clinicians interact with more TNG older adults, it is important to note that patients may be in differing stages of social or medical transition (Fabbre 2014). As a result, TNG patients will differ in terms of gender presentation and expression. Moreover, many TNG individuals convey signs of medical mistrust (D'Avanzo et al. 2019; Ho et al. 2021). This is understandable, especially as many TNG older adults have experienced poor care, maltreatment, and discrimination throughout their lifetimes (Willis et al. 2020; Witten 2016). Clinicians should anticipate potential mistrust and work toward establishing a warm patient-clinician relationship at the outset. For example, clinicians should introduce themselves with their own name and pronouns, ask if the patient would like to share the same information, and explain the intent behind each question throughout the interview. Clinicians should also ensure that they use a patient's chosen name and pronouns in documentation, including electronic health records (EHRs), if the patient consents.

One way of implementing comprehensive, gender-affirming psychiatric care is through an interdisciplinary collaborative care (ICC) model (Ducheny et al. 2017). ICC transcends institutionalized models of health care by centering ICC teams that contain individuals of varying professional backgrounds (e.g., psychiatrist, internist, social worker) to foster mutual exchange of knowledge, which improves the ability of each team member to address patients' needs comprehensively. An example ICC team caring for a TNG older adult may consist of a psychiatrist, primary care clinician, palliative care nurse, and legal advocate. This team works together to establish affirmative care pathways to successfully provide gender-affirming primary and psychiatric care, as well as referrals to gender-affirming specialty procedures (e.g., electrolysis, facial gender-affirming surgery), nursing homes, or hospice care while considering multiple axes of TNG older adult care and personhood. In building these affirmative-care pathways, ICC teams share knowledge of gender-affirming care and resources between team members who have more or less experience in the field, resulting in more effectual care for TNG older adults.

This model of care has been implemented in several hospitals and community health care centers that serve TNG adults, such as Fenway Health in Boston (Reisner et al. 2015); Howard Brown Health in Chicago; Legacy Community Health in Houston; the Los Angeles LGBT Center; and the Mount Sinai Center for Transgender Medicine and Surgery in New York

(Shin et al. 2021). Clinicians at Columbia University Medical Center have successfully implemented the Elder LGBT Interprofessional Collaborative Care Program, which provides interdisciplinary care for Two-Spirit, lesbian, gay, bisexual, transgender, queer, intersex, asexual, and more (2SLGBTQIA+) older adults in New York (Kwong et al. 2017). Although too few programs specifically address the multifaceted needs of TNG older adults, systematic assessment of those needs is ongoing in urban and rural settings (Dakin et al. 2020; Niemet and Rice 2022). We are optimistic that health centers can build on existing infrastructures to seamlessly incorporate ICC models for TNG older adults in the near future (Gruss and Hasnain 2021).

In some cases, clinicians may find that TNG older adults strongly advocate for their health care choices and treatment plans. Although some clinicians may perceive this as a sign of unwillingness for collaboration or resistance to care, we encourage clinicians to understand this behavior as a protective mechanism in the context of long-standing health care structures that have been historically damaging to TNG communities. Additionally, TNG older adults facing ageism in many settings may perceive younger clinicians as disrespectful of their age and lived experiences. Clinicians are encouraged to consider the self-determination of TNG older adults and support their active participation in their own care.

Many clinicians of older adults protest that sexuality is outside of their scope of practice (Haesler et al. 2016), but sexual intimacy is pertinent to older adult experiences and warrants clinical consideration. Indeed, positive sexual behaviors are related to decreased anxiety and distress and increased self-esteem and quality of life (Holt et al. 2021; Srinivasan et al. 2019). The literature on sexual intimacy among TNG older adults is scant, but guidelines for TNG adults can be extrapolated from studies on intimacy among aging sexual minority populations (Lawton et al. 2014). Open, nonjudgmental communication between mental health clinicians, TNG older adult patients, and their sexual partners is pivotal for addressing intimacy concerns. For TNG older adults who have undergone gender-affirming procedures, ICC teams inclusive of psychiatrists, urologists, plastic surgeons, gynecologists, and sex therapists may be most effective in comprehensively meeting sexual intimacy needs and providing sexual health care.

MENTAL HEALTH CARE ACROSS ELDER CARE SETTINGS

As adults become more infirm with age, many clinicians refer them to community-based (e.g., residential) supportive or long-term care settings to facilitate activities of daily living and provide social support. Some older adults prefer to "age in place," receiving supportive services and clinical care in their home; yet 2SLGBTQIA+ older adults describe internal and/or external pressure to "straighten up" their homes (e.g., remove photos and books, wear different clothing) for clinician visits, fearing mistreatment if clinicians were to discover their sexual orientation or gender identity.

Most older adults wish to avoid nursing homes and long-term care facilities, and many TNG older adults are particularly reluctant, as they can be sites of immense anti-TNG discrimination and prejudice. Indeed, several systematic and integrative reviews have highlighted that most medical staff in such facilities are untrained and ill-equipped to provide affirming care for TNG older adults, toward whom they often retain negative attitudes (Caceres et al. 2020; Fasullo et al. 2021). Egregiously unaffirming practices can result, such as a transgender woman being assigned to the same room as a cisgender man. This was exemplified in a 2022 court case in which a transgender woman was refused care at an assisted living facility in Maine. The plaintiff and defendant reached a settlement consisting of new comprehensive transgender nondiscrimination policies to be adopted at all facilities operated by Adult Family Care Homes of Maine, as well as LGBT-competency training for all employees (GLBTQ Legal Advocates and Defenders 2022).

Many TNG older adults feel pressure to detransition (i.e., cease or reverse an already-initiated social or medical gender affirmation process) or actively conceal their identities out of fear of being misgendered, verbally ridiculed, or abused (Arthur 2015). In one internationally distributed study of 1,963 TNG adults (922 of whom were older than 50), a large proportion of respondents noted fear of future illness and involuntary disclosure of their TNG identities that would result in withdrawal or refusal of care at the end of their lives (Witten 2014a). Many TNG older adults also expressed concern about being grouped with sexual minority older adults, without specific care for their distinct TNG identities (Witten 2014a). These fears result in material effects on mental and physical health (Hendricks and Testa 2012): it has been shown that fear of accessing health care services (e.g., transitional and long-term care) is associated with increased levels of depressive symptoms and stress (Fredriksen-Goldsen et al. 2014).

Research comprehensively demonstrates that there are significant gaps in caring for TNG older adults in long-term-care settings, which results in anticipatory fear and damage to mental and physical well-being. Clinicians are encouraged to advocate for and incorporate gender-affirming approaches to transitional and long-term care, especially as a growing number of TNG individuals reach later life. This includes development of staff training, instatement of institutional policies and protections for TNG older adults, and equitable ombudsman structures that protect against TNG discrimination and abuse.

ADVANCE CARE PLANNING AND END-OF-LIFE PREPARATIONS

A common concern for all aging patients is advance care planning: the verbal and legal documentation of one's care preferences in the event of life-limiting illnesses or the inability to speak for oneself (e.g., dementia, comatose state). Without formal documentation of a patient's wishes for care or the appointment of a health care proxy, the law identifies next of kin (usually spouse, children, or other biological family) for substituted decision-making. This can be very stressful for LGBQ+ and TNG older adults, who may not have a spouse or children or may be estranged from their biological family. Studies have shown that TNG older adults are largely unaware of how to undertake advanced care planning (Witten 2014a), and along with most patients are generally uncomfortable in initiating end-of-life discussions with clinicians (Hughes and Cartwright 2014). To ensure patient autonomy, psychiatrists and mental health clinicians should facilitate such discussions early on, before patients experience possible cognitive decline.

Although there is a dearth of literature on TNG older adult experiences in navigating end-of-life and palliative care, commonalities can be derived from literature on the experiences of older sexual minority people. Multiple studies demonstrate the importance of nonjudgmental clinician-patient communication, an emphasis on spirituality and palliative care options rather than extensive life-extending treatments, hesitance toward institution-based care owing to anticipated discrimination, and inclusion of significant others to provide logistical and emotional support (Harding et al. 2012; Stinchcombe et al. 2017).

Additionally, TNG hospice patients have expressed concern about how their gender identity will be respected and honored in death certificates, burial practices, and headstones, particularly among family members or institutions that are not TNG affirming. Clinicians can support their patients by exploring these issues and ensuring that the patient has legally recognized documents identifying their final wishes.

CASE STUDIES

Case Example: Michael

Michael (he/him) was born in 1951 and assigned female at birth. Growing up in a small, Midwestern town, he gravitated toward boys' clothing and activities and was considered a "tomboy." Michael recalled the moment he heard about Christine Jorgensen: he felt, for the first time, that there was someone else like him. At the age of 20, with his family's support, Michael underwent "sex reassignment surgery" at a Midwestern hospital. During the subsequent decades, he moved to a different state, pursued a career, married, and raised a family. He kept his past a secret from everyone but his wife, seeing only negative public attention of transgender issues during the rare moments they were discussed. When his children were adults, he shared his gender journey with them, which was difficult for them to acknowledge. Two of his children became estranged from him, but the other two have come to understand and support his identity. Today, in his 70s, Michael is successfully aging and is out as a transgender man in many aspects of his life.

Case Example: Miranda

Miranda (she/her) was born in 1956 in New York. Assigned male at birth, she knew early on that others' expectations of her gender did not align with her internal identity as a girl. At that young age, she knew she would be teased if she acted like a girl, so she worked to develop the "boy side" for all to see. From her teenage years to young adulthood, she was plagued by alcohol use disorder and depression, and she often thought that taking her own life was her only option. To better understand her persistent feeling of being a woman, she sought people and communities with similar experiences, but she was unable to identify any that fit. Miranda felt that drag queens were performers, transvestites were cross-dressing for pleasure, and although "transsexual" seemed to be the closest identity that resonated with how she felt internally, the term felt too surgery focused. Miranda faced intense gender dysphoria for years, until she came out as transgender in 2016 at the age of 60 and embraced her womanhood legally, medically, and socially. Invigorated by her newfound gender affirmation, she also worked to become sober and experienced a more hopeful lens for her future. Today, she works with a health care organization helping older TNG people. No more secrets: simply a proud woman, happy to finally be herself.

When clinicians engage with TNG older adults, it is important to consider their age, lived experiences, stages of TNG identity and expression, and the intersections of these characteristics. In the first case example, Michael transitioned at the age of 20 as a young adult and was thus able to integrate his TNG identity into his emerging sense of self. He pursued a meaningful career, cared for his family, and lived the next 50 years as his authentic self.

Comparatively, for Miranda, who was 60 years old when she came out as transgender, much of her adult life was overshadowed by her gender dysphoria, which contributed to her depression, suicidality, and alcoholism. At a time when many peers were thinking about retirement, Miranda was developing her newfound identity as a woman, a process most had done much earlier in their lives. It is clear from these examples that the experiences of older TNG adults are highly heterogeneous; thus, psychiatric care for this population must be individualized.

RESILIENCE OF TNG OLDER ADULTS

TNG older adults have endured—and continue to endure—long-standing adversities across their life span with respect to health care, social services, employment, housing, and education. In spite of this, TNG older adults demonstrate immense resilience and resourcefulness in navigating their lives and aging successfully (McFadden et al. 2013; Witten 2014b). Indeed, one study has shown that suicidal ideation seems to lessen as TNG individuals age, which is posited to be associated with increased resilience and coping skills (Nuttbrock et al. 2010).

Multiple factors foster resilience among TNG older adults, including social support and community connectedness, which are both associated with positive mental health and well-being among this population (Fredriksen-Goldsen et al. 2014). Many TNG older adults cultivate social support through their *chosen family*, a group of individuals who choose each other, whether implicitly or explicitly, to provide mutual emotional, physical, and financial support (Knauer 2016). This is uniquely important for 2SLGBTQIA+ older adults, especially those who face rejection from their family of origin or society at large.

Programs and organizations, such as the Transgender Aging Network, can also serve as the foundation for building community among TNG older adults. In addition to providing culturally responsive training to health care professionals on affirming care for TNG older adults, the LGBTQIA+ Aging Project at the Fenway Institute offers community programming for LGBQ+ and TNG older adults. These programs all foster resilience and social support, thereby benefiting the mental health and well-being of TNG older adults. Psychiatrists and mental health clinicians ought to consider the positive impact of social support and community connectedness and refer TNG older adult patients to community organizations accordingly.

CONCLUSION

In this chapter, we provide a broad overview of considerations for clinicians providing comprehensive gender-affirming psychiatric care to TNG older adults, including 1) self-awareness regarding one's cultural responsiveness (or lack thereof) with respect to gender-affirming psychiatric care; 2) continuing education on psychiatric care needs for TNG patients; 3) attending to community-centered engagement with TNG individuals; and 4) continually challenging societal prejudice against TNG older adults at individual, interpersonal, and structural levels.

REFERENCES

Adams N, Hitomi M, Moody C: Varied reports of adult transgender suicidality: synthesizing and describing the peer-reviewed and gray literature. Transgend Health 2(1):60–75, 2017 28861548

Aldwin CM, Spiro A III, Park CL: Health, behavior, and optimal aging: A life span developmental perspective, in Handbook of the Psychology of Aging. Edited by Birren JE, Schaie KW, Abeles RP, et al. Cambridge, MA, Academic Press, 2006, pp 85–104

Aldwin CM, Igarashi H, Gilmer DF, Levenson MR: Health, Illness, and Optimal Aging: Biological and Psychosocial Perspectives. Berlin, Springer, 2017

American Psychiatric Association: Diagnostic and Statistical Manual of Mental Disorders, 3rd Edition. Washington, DC, American Psychiatric Association, 1980

American Psychological Association: Guidelines for psychological practice with transgender and gender nonconforming people. Am Psychol 70(9):832–864, 2015 26653312

Arthur DP: Social work practice with LGBT elders at end of life: developing practice evaluation and clinical skills through a cultural perspective. J Soc Work End Life Palliat Care 11(2):178–201, 2015 26380926

Bowleg L: Evolving intersectionality within public health: from analysis to action. Am J Public Health 111(1):88–90, 2021 33326269

Brevard A: Woman I Was Not Born to Be: A Transsexual Journey. Philadelphia, PA, Temple University Press, 2011

Brown A: About 5% of young adults in the U.S. say their gender is different from their sex assigned at birth. Pew Research Center, June 7, 2022. Available at: https://www.pewresearch.org/fact-tank/2022/06/07/about-5-of-young-adults-in-the-u-s-say-their-gender-is-different-from-their-sex-assigned-at-birth/. Accessed June 19, 2022.

Caceres BA, Travers J, Primiano JE, et al: Provider and LGBT individuals' perspectives on LGBT issues in long-term care: a systematic review. Gerontologist 60(3):e169–e183, 2020 30726910

Cook-Daniels L: Understanding transgender elders, in Handbook of LGBT Elders: An Interdisciplinary Approach to Principles, Practices, and Policies. Berlin, Springer, 2016, pp 285–308

Dakin EK, Williams KA, MacNamara MA: Social support and social networks among LGBT older adults in rural southern Appalachia. J Gerontol Soc Work 63(8):768–789, 2020 32558626

D'Avanzo PA, Bass SB, Brajuha J, et al: Medical mistrust and PrEP perceptions among transgender women: a cluster analysis. Behav Med 45(2):143–152, 2019 31343968

Davy Z: The DSM-5 and the politics of diagnosing transpeople. Arch Sex Behav 44(5):1165–1176, 2015 26054486

Downing JM, Przedworski JM: Health of transgender adults in the U.S., 2014–2016. Am J Prev Med 55(3):336–344, 2018 30031640

Ducheny K, Hendricks ML, Keo-Meier CL: TGNC-affirmative interdisciplinary collaborative care, in Affirmative Counseling and Psychological Practice With Transgender and Gender Nonconforming Clients. Edited by Singh A, Dickey LM. Washington, DC, American Psychological Association, 2017

Elder GH Jr: Time, human agency, and social change: perspectives on the life course. Soc Psychol Q 57:4–15, 1994

Fabbre VD: Gender transitions in later life: the significance of time in queer aging. J Gerontol Soc Work 57(2-4):161–175, 2014 24798691

Factor RJ, Rothblum ED: A study of transgender adults and their non-transgender siblings on demographic characteristics, social support, and experiences of violence. J LGBT Health Res 3(3):11–30, 2007 19042902

Fasullo K, McIntosh E, Buchholz SW, et al: LGBTQ older adults in long-term care settings: an integrative review to inform best practices. Clin Gerontol 45(5):1087–1102, 2021 34233601

Fredriksen-Goldsen KI, Cook-Daniels L, Kim H-J, et al: Physical and mental health of transgender older adults: an at-risk and underserved population. Gerontologist 54(3):488–500, 2014 23535500

Gaveras EM, Fabbre VD, Gillani B, Sloan S: Understanding past experiences of suicidal ideation and behavior in the life narratives of transgender older adults. Qualitative Social Work 22(1), 2021

GLBTQ Legal Advocates and Defenders: Transgender woman reaches landmark settlement with Maine assisted living facility that denied her a room. GLAD, June 13, 2022. Available at: https://www.glad.org/post/transgender-woman-reaches-landmark-settlement-with-maine-assisted-living-facility-that-denied-her-a-room/. Accessed July 1, 2022.

Gruss V, Hasnain M: Building the future geriatrics workforce through transformative interprofessional education and community-engaged experiential learning. J Interprof Educ Pract 22:100389, 2021

Haesler E, Bauer M, Fetherstonhaugh D: Sexuality, sexual health and older people: a systematic review of research on the knowledge and attitudes of health professionals. Nurse Educ Today 40:57–71, 2016 27125151

Harding R, Epiphaniou E, Chidgey-Clark J: Needs, experiences, and preferences of sexual minorities for end-of-life care and palliative care: a systematic review. J Palliat Med 15(5):602–611, 2012 22401314

Hendricks ML, Testa RJ: A conceptual framework for clinical work with transgender and gender nonconforming clients: an adaptation of the minority stress model. Prof Psychol Res Pr 43(5):460–467, 2012

Herman JL, Brown TN, Haas AP: Suicide thoughts and attempts among transgender adults: findings from the 2015 U.S. Transgender Survey. 2019. Available at: https://escholarship.org/uc/item/1812g3hm. Accessed July 17, 2023.

Ho IK, Sheldon TA, Botelho E: Medical mistrust among women with intersecting marginalized identities: a scoping review. Ethn Health 27:1733–1751, 2021 34647832

Holt M, Broady T, Callander D, et al: Sexual experience, relationships, and factors associated with sexual and romantic satisfaction in the first Australian Trans and Gender Diverse Sexual Health Survey. International Journal of Transgender Health 24(1):38–48, 2021

Hughes M, Cartwright C: LGBT people's knowledge of and preparedness to discuss end-of-life care planning options. Health Soc Care Community 22(5):545–552, 2014 24935483

Jarrett BA, Peitzmeier SM, Restar A, et al: Gender-affirming care, mental health, and economic stability in the time of COVID-19: a multi-national, cross-sectional study of transgender and nonbinary people. PLoS One 16(7):e0254215, 2021 34242317

Kcomt L: Profound health-care discrimination experienced by transgender people: rapid systematic review. Soc Work Health Care 58(2):201–219, 2019 30321122

Knauer NJ: LGBT older adults, chosen family, and caregiving. J Law Relig 31(2):150–168, 2016

Kwong J, Bockting W, Gabler S, et al: Development of an interprofessional collaborative practice model for older LGBT adults. LGBT Health 4(6):442–444, 2017 28170293

Lawton A, White J, Fromme EK: End-of-life and advance care planning considerations for lesbian, gay, bisexual, and transgender patients #275. J Palliat Med 17(1):106–108, 2014 24351127

Linscott B, Krinsky L: Engaging underserved populations: outreach to LGBT elders of color. Generations 40(2):34–37, 2016

McFadden SH, Frankowski S, Flick H, Witten TM: Resilience and multiple stigmatized identities: Lessons from transgender persons' reflections on aging, in Positive Psychology: Advances in Understanding Adult Motivation. Berlin, Springer Science + Business Media, 2013, pp 247–267

Meyerowitz J: How Sex Changed: A History of Transsexuality in the United States. Cambridge, MA, Harvard University Press, 2004

Niemet CJ, Rice K: LGBTQ&A: development of a needs assessment to define access, needs, and barriers to health care services among LGBTQ older adults. J Prev Interv Community 50(1):8–22, 2022 34605360

Nuttbrock L, Hwahng S, Bockting W, et al: Psychiatric impact of gender-related abuse across the life course of male-to-female transgender persons. J Sex Res 47(1):12–23, 2010 19568976

Reisner SL, Bradford J, Hopwood R, et al: Comprehensive transgender healthcare: the gender affirming clinical and public health model of Fenway Health. J Urban Health 92(3):584–592, 2015 25779756

Scarpella KM: Male-to-female transsexual individuals' experience of clinical relationships: A phenomological study, in Electronic Theses and Dissertations. Denver, CO, University of Denver, 2010

Shin SJ, Pang JH, Tiersten L, et al: The Mount Sinai interdisciplinary approach to perioperative care improved the patient experience for transgender individuals. Transgend Health 7(5):449–452, 2022 36644486

Siverskog A: Ageing bodies that matter: age, gender and embodiment in older transgender people's life stories. NORA-Nordic J Feminist Gend Res 23(1):4–19, 2015

Slagstad K: The political nature of sex: transgender in the history of medicine. N Engl J Med 384(11):1070–1074, 2021 33534975

Srinivasan S, Glover J, Tampi RR, et al: Sexuality and the older adult. Curr Psychiatry Rep 21(10):97, 2019 31522296

Stinchcombe A, Smallbone J, Wilson K, Kortes-Miller K: Healthcare and end-of-life needs of lesbian, gay, bisexual, and transgender (LGBT) older adults: a scoping review. Geriatrics (Basel) 2(1):13, 2017 31011023

Wernick JA, Busa S, Matouk K, et al: A systematic review of the psychological benefits of gender-affirming surgery. Urol Clin North Am 46(4):475–486, 2019 31582022

White Hughto JM, Reisner SL: Social context of depressive distress in aging transgender adults. J Appl Gerontol 37(12):1517–1539, 2018 28380703

Willis P, Dobbs C, Evans E, et al: Reluctant educators and self-advocates: older trans adults' experiences of health-care services and practitioners in seeking gender-affirming services. Health Expect 23(5):1231–1240, 2020 32677100

Wilson EC, Chen Y-H, Arayasirikul S, et al: Connecting the dots: examining trans-gender women's utilization of transition-related medical care and associations with mental health, substance use, and HIV. J Urban Health 92(1):182–192, 2015 25476958

Witten TM: Graceful exits: intersection of aging, transgender identities, and the fam-ily/community. J GLBT Fam Stud 5(1–2):35–61, 2009

Witten TM: End of life, chronic illness, and trans-identities. J Soc Work End Life Pal-liat Care 10(1):34–58, 2014a 24628141

Witten TM: It's not all darkness: robustness, resilience, and successful transgender aging. LGBT Health 1(1):24–33, 2014b 26789507

Witten TM: The intersectional challenges of aging and of being a gender non-con-forming adult. Generations 40(2):63–70, 2016

Witten TM: Health and well-being of transgender elders. Annu Rev Gerontol Geriatr 37(1):27–41, 2017

World Professional Association for Transgender Health: Standards of Care for the Health of Transsexual, Transgender, and Gender Nonconforming People, 7th Version. East Dundee, IL, World Professional Association for Transgender Health, 2012. Available at: https://www.wpath.org/publications/soc. Accessed July 1, 2022.

CHAPTER 15

Eating Disorders and Body Image Satisfaction in Transgender, Non-binary, and/or Gender-Expansive (TNG) People

Teddy G. Goetz, M.D., M.S.
Scout Silverstein, M.P.H.
Melissa Simone, Ph.D.

TO begin this chapter, we clarify a few terms we use with intention:

- *Eating disorders:* clusters of behaviors around feeding and food that cause distress or harm to the individual; includes various disorders as defined by DSM-5 (American Psychiatric Association 2013).
- *Disordered eating:* behaviors around feeding and food that cause distress or harm to the individual, but do not meet DSM-5 criteria for an eating disorder.
- *Gender dysphoria:* distress related to incongruence between internal sense of gender and external embodiment; can refer to specific body parts or overall embodiment.
- *Body dysmorphia:* a sensation of distress related to perceived defect in appearance that is not perceptible to others, often at an obsessive level.

In this chapter, we aim to a) describe body image concerns among TNG groups; b) contextualize eating disorder risk factors in TNG groups; and c) provide recommendations for effective eating disorder treatment.

BODY IMAGE CONCERNS IN TNG GROUPS.

Recent findings suggest that TNG people have a risk of experiencing eating disorders up to eight times that of cisgender peers (Diemer et al. 2015, 2018; Guss et al. 2017; Simone et al. 2020). Such disparities are prominent in the context of unsafe weight control behaviors, such as fasting (nearly three times greater odds) or misusing laxatives (>26 times greater odds) (Guss et al. 2017). Eating disorders have the second highest mortality rate of all psychiatric illnesses (Chesney et al. 2014), so these findings are cause for concern; adequate prevention, detection, and treatment of eating disorders in TNG people is needed. Past-year self-injury, suicidal ideation, and suicide attempts occur at strikingly high rates for TNG people with eating disorders (74.8%, 75.2%, and 74.8%, respectively); for suicidal behavior, the disparity is notable: 24 times higher than cisgender women with eating disorders and 21 times higher than TNG people without eating disorders (Duffy et al. 2019).

TNG people have diverse experiences with their relationship to food and body. *Trans broken arm syndrome* is a phenomenon "wherein trans people seek care for a health concern unrelated to gender, but clinicians dismiss the concern as a consequence of being trans" (Paine 2021, p. 7). Gender dysphoria is not a universal experience, even though trans broken arm syndrome may have people believing otherwise through overdiagnosis and misdiagnosis. Analogous to trans broken arm syndrome, *fat broken arm syndrome* occurs when clinicians decline to properly investigate an obese patient's health concern, automatically assuming the patient's weight is the whole reason for the reported health concern.

Certain secondary sex characteristics (e.g., breast tissue, peri-hip tissue, general fat distribution) are partially mutable and specifically fluctuate with body size and composition. Patients may use disordered eating to reduce their dysphoria and psychological distress regarding mainstream gendered body image ideals. We affirm the adaptive function of such a form of coping. Table 15–1 shows some examples of ways that clinicians might support patients in less harmful symptomatic management of dysphoria.

Social and Environmental Factors Contributing to Eating Disorders and Body Image Concerns in TNG Populations

Minority stress theory (see Chapter 2, "Stigma and Mental Health Inequities") posits that exposure to and internalization of identity-based stigma, discrimination, and prejudice increase the risk for psychiatric pathology underlying documented health disparities (Brooks 1981), such as eating disor-

TABLE 15–1.	Physical presentations and sources of distress of gender dysphoria and associated actions		
Dysphoria item	**Source of distress**	**Patient action**	**Clinician opportunities (as desired by patient and clinically appropriate)**
Menses	Present	Restrictive eating to induce amenorrhea or oligomenorrhea	Optimize GAHT and discuss timeline for anticipated changes
			Prescribe oral contraceptives without withdrawal period
			Use progesterone-releasing intrauterine device to reduce menses
			Refer for hysterectomy (with recommendation to leave ovaries intact if not on testosterone long term, to circumvent the need for estrogen replacement)
Chest, breasts	Too large	Restrictive eating	Optimize GAHT and discuss timeline for anticipated changes
			Refer for top surgery
			Refer to physical therapy if significant back pain from binding
	Too small	Attempting weight gain, weight cycling	Optimize GAHT and discuss timeline for anticipated changes
			Refer for breast augmentation
			Refer to breast-enhancing clothing options
Hips	Too large	Restrictive eating	Optimize GAHT and discuss timeline for anticipated changes
			Refer for liposuction
			Set realistic goals (bone structure cannot change)
			Suggest targeted exercises to increase shoulder, chest, and back muscles to offset hips, under supervision of physical therapy or personal trainer, as able

TABLE 15–1. Physical presentations and sources of distress of gender dysphoria and associated actions *(continued)*

Dysphoria item	Source of distress	Patient action	Clinician opportunities (as desired by patient and clinically appropriate)
	Too small	Attempting weight gain, weight cycling	Optimize GAHT and discuss timeline for anticipated changes
			Refer for plastic surgery consult
			Refer to hip-enhancing clothing options
Face	Too round, soft	Restrictive eating	Optimize GAHT and discuss timeline for anticipated changes
			Discuss makeup techniques
			Refer for facial masculinization surgery
	Too sharp, angular	Attempting weight gain, weight cycling	Optimize GAHT and discuss timeline for anticipated changes
			Discuss makeup techniques
			Refer for facial feminization surgery
Stomach	Hourglass body shape	Attempting weight gain, weight cycling	As above for hips/chest
	Lack of hourglass body shape	Restrictive eating	As above for hips/chest
Genitals	Incongruent	Trying to increase size of pannus to not see genitals	Refer for genital gender-affirming surgery

Note. GAHT=gender-affirming hormone therapy.

der disparities among TNG young people. Relatedly, the sociocultural model for eating disorder etiology posits that socialized body image ideals in the dominant culture may be internalized and canonized, which in turn may increase the risk of unsafe weight control practices to attain a socially sanctioned body shape (Thompson et al. 1999). Existing ideals in Western cultures are Anglocentric and gendered, wherein there exists a "thin ideal" for feminine individuals and a "muscular ideal" for masculine individuals (Thompson and Cafri 2007; Thompson and Stice 2001); a model of "androgyny" signifying "very thin, white, and able-bodied" (White 2019, pp. 118) has emerged as a non-binary ideal (Yeadon-Lee 2016). The sociocultural eating disorders model has historically centered on cisgender women; however, the notion of an idealized body shape and socially sanctioned body shapes has been shown to contribute to body image concerns among TNG people (Brewster et al. 2019; Gordon et al. 2019).

Experiences of minority stress and constraining sociocultural norms differ across subgroups of TNG people, as a result of divergent forms of oppression and marginalization. Different subgroups of gender identities often experience distinct forms of sociocultural pressure, access to resources, manifestations of stigma-related stressors, and idealized body shapes (Brewster et al. 2014; Crenshaw 1991). Accordingly, case studies have described how eating disorder behaviors can function differently across subgroups of TNG young people. For example, eating disorder symptoms may emerge in trans men to suppress characteristics associated with sex predicted at birth, whereas trans women may develop eating disorder patterns similar to cisgender women striving to attain a thin ideal (Hepp and Milos 2002; Strandjord et al. 2015). Moreover, some research suggests that genderqueer and non-binary individuals exhibit higher rates of eating disorders than their peers who identify along the gender binary (Goldberg et al. 2019); this may be partially attributed to more frequent experiences of being misgendered (Goldberg et al. 2019) or efforts to attain an androgynous, narrow body (Galupo et al. 2021; Rankin and Beemyn 2012).

Physical and personal safety make up another domain that may be attributed to eating disorder risk among TNG groups. Violence, discrimination, and harassment are more likely to be endured by transgender people, particularly transgender women of color, and these experiences can impact the relationship to food and body (Gordon et al. 2016). Other factors that can influence the likelihood of a TNG person developing an eating disorder or the acuity of an already existing eating disorder: isolation from Two-Spirit, lesbian, gay, bisexual, transgender, queer, intersex, asexual, and more (2SLGBTQIA+) community spaces; identity erasure in media and physical surroundings; housing and employment discrimination; rejection from support systems upon disclosure of TNG identity; and increased rates of suicidal ideation.

Transgender youth who experience significant minority stress are more likely to develop eating disorders (Watson et al. 2017). There is also a growing body of research correlating financial insecurity and consequential food scarcity with increased eating disorder symptomatology among 2SLGBTQIA+ young adults (Arikawa et al. 2021). Underscoring much of this health disparity are gendered body, exercise, and eating ideals. It is important to understand that gender dysphoria is often foundationally a reaction to rigid and oppressive gender ideals that are rooted in cissexism, ableism, and white supremacy (Harrison 2021).

Social media can serve as an important tool for prevention and care by increasing visibility, promoting health education materials, serving as a space for recovery communities, and facilitating communication and coalition-building. Social media enables TNG people with eating disorders to engage with a wider range of eating disorder clinicians and people living with or in recovery from eating disorders. Few resources are specifically designed for TNG and intersex people with eating disorders, so social media enables these communities to feel seen and understood. Safety, comfort, and community belonging can be generated by "bite-sized" content.

Simultaneously, societal gender norms and Anglocentric beauty ideals are coded into these platforms (Marino 2006; Noble 2018), including whichever implicit biases the programmers hold (likely anti-TNG) (Axt et al. 2021; Wang-Jones et al. 2017). Such *algorithms of oppression*, as coined by critical race and information scholar Safiya Umoja Noble (2018), shape the ways that social media platforms code, force, and thus reinforce cisnormative binary gender norms that erase transness and gender diversity. This manifests in the popular social media digital filters (e.g., Snapchat, Instagram) that distort facial features, offering users a way to interact with and manipulate their own image. Such filters can be particularly fraught for TNG persons and those with body image concerns.

So-called gender-swap filters offer a particularly rich opportunity for considering the emotional impacts of cisnormative facial gender signifiers. Indeed, a mixed-methods study explored the emotional impact of cisnormative facial gender signifiers, through the literal lens of the Snapchat gender-swap filters, with 27 TNG adults. Participants' descriptions of gendered legibility markers for "men" and "women" were consistent with one another and with their descriptions of and measurements from the filtered gender-swap selfies (e.g., for men: wide jaw, forehead, and neck; thick eyebrows; beard; for women: large eyes and lips; lower hairline; long hair; makeup) (Goetz 2021). Notably, there was a clear disjunction between TNG participants' fantasies for their gendered features and legibility and the discomfort associated with filters accentuating such stereotyped features, which suggests that fantasy around digitally altered images and social media is not predictive of real-life satisfaction

(Goetz 2021). More work is clearly needed during this era of widespread engagement with filter use, and social media use more broadly.

Gender-Affirming Care and Body Dysphoria

Although access to gender-affirming care is understood to be a protective factor, it is essential to recognize how gender dysphoria can intensify or shift with gender-affirming care. It can be very destabilizing if undesired effects of otherwise-desired gender-affirming hormone therapy (GAHT) occur. A person seeking gender-affirming surgery may experience heightened distress around the appearance of their surgical results or, upon alleviation of one source of dysphoria, subsequently develop more pronounced distress about a part of their body toward which they were previously ambivalent.

Recent literature suggests that engagement in gender-affirming health care often reduces disordered eating (e.g., Nagata et al. 2020), but there are likely limitations to existing studies. Additionally, TNG persons may experience ambivalence about undergoing gender-affirming health care amid uncertainty about outcomes, particularly individuals who have been striving for a sense of control through disordered eating.

For example, GAHT outcomes are largely genetic (e.g., facial hair, vocal range, muscle development, acne, balding, breast/hip growth), which can make starting GAHT feel like a game of chance. If an individual desires some changes that will alleviate dysphoria (e.g., lower voice, higher muscle mass) but would be upset by others (e.g., balding, back hair), decisions around GAHT can be extremely fraught, particularly for someone already struggling to relinquish the sense of control they had found through eating disorder behaviors. Similarly, top surgery results can be asymmetrical, with some individuals developing hypertrophic or keloid scarring; many lose nipple sensation. Regarding hysterectomy, concerns might include scarring or reduced pleasure from front-hole sex. Thus an intervention intended to support recovery from disordered eating practices could still induce substantial fear in someone who nonetheless desires to change. As clinicians, we can provide space for discussing such ambivalence without judgment and with a harm-reduction approach, prioritizing patient-driven care.

When considering GAHT, TNG persons with a history of disordered eating may experience anxiety and ambivalence around the possibility of weight gain, which is a very common side effect of both estradiol and testosterone GAHT. It is important to counsel patients that the weight gain will likely be different from that experienced in their first puberty (e.g., increased muscle on testosterone and breast/hip development with estradiol) and may counterintuitively offer some alleviation of dysphoria rather than worsening it. That reduced distress regarding dysphoric fat distribution may additionally support recovery from eating disorders.

For clinicians treating TNG patients who report a history of disordered eating, and who have not previously sought treatment, we recommend taking a holistic review of the patient's health history and tailoring tests to individual needs. If possible and appropriate, clinicians can obtain a detailed laboratory and vital sign history, including weight history, from the patient's primary care clinician. If the patient has a uterus and ovaries during the period of disordered eating and reports irregular periods for that time, the possibility of functional hypothalamic amenorrhea or polycystic ovarian syndrome (PCOS) should be considered. Minimal published work specifically considers functional hypothalamic amenorrhea in TNG populations, so for the sake of adapting clinical guidelines, the conjecture can be likened to the (cisnormatively named) *female athlete triad*, which is marked by insufficient caloric intake paired with excessive exercise, resulting in functional hypothalamic amenorrhea and decreased bone density. PCOS can be a cause of oligomenorrhea without disordered eating behaviors, but it often is comorbid with eating disorders. PCOS has been shown to increase eating disorder risk and should be part of the differential diagnosis for persistent oligomenorrhea when weight is restored (Lee et al. 2017).

The two main health concerns associated with oligomenorrhea or amenorrhea for prolonged periods are endometrial hyperplasia (which may progress to endometrial cancer) and osteoporosis. If the patient is not currently menstruating without clear explanation, it is prudent to treat with a short course of progesterone to prevent endometrial hyperplasia. If the endometrium (uterine lining) has been exposed to sufficient estrogen in the preceding months to develop at all, this should induce menstruation, as would occur in causes of oligomenorrhea without low estrogen, such as PCOS. If progesterone fails to induce menstruation, recent body-wide endogenous estrogen levels may have been too suppressed to support any endometrial development, which supports a diagnosis of functional hypothalamic amenorrhea, in the absence of clinical findings suggesting much rarer pathology (e.g., a pituitary tumor). Such progesterone dosing should be completed at minimum every 6 months, as long as the patient remains in an estrogen-dominant hormonal milieu and remains amenorrheic. We acknowledge that patients with menstruation dysphoria may struggle with such a treatment plan, and each patient's care plan should be tailored to clinical context (see Table 15–1). If irregular spotting begins to occur after a prolonged history of functional hypothalamic amenorrhea, an endometrial biopsy would be reasonable to rule out endometrial cancer. Such a procedure might be difficult for patients with front-hole dysphoria; clinicians should appropriately counsel patients and consider setting aside additional time for the appointment to ensure that the patient is as comfortable as possible with the procedure.

Regarding osteoporosis, clinical guidelines from the leading endocrine societies suggest obtaining a bone mineral density scan via dual-energy x-ray absorptiometry (DXA) for a patient with ≥6 months of amenorrhea (Gordon et al. 2017). DXA scans are also typically indicated at least every 2 years for patients with severe and enduring anorexia or a documented history of malnutrition. Patients who are athletes may be asked about history of stress fractures to assess bone health, but this is a much less sensitive and specific metric.

The need for clinicians who are well trained in the nuances of treating TNG patients with eating disorders or disordered eating is immense, but there is an extreme shortage of dually competent clinicians. To address this training gap, we reiterate the importance of continuing education options in 1) gender-affirming care and basic ways to be an affirming clinician for TNG patients, and 2) eating disorders and disordered eating, particularly among those who are not cisgender women. TNG people may initiate disordered eating behaviors (e.g., dietary restriction or purging) for an array of reasons. Gender-affirming medical care has been shown to improve the quality of life for TNG people who desire medical transition (Ives et al. 2019). There are numerous common barriers to accessing such care, including legal restrictions, lack of insurance coverage, inability to secure clinician letters of support, and clinicians instituting arbitrary body mass index (BMI) limits that restrict patient eligibility for care. BMI limits are not evidence-based; of note, research has actually demonstrated that patients with increased BMI can safely pursue surgery and that BMI alone should not be a deciding factor for surgical candidacy (Ives et al. 2019). Often, prescriptive weight loss is coupled with surgical denial without the clinician screening for the presence of current or past eating disorders. To avoid causing further harm to TNG patients, clinicians should use an individualized approach to assess each patient's health using indicators such as vitals, laboratory values, and health histories (Brownstone et al. 2021).

Regrettably, it is legally permissible in many places to refuse medical care to TNG people, and current political and legal efforts aim to criminalize clinicians who treat TNG people. Fear of discrimination in health care environments can deter TNG people from seeking treatment or disclosing the severity of behaviors related to an eating disorder. This cycle of harm and avoidance leads to underdiagnosis of eating disorders in TNG populations. Much of the current literature reports diagnostic prevalence, and such statistics do not reflect the lived experience of TNG people.

TREATMENT CONSIDERATIONS

Substantial barriers to physical and mental health care services in TNG populations are well documented (James et al. 2016). Thus, TNG people with clinically significant eating disorder symptomatology may not have access to services and may go undiagnosed and untreated. Moreover, the historical emphasis on cisgender women in eating disorder etiology and treatment research has largely shaped the perceptions of eating disorders among clinicians and existing eating disorder assessments, to the detriment of TNG people struggling with eating and weight concerns. Access to an eating disorder diagnosis may increase an individual's awareness of their own eating- and weight-related concerns and provide a pathway to treatment. As such, it is imperative that clinicians attend to the unique concerns of TNG people presenting with eating- or weight-related concerns. Notably, eating disorder prevention and treatment efforts have been established to deconstruct the "thin ideal" in the media that is often internalized among cisgender women. The functions of weight control behaviors and the ideals of body image experienced among TNG people, however, do not parallel those experienced by cisgender women. Increasing evidence suggests that TNG people are at heightened risk for developing eating disorders and body image concerns, so a shift in the public perception of what an eating disorder looks like is long overdue.

TNG people may struggle to navigate eating disorder treatment environments. There is a long-perpetuated stereotype that eating disorders primarily affect white, thin, cisgender young women—in part because such demographics reflect those who have historically been able to access (typically extremely costly) treatment. When TNG people do enter treatment, their treatment teams usually lack knowledge and training about the intersection between eating disorders and TNG experience; this leads TNG patients to avoid self-disclosure of their gender identity in an effort to circumvent discrimination or backlash from staff (Thapliyal et al. 2018). In one research study, "even when a therapist was experienced as 'excellent,' there was evidence of an unexamined world view that was underpinned by the dominance of both heterosexual and dualistic gender norms" (Thapliyal et al. 2018, p. 9). For treatment environments to reach a level of cultural sensitivity that allows TNG people to attain meaningful recovery, eating disorder clinicians must engage in critical reflection, training, and continued (un)learning about how gender, race, class, body size, and disability inform the development of an eating disorder.

To meet these challenges, gender-affirming eating disorder resources specifically designed to meet TNG patients' needs, including "meal support groups, psychoeducation, family and caregiver support, crisis tools, and peer connection/coaching," can be extremely beneficial (Geilhufe et al. 2021, p. e377). Additionally, peer support, historically used in substance use disorder treatment, is an emerging treatment approach in eating disorders. In eating disorder care, it is common practice to focus on combating negative body image (Danielsen and Rø 2012). Frequently, clinicians incorporate somatic experiences through approaches that foster radical acceptance, mindfulness, and intuitive eating (Pellizzer et al. 2018). These practices may be contraindicated for people with experiences of gender dysphoria, disability, chronic illness, or other factors that jeopardize the ability to feel safe with accessing *embodiment* (inhabiting one's bodily processes). A shift from embodiment toward *attunement* (observing one's bodily processes) may be more appropriate. Methods for approaching this may include brief check-in exercises rather than dedicated, focused, and prolonged exercises to gauge hunger, discomfort, tiredness, stress responses, and other sensations. Introducing exposures that are easier to observe and tolerate may help in working toward building the capacity to tolerate more difficult emotions and sensations (Reilly et al. 2017).

In light of the current limitations of the field, following are brief descriptions of possible future directions.

- *Integrated care model:* For TNG people whose disordered eating is at least partially rooted in gender dysphoria, integrating care could offer overall higher-quality treatment and improved patient experience. Integrating care involves coordination and transparency between the clinicians providing mental health care, GAHT, and gender-affirming surgery (as applicable), with specific attention to developing alternative coping mechanisms and a more congruent and affirmed self-image. Further research is needed to develop and test such treatment structures.
- *Tailored interventions:* Most current interventions for eating disorders are designed for cisgender women—or more specifically, young, white, cisgender women. Research is needed to develop evidence-based interventions for TNG populations specifically.
- *Gender-expansive treatment standards:* The current treatment guidelines for weight restoration are divided according to a binary understanding of gender. Such paradigms cause confusion and limit the targeted care for TNG patients, from puberty blockers to GAHT and gender-affirming surgery. Research is needed to define best practices to offer equitable health care for TNG patients.

REFERENCES

American Psychiatric Association: Diagnostic and Statistical Manual of Mental Disorders, 5th Edition. Arlington, VA, American Psychiatric Association, 2013

Arikawa AY, Ross J, Wright L, et al: Results of an online survey about food insecurity and eating disorder behaviors administered to a volunteer sample of self-described LGBTQ+ young adults aged 18 to 35 years. J Acad Nutr Diet 121(7):1231–1241, 2021 33158800

Axt JR, Conway MA, Westgate EC, Buttrick NR: Implicit transgender attitudes independently predict beliefs about gender and transgender people. Pers Soc Psychol Bull 47(2):257–274, 2021 32608330

Brownstone LM, DeRieux J, Kelly DA, et al: Body mass index requirements for gender-affirming surgeries are not empirically based. Transgend Health 6(3):121–124, 2021 34414267

Brewster ME, Velez BL, Esposito J, et al: Moving beyond the binary with disordered eating research: a test and extension of objectification theory with bisexual women. J Couns Psychol 61(1):50–62, 2014 24188653

Brewster ME, Velez BL, Breslow AS, Geiger EF: Unpacking body image concerns and disordered eating for transgender women: the roles of sexual objectification and minority stress. J Couns Psychol 66(2):131–142, 2019 30702325

Brooks VR: Minority Stress and Lesbian Women. Blue Ridge Summit, PA, Lexington Books, 1981

Chesney E, Goodwin GM, Fazel S: Risks of all-cause and suicide mortality in mental disorders: a meta-review. World Psychiatry 13(2):153–160, 2014 24890068

Crenshaw K: Mapping the margins: intersectionality, identity politics, and violence against women of color. Stanford Law Rev 43(6):1241–1299, 1991

Danielsen M, Rø Ø: Changes in body image during inpatient treatment for eating disorders predict outcome. Eat Disord 20(4):261–275, 2012 22703568

Diemer EW, Grant JD, Munn-Chernoff MA, et al: Gender identity, sexual orientation, and eating-related pathology in a national sample of college students. J Adolesc Health 57(2):144–149, 2015 25937471

Diemer EW, White Hughto JM, Gordon AR, et al: Beyond the binary: differences in eating disorder prevalence by gender identity in a transgender sample. Transgend Health 3(1):17–23, 2018 29359198

Duffy ME, Henkel KE, Joiner TE: Prevalence of self-injurious thoughts and behaviors in transgender individuals with eating disorders: a national study. J Adolesc Health 64(4):461–466, 2019 30314865

Galupo MP, Pulice-Farrow L, Pehl E: "There is nothing to do about it": nonbinary individuals' experience of gender dysphoria. Transgend Health 6(2):101–110, 2021 34414266

Geilhufe B, Tripp O, Silverstein S, et al: Gender-affirmative eating disorder care: clinical considerations for transgender and gender expansive children and youth. Pediatr Ann 50(9):e371–e378, 2021 34542335

Goetz TG: Swapping gender is a Snap(chat): limitations of (trans) gendered legibility within binary digital and human filters. Catalyst 7(2):1–31, 2021

Goldberg AE, Kuvalanka KA, Budge SL, et al: Health care experiences of transgender binary and nonbinary university students. Couns Psychol 47(1):59–97, 2019

Gordon AR, Austin SB, Krieger N, et al: "I have to constantly prove to myself, to people, that I fit the bill": perspectives on weight and shape control behaviors among low-income, ethnically diverse young transgender women. Soc Sci Med 165:141–149, 2016

Gordon AR, Austin SB, Pantalone DW, et al: Appearance ideals and eating disorders risk among LGBTQ college students: the being ourselves living in diverse bodies (BOLD) study. J Adolesc Health 64:2,S43–S44, 2019

Gordon CM, Ackerman KE, Berga SL, et al: Functional hypothalamic amenorrhea: an Endocrine Society Clinical Practice Guideline. J Clin Endocrinol Metab 102(5):1413–1439, 2017 28368518

Guss CE, Williams DN, Reisner SL, et al: Disordered weight management behaviors, nonprescription steroid use, and weight perception in transgender youth. J Adolesc Health 60(1):17–22, 2017 28029539

Harrison DS: Belly of the Beast: The Politics of Anti-Fatness as Anti-Blackness. Berkeley, CA, North Atlantic Books, 2021

Hepp U, Milos G: Gender identity disorder and eating disorders. Int J Eat Disord 32(4):473–478, 2002 12386912

Ives GC, Fein LA, Finch L, et al: Evaluation of BMI as a risk factor for complications following gender-affirming penile inversion vaginoplasty. Plast Reconstr Surg Glob Open 7(3):e2097, 2019

James S, Herman J, Rankin S, et al: The Report of the 2015 U.S. Transgender Survey. Washington, DC, National Center for Transgender Equality, 2016

Lee I, Cooney LG, Saini S, et al: Increased risk of disordered eating in polycystic ovary syndrome. Fertil Steril 107(3):796–802, 2017 28104244

Marino MC: Critical code studies, in Electronic Book Review. Cambridge, MA, MIT Press, 2006

Nagata JM, Murray SB, Compte EJ, et al: Community norms for the Eating Disorder Examination Questionnaire (EDE-Q) among transgender men and women. Eat Behav 37:101381, 2020 32416588

Noble SU: Algorithms of Oppression: How Search Engines Reinforce Racism. New York, NYU Press, 2018

Paine EA: "Fat broken arm syndrome": negotiating risk, stigma, and weight bias in LGBTQ healthcare. Soc Sci Med 270:113609, 2021 33401217

Pellizzer ML, Tiggemann M, Waller G, Wade TD: Measures of body image: confirmatory factor analysis and association with disordered eating. Psychol Assess 30(2):143–153, 2018 28277693

Rankin S, Beemyn G: Beyond a binary: the lives of gender-nonconforming youth. About Campus 17(4):2–10, 2012

Reilly EE, Anderson LM, Gorrell S, et al: Expanding exposure-based interventions for eating disorders. Int J Eat Disord 50(10):1137–1141, 2017 28815659

Simone M, Askew A, Lust K, et al: Disparities in self-reported eating disorders and academic impairment in sexual and gender minority college students relative to their heterosexual and cisgender peers. Int J Eat Disord 53(4):513–524, 2020 31943285

Strandjord SE, Ng H, Rome ES: Effects of treating gender dysphoria and anorexia nervosa in a transgender adolescent: lessons learned. Int J Eat Disord 48(7):942–945, 2015 26337148

Thapliyal P, Hay P, Conti J: Role of gender in the treatment experiences of people with an eating disorder: a metasynthesis. J Eat Disord 6(1):18, 2018 30123504

Thompson JK, Cafri G: The Muscular Ideal: Psychological, Social, and Medical Perspectives. Washington, DC, American Psychological Association, 2007

Thompson JK, Stice E: Thin-ideal internalization: mounting evidence for a new risk factor for body-image disturbance and eating pathology. Curr Dir Psychol Sci 10(5):181–183, 2001

Thompson JK, Heinberg LJ, Altabe M, Tantleff-Dunn S: Exacting Beauty: Theory, Assessment, and Treatment of Body Image Disturbance. Washington, DC, American Psychological Association, 1999

Wang-Jones T, Alhassoon OM, Hattrup K, et al: Development of gender identity implicit association tests to assess attitudes toward transmen and transwomen. Psychol Sex Orientat Gend Divers 4(2):169–183, 2017

Watson RJ, Veale JF, Saewyc EM: Disordered eating behaviors among transgender youth: probability profiles from risk and protective factors. Int J Eat Disord 50(5):515–522, 2017 27862124

White FR: Embodying the fat/trans intersection, in Thickening Fat. Boston, MA, Routledge, 2019, pp 110–121

Yeadon-Lee T: What's the story? Exploring online narratives of non-binary gender identities. Int J Interdisciplinary Soc Commun Stud 11(2):19–34, 2016

Substance Use Disorders Within Transgender, Nonbinary, and/or Gender-Expansive (TNG) Communities

Kevin Johnson, M.D.
Laura Erickson-Schroth, M.D.
Alann Weissman-Ward, M.D.

SUBSTANCE use disorders (SUDs), also known as addiction, refer to the use of substances in a way that can cause significant disruptions or problems. Those with SUDs may struggle to reduce or stop their use despite repeated efforts, even though they see the harm inflicted by use. They may require escalating doses to get the same effect or to curb debilitating withdrawal symptoms. They may compulsively use the drug or spend significant time acquiring, using, or recovering from it. Cravings may induce severe distraction or drive to use (American Psychiatric Association 2022). Many individuals with SUDs are not aware of it or do not connect their problems to drug use (Galanter et al. 2015).

Transgender, nonbinary, and gender-expansive (TNG) youth and adults are more likely to use substances or develop SUDs than their cisgender peers (Connolly and Gilchrist 2020; Day et al. 2017; de Freitas et al. 2020; Frost et al. 2021; Hughto et al. 2021; Keuroghlian et al. 2015; Ruppert et al. 2021). According to one large survey (James et al. 2016), TNG adults were three times more likely to report illicit drug, marijuana, or nonmedical prescription drug use (NMPDU) than the general population (29% vs. 10%). Compared with cisgender peers, in a 2022 meta-analysis, TNG participants were 1.4–1.5 times more likely to report lifetime substance use and 1.8–2.1 times more likely to report current use of substances other than tobacco or alcohol (Cotaina et al. 2022). Substance use prevalence was 2.5–4 times higher for TNG youth compared with their cisgender peers in a sample of California middle and high school students (Day et al. 2017).

Individuals with SUDs—regardless of gender modality—often experience stigma and discrimination in health care settings, the legal system, the workplace, and other environments. In health care settings, many are refused medical treatment or inappropriately blamed for their medical problems (Kelly and Westerhoff 2010). This discrimination can prevent those with SUDs from seeking medical care, thus leading to poorer health outcomes. Substance use can also increase the risk of contracting HIV or hepatitis, both of which are already prevalent in TNG communities (James et al. 2016). In this chapter, we review what is known about substance use in TNG communities, why SUDs are so prevalent, and the available best practices regarding treatment and recovery.

SO WHAT DO WE CALL IT? DEFINING ADDICTION

Many terms describe substance use and addiction in research, clinical settings, and general parlance (Babor and Hall 2007; Galanter et al. 2015; Miller et al. 2019). Correct terminology makes it easier to communicate accurate clinical information, avoids undue stigma, and distinguishes a clinical disorder from any general use of a substance. Although many use the terms *addiction* or *alcoholism*, DSM-5-TR uses *substance use disorder* (American Psychiatric Association 2022; Galanter et al. 2015), because the word "addiction" has an overly negative connotation. ICD-11 similarly uses *disorders due to substance use* (World Health Organization 2019).

Other descriptors include *unhealthy, hazardous, at-risk,* or *harmful* use, which describe substance use that is excessive or that places one at risk for negative health consequences—such as heavy drinking or using more medications than prescribed—which can occur whether or not one has an SUD. *Dependency* refers to physical reliance on a substance, that is, requiring larger amounts of the substance to achieve the same effect (a.k.a. *tolerance*) or experiencing withdrawal symptoms if the substance is suddenly stopped. This can happen with prescription medications that, even if used appropriately, can become *habit forming.* NMPDU (or *prescription drug misuse*) refers to inappropriate use of prescription medications, by taking more than prescribed or for an unintended indication or taking medications prescribed to other people (Kidd et al. 2021).

Because of addiction-related stigma, terminology and language should be used mindfully in both clinical and nonclinical settings (Babor and Hall 2007; Botticelli and Koh 2016; Broyles et al. 2014; Miller et al. 2019). Patients may perceive stigmatizing language as pathologizing, labeling, or demeaning. Such language can discourage patients from seeking treatment and enforce a clinician's unconscious bias. When patients are labeled as having "substance abuse" rather than a *substance use disorder*, clinicians are more likely to recommend punitive clinical approaches (Kelly and Westerhoff 2010). Some outdated or problematic terms include "substance abuser," as the word "abuse" can also have negative connotations (Babor and Hall 2007). The terms "inappropriate use" or "problem use" may perpetuate stigma in conversations with patients (e.g., "you are inappropriate," "you are a problem") (Miller et al. 2019). Stigmatizing epithets like "junkie," "drunkard," or "drug-seeker" can also cause harm and should be avoided (Table 16–1).

Some may self-identify as "addicts" or "alcoholics" in recovery groups or other nonmedical settings, which can be an affirming or empowering reclamation of the language (Johnson and Weissman-Ward 2022); in clinical settings, however, it is more appropriate to stick with people-first language (e.g., *person with alcohol use disorder*, not "alcoholic") (Broyles et al. 2014). *SUD* and *addiction* are used interchangeably in this chapter, and we include alcohol use in the term *substance use*.

DRUGS OF ABUSE: A BRIEF PRIMER

Drugs of abuse refer to psychoactive substances that have addictive potential or carry risk of causing an SUD in users (Center for Drug Evaluation and Research 2017). They can be classified based on metrics such as chemical structure or pharmacodynamic effects.

Tobacco and Other Nicotine-Based Products

Of commonly used substances, nicotine has the highest risk of dependence (Meyer and Quenzer 2005) and the deadliest long-term sequelae (Centers for Disease Control and Prevention 2005). Half of smokers die from tobacco-related disease, including those who smoke fewer than five cigarettes a day (Bjartveit and Tverdal 2009). Nicotine is largely ingested as tobacco (e.g., cigarette, snuff, chew), although addiction via flavored vape pen is on the rise (Galanter et al. 2015). Tobacco use is a relative contraindication to estrogen gender-affirming hormone therapy (GAHT) because of the increased risk for

TABLE 16-1. Recommendations for using nonstigmatizing language

Avoid	Instead Use
Substance abuse	Substance use
	At-risk use
	Unhealthy use
	Hazardous use
	Harmful use
	Substance misuse
Drug habit, drug problem	Substance use disorder (DSM-5-TR)
	Disorders due to substance use (ICD-11)
	Substance dependency
Polysubstance abuse	Multiple substance use disorders
Addict, user, abuser, alcoholic, drunkard, crackhead, pothead, dope fiend, junkie, drug seeker	Person with addiction
	Person with a substance use disorder
Binge	Heavy drinking episode
Dirty vs. clean (drug test)	Positive or negative screen
	Detected or not detected
Clean (individual), former/reformed addict	Person in recovery
	Abstinent
	Not drinking or taking drugs
Substitution or replacement therapy, medication-assisted treatment	Treatment or medication for addiction
	Medication for addiction treatment
	Medication-assisted recovery
Addicted baby, born addicted	Baby experiencing substance withdrawal
	Babies with neonatal abstinence syndrome
Drunk, smashed, messed up	Intoxicated
	Under the influence

blood clots (Hembree et al. 2017). Surgeons highly encourage smoking cessation owing to tobacco's clear association with surgical complications including morbidity; infections; wound, pulmonary, and neurological complications; and admission to an intensive care unit (Grønkjær et al. 2014).

Tobacco use is highly prevalent in TNG communities, although subgroup prevalence is inconclusive. For example, studies conflict on whether there is more tobacco use among trans men (Buchting et al. 2017) or trans women (Gómez-Gil et al. 2018). Research on nonbinary samples has reported smoking risk comparable to that of binary TNG peers (Ruppert et al. 2021) but also a slightly increased risk (Kcomt et al. 2020). A 2022 meta-analysis of 20 different studies observed a higher odds ratio for tobacco use in TNG people, who were 1.65 times more likely to report current tobacco use compared with the cisgender population and 1.52 times more likely to report a current tobacco use disorder (Cotaina et al. 2022). Rates of cigar, e-cigarette, and other forms of nicotine use were also elevated among TNG individuals compared with their cisgender peers (Buchting et al. 2017). One study found that TNG youth were three times more likely to use cigarettes in school (De Pedro et al. 2017), but others found minimal or no difference in tobacco use between TNG and cisgender populations (Cotaina et al. 2022; James et al. 2016).

Alcohol

After caffeine, alcohol is the most commonly used psychoactive substance. Acute alcohol intoxication increases risk of violence and traffic accidents and exacerbates depression (Galanter et al. 2015). In addition to dependence, chronic alcohol use can cause numerous negative effects on most organ systems of the body, including liver cirrhosis, dementia, cardiovascular disease, and other chronic conditions. TNG people report increased rates of heavy alcohol use compared with cis peers, and trans men report higher levels of heavy drinking than trans women (Ruppert et al. 2021). Nonbinary individuals—particularly those assigned male gender at birth (AMAB)—report higher rates of heavy drinking than binary TNG peers (Ruppert et al. 2021). Gender-related psychological and physical abuse has been associated with a 3.7 times greater odds of heavy drinking among TNG adults (Nuttbrock et al. 2014). TNG high school students who identified as heterosexual or questioning their sexual orientation were at greatest risk for early initiation of alcohol use and heavy drinking in one sample (Gerke et al. 2022).

Opioids

Opioids include a combination of synthetic, endogenous, or plant-derived substances that target opioid receptors, which are also the target for endogenous opioids such as endorphins. Diacetylmorphine, also known as heroin, is also an opioid. TNG middle and high school students were more than twice as likely as cisgender peers to report use of prescription analgesics, including morphine, oxycodone, hydromorphone, and fentanyl, within the previous 30 days (De Pedro et al. 2017).

Stimulants

Stimulants refer to a class of drugs that cause an activating effect, usually through the increase of catecholamine levels. Typical stimulants are cocaine, amphetamines, methamphetamines, and methylenedioxy-methamphetamine (MDMA), although caffeine and nicotine are also classified as stimulants. Among transfeminine individuals, methamphetamine use is often associated with high-risk sexual behavior and more cocaine use within the past year than trans men (Ruppert et al. 2021). One study estimated that TNG students were more than twice as likely to use cocaine or amphetamines than cisgender peers (De Pedro et al. 2017), and another study reported higher rates of stimulant use among young trans women compared with nonbinary AMAB youth (Newcomb et al. 2020).

Sedatives and Hypnotics

Sedatives include benzodiazepines, barbiturates, and selective nonbenzodiazepine hypnotics (such as zolpidem). One study in the national Veterans Health Administration showed that TNG veterans were 50% more likely to report having a sedative use disorder than non-TNG peers (Frost et al. 2021).

Hallucinogens and Inhalants

Hallucinogens (such as LSD, PCP, ketamine, and dextromethorphan) are compounds that induce unique alteration of consciousness. TNG middle and high school students were nearly three times more likely to report use of inhalants within the previous 30 days than non-TNG peers (De Pedro et al. 2017).

Cannabis

Cannabis refers to the cannabis plant and its derivatives. Its psychoactive properties come from a variety of cannabinoids, including THC. One may smoke the plant or ingest it from a vape pen, edible, or other products. All use, whether for intoxication or medicinal purposes, poses a risk for developing cannabis use disorder. Several studies show higher rates of cannabis use among TNG people than cisgender peers (Newcomb et al. 2020; Ruppert et al. 2021). A quarter of TNG respondents in one study reported past-month marijuana use, compared with 8% of the U.S. population (James et al. 2016). Research suggests greater cannabis use among trans men than trans women; AMAB nonbinary individuals reported more cannabis use than trans men, trans women, or nonbinary individuals who were assigned female gender at birth (AFAB) (Newcomb et al. 2020).

Anabolic Steroids

Anabolic-androgenic steroids (AASs) are a family of hormones that include testosterone and > 100 of its synthetic relatives (Kanayama et al. 2010). AASs are largely legal and available without a prescription, online or outside the

United States. Hazardous AAS use among TNG people is presumed to be common, although limited data exist. Hazardous AAS is distinct from GAHT in key ways. Most AAS users primarily seek a more muscular appearance or better athletic performance, rather than to alleviate gender dysphoria. AAS doses are usually 10–100 times higher than those used for GAHT (Ip et al. 2011) and may yield serum levels 50 times the physiological range for cisgender men (Kanayama and Pope 2012). In one study, TNG youth were >7 times more likely than cisgender peers to report using "bodybuilding hormones" (Guss et al. 2017); the authors did not specify whether they were used for gender dysphoria.

Behavioral Addictions

Some develop *behavioral addictions*, or *process addictions*, which refer to behaviors that lead to *mood-altering events*, which themselves can cause pleasure and eventual dependency through repetitive or compulsive engagement in that behavior (Miller et al. 2019; Sussman et al. 2011). Identified behavioral addictions include internet use, love, sex, exercise, work, gambling, tanning, kleptomania, and compulsive spending (Miller et al. 2019; Sussman et al. 2011). Up to 47% of the U.S. adult population may suffer from a behavioral addiction with serious negative consequences (Sussman et al. 2011), and many co-occur with SUDs (Miller et al. 2019). There is a limited but revealing body of research regarding behavioral addictions or compulsive behaviors in TNG individuals (Ruppert et al. 2021). Pathological gambling was found to be three times more prevalent in a TNG sample, particularly trans women, than in cisgender peers (Rider et al. 2019). One study reported a 15.1% lifetime incidence of sex addiction among TNG participants (Mathy 2003), three to five times the national average (Derbyshire and Grant 2015). In a study of 484 TNG adults, 8% of trans men and 8.1% of trans women reported a recent history of compulsive exercise (Nagata et al. 2020). In another, 17.8% of TNG participants reported compulsive work problems, 20% food addiction, and 37% a compulsive spending problem (Mathy 2003); notably, these data were not directly compared with a cisgender control group.

MODELS OF ADDICTION: WHY ARE TNG INDIVIDUALS AT RISK?

Many people who use substances do not develop an SUD, and contrary to common misconception, drugs such as cocaine and heroin are not instantly addictive (Meyer and Quenzer 2005). So why do some people develop an SUD while others do not? And why are some groups, including TNG communities, at higher risk? Such questions have shaped development of models of addiction, over years of research and clinical practice.

Addiction models vastly differ and even conflict at some important points (Thombs 1999). Many can be incorporated into a biopsychosocial model of addiction, which incorporates a wide range of biological, psychological, and social factors that contribute to the development of an SUD (Meyer and Quenzer 2005). Biological factors include genetic vulnerabilities and the long-term effects of increased use of substances, leading to neurobiological dependence.

Psychological factors include the internalized effects of *minority stress theory*, an evidence-based framework describing how the negative impacts of discrimination can affect mental health and self-image (Hendricks and Testa 2012; Meyer and Quenzer 2005; National LGBT Health Education Center 2018) (see Chapter 2, "Stigma and Mental Health Inequities"). Among TNG populations, substance use has been correlated with numerous sequelae of minority stress: gender-related discrimination, high visual gender nonconformity, and intersectional identities, including sexual minority status (Connolly and Gilchrist 2020; Gerke et al. 2022; Keuroghlian et al. 2015; Kidd et al. 2021). Those who reported NMPDU were also more likely to report lower self-esteem, more gender-identity-based discrimination, and higher levels of anxiety, depression, and somatic distress (Benotsch et al. 2013). These psychological factors highlight the importance of learning more adaptive ways to cope with discrimination, stigma, and stress without resorting to substance use.

Substance use is associated with social factors that disproportionately affect TNG communities, including unemployment, intimate partner violence, incarceration, sex work, homelessness, or comorbid diagnoses. Structural discrimination is one of the reported factors motivating higher tobacco consumption among TNG individuals (Shires and Jaffee 2016). Interventions are often needed at an institutional or legal level to address gender-related discrimination, violence, homelessness, and abuse (Gerke et al. 2022), and there are calls for more intervention with TNG youth to provide support, education, and early intervention.

Social factors within TNG communities can also perpetuate substance use. Many studies have found that substance use can promote group solidarity within marginalized communities (Thombs 1999) and places individuals at greater risk of developing an SUD. For example, TNG social gatherings often occur in bars or places with access to substances (Cochran et al. 2007), and the relative safety and opportunity to socialize without discrimination may encourage or normalize consumption and inappropriate use (Peacock et al. 2015). Alcohol and tobacco advertisements capitalize on this by targeting TNG communities (Drabble 2000; Hunt 2012).

INTERVENTION, TREATMENT, AND MANAGEMENT

Many TNG individuals avoid seeking SUD treatment for fear of discrimination (Matsuzaka 2018). In a survey based in the District of Columbia, only 36% of participants who believed their drinking was a problem, and only 53% of those who believed they had a drug problem, sought treatment (Xavier 2000). Even when TNG people do seek treatment, there are limited effective options that meet their needs. In a small sample of people who had received SUD treatment in New York City, TNG participants reported lower therapeutic support, ability to be honest and open, feelings of connection, treatment satisfaction, current abstinence, and program completion than cisgender peers, whether LGB or straight (Senreich 2011).

Those who seek treatment may have distinct goals for recovery. Many aim for abstinence from all substances; others seek to reduce use to a more manageable level. Those who are abstinent or in treatment may consider themselves in recovery. The definition of *recovery* is context dependent, yet most agree that achieving recovery requires more than abstinence from a substance. Per a report from the U.S. Surgeon General (U.S. Department of Health and Human Services 2016), recovery "goes beyond the remission of symptoms to include a positive change in the whole person." People choose their path to recovery based on their cultural values, socioeconomic status, access to health care, psychological needs, and personal experience of SUD. Other terms include *sobriety*, often used in 12-step groups. *Clean* refers to having no substances in one's system, but this term should be avoided, as it implies those who are in active addiction are "dirty."

Assessing TNG Patients for Treatment

Addiction treatment should be person-centered. The American Society of Addiction Medicine (ASAM) suggests using six assessment dimensions to identify patient needs (Miller et al. 2019): acute intoxication and/or withdrawal; biomedical conditions and complications; emotional, behavioral, or cognitive conditions and complications; readiness to change; relapse, continued use, or continued problem potential; and recovery/living environment. This model encourages clinicians to consider how various environmental factors impact mental health, impede safe living conditions, or affect treatment retention. Such factors may include the effects of transphobia or homophobia (both internal and societal), lack of access to gender-affirming care, violence, family issues, and social isolation and may need to be addressed during treatment (Lombardi and van Servellen 2000). The dimensions also encourage the treatment of co-occurring medical and mental health conditions, which may include gender-affirming care (de Freitas et al. 2020).

These factors also assist with determining the level of care at which treatment should be initiated or adjusted. For example, some may safely begin treatment in the outpatient setting; for some, inpatient treatment may be more appropriate or necessary because of medical or environmental factors. TNG individuals can face unique challenges at all levels of care. Many programs approach treatment with the primary intent to reduce harm—commonly known as *harm reduction*—which has been known to help patients stay in treatment by increasing engagement and access to medical treatment and reducing the risk of life-threatening issues (e.g., overdose; infection with HIV or hepatitis) (Miller et al. 2019).

Inpatient Treatment

Although many TNG people seek inpatient addiction treatment services, little formal research has explored their experiences (Flentje et al. 2014). Treatment centers typically have gender-segregated housing and bathroom arrangements, and many expect participants to stay in living quarters corresponding with their gender assigned at birth. Group therapy is often divided by gender and enforced by gender assigned at birth; staff may fail to honor patients' names and pronouns. Patients also may be denied access to GAHT in inpatient addiction settings (Lyons et al. 2015; Matsuzaka 2018; Senreich 2011). In a small qualitative study of TNG people who had participated in inpatient SUD programs, those who reported having experienced stigma and violence were more likely to leave treatment prematurely than those who had support during treatment (Lyons et al. 2015). Other studies highlight the importance of having TNG clinicians or peer advocates directly involved with treatment (Glynn and van den Berg 2017; Nemoto et al. 2005). In addition, better access to gender-affirming care can enhance SUD treatment. For example, after starting GAHT, trans women report higher rates of smoking cessation (64%) compared with the national average (6.2%) (Myers and Safer 2017).

Outpatient Treatment

Outpatient treatment may refer to group therapy, individual psychotherapy, case management, or intensive outpatient treatment. Many outpatient treatment facilities segregate treatment based on gender assigned at birth and include staff who have little to no training specific to TNG individuals. Some forms of outpatient treatment can be adjusted to better meet TNG communities' needs, however. For example, *cognitive-behavioral therapy* (CBT) can be adjusted to focus on building healthier strategies for coping with TNG-specific triggers for cravings (e.g., nonconformity-related discrimination, expectations of rejection, identity concealment, internalized transphobia) (Pachankis 2015).

Relapse and Resumed Use

Relapse refers to an acute worsening of a patient's SUD, which may or may not involve returning to substance use. SUDs are considered relapsing-remitting conditions; relapse is often accepted as part of the progress toward recovery. There is a common misconception that SUDs are harder to treat than other relapsing-remitting conditions; rather, SUD relapse rates are ~10% lower than rates associated with other chronic conditions, such as hypertension and asthma (McLellan et al. 2000). Relapse carries significant overdose risk, especially for opioids or alcohol. It is important to ensure that all patients with opioid use disorders, despite their length of time without use, have access to naloxone and know how to use it.

Medication Treatment

Medication treatment (or *medication for addiction treatment*, MAT) describes therapies that ease cravings, promote abstinence, or prevent relapse. When considering medication treatment, consider possible interactions with endogenous hormone levels, GAHT, or other medications.

Methadone and Buprenorphine

Methadone and *buprenorphine* target opioid cravings. Both medications have been shown to reduce rates of opioid relapse, HIV transmission, overall mortality, and criminality (Fullerton et al. 2014). Methadone is heavily regulated because of its potentially deadly side effects. Buprenorphine, which is safer, can be prescribed in office settings (Substance Abuse and Mental Health Services Administration 2021). As opioid agonists, both medications may enhance the adverse effects of diuretics such as spironolactone, which is often used as an androgen blocker in GAHT. Conversely, spironolactone, a weak CYP3A4 inducer, may decrease methadone and buprenorphine levels (PDR Network 2022b; Substance Abuse and Mental Health Services Administration 2021). Estrogen and progestins compete with buprenorphine for the CYP3A4 enzyme and may increase buprenorphine levels (Substance Abuse and Mental Health Services Administration 2021). With chronic use, methadone can lower endogenous testosterone levels (Bawor et al. 2014). Methadone can also prolong the QTc interval and should be used in caution with leuprolide, which poses similar risks (PDR Network 2022a).

Naloxone and Naltrexone

Naloxone and *naltrexone* block opioid receptors. Naloxone (Narcan) is shorter-acting and can be administered in response to an opioid overdose (Galanter et al. 2015; Miller et al. 2019). Naltrexone can be administered daily in oral form or as a monthly long-acting injectable (Vivitrol) to reduce the rate of relapse for those with opioid use disorder or alcohol use disorder (Galanter et al. 2015; Miller et al. 2019; Substance Abuse and Mental Health Services Administration 2021). Both medications are considered safe in conjunction with GAHT; because they block the effects of opioid analgesics, use must be carefully considered in all patients approaching gender-affirming surgery (GAS).

Bupropion

Bupropion, while most commonly used to treat depression, has been shown to reduce cravings for tobacco, cocaine, and methamphetamines (Galanter et al. 2015). It is considered generally safe, though it increases seizure risk, as do estrogen (Johnson and Kaplan 2017) and one metabolite of testosterone (Reddy 2004), yet there is no evidence that seizure history is an absolute contraindication to starting GAHT. Bupropion is contraindicated in those with a history of some eating disorders more prevalent among TNG individuals, such as anorexia nervosa.

Disulfiram

Disulfiram is an alcohol-sensitizing agent that works by inhibiting the enzyme aldehyde dehydrogenase, which assists with alcohol metabolism (Galanter et al. 2015). Drinking while taking this medication can lead to high levels of alcohol in the system and a disulfiram-ethanol reaction: flushing, increased heart rate, nausea, vomiting, and other uncomfortable symptoms (Galanter et al. 2015). There is also some evidence that disulfiram can help with stimulant use disorder (Galanter et al. 2015). Those taking this medication should discontinue it at least a week before surgery to minimize risk of potential interactions with medications administered in the perioperative setting (University of Wisconsin Hospitals and Clinics Authority 2020).

Acamprosate

Acamprosate reduces alcohol cravings and, for those who return to drinking, reduces the risk of heavy drinking (Galanter et al. 2015). There are no known interactions between acamprosate and GAHT.

Varenicline

Varenicline binds nicotinic receptors and has been shown to encourage smoking cessation by reducing cravings for nicotine and assisting with nicotine withdrawal symptoms. In 2009, the U.S. Food and Drug Administration (FDA) issued a public health advisory for suicidal thoughts and behavioral changes in those taking varenicline; however, a reanalysis of 17 clinical trials found no evidence that varenicline is associated with adverse psychiatric events (Gibbons and Mann 2013). There are no known interactions between varenicline and GAHT; in fact, smoking cessation is highly encouraged, especially for those taking estrogen (Hembree et al. 2017).

Nicotine Replacement Therapy
Five nicotine replacements are approved by the FDA to treat tobacco use disorder: patches, nasal spray, lozenges, gum, and vapor inhalers. None has known interactions with GAHT.

12-Step Programs and Other Mutual Help Organizations

Those in recovery often benefit from peer-led, community-based recovery groups such as Alcoholics Anonymous (AA). AA is known for its 12-step model, which is designed to help people abstain from substances or compulsive behaviors. The 12 steps of AA have propagated similar 12-step fellowships such as Narcotics Anonymous, Crystal Meth Anonymous, Sex Addicts Anonymous, Overeaters Anonymous, and many others. One of the critiques of 12-step programs involves the strong suggestion to seek a "higher power" and the use of the word "God" during meetings, which many interpret as a form of religiosity or proselytizing and can be triggering for TNG people with a history of spiritual trauma. There is an understandable fear of encountering transphobic, sexist, or homophobic members, and many have reported feeling left out or overlooked during meetings on the basis of their gender modality (Horgos 2019; Lucky 2019). To compensate for this, many groups specifically cater to those who are 2SLGBTQIA+ or TNG.

In addition to 12 steps, the 12 traditions outline the fellowship's guidelines. Many who fear discrimination or exclusion may find solace in the third tradition of AA, which states that "the only requirement for membership is a desire to stop drinking [or using]" (Alcoholics Anonymous World Services, Inc. 1982; Jane 2019). That means that as long as a person has a desire to move forward in recovery, they are welcome, regardless of gender modality. The 12-step groups are not a substitute for therapy with qualified professionals, but many TNG people have credited 12-step recovery programs for keeping them sober in a way that helps them come out, build self-esteem, or start gender-affirming care (Mooney and Dold 1992).

There are alternative recovery-oriented fellowships, such as LifeRing and Secular Organizations for Sobriety (SOS). Both take a more secular approach to recovery. Refuge Recovery takes a Buddhist approach; and SMART Recovery uses strategies rooted in CBT.

CONSIDERATIONS REGARDING GENDER-AFFIRMING CARE

Little research covers best practices for helping someone with an SUD to seek gender-affirming care. Multiple studies across various populations have shown that ensuring access to GAHT and surgical treatment while in substance use treatment improves quality of life and decreases depression and anxiety (Allen et al. 2019; Dhejne et al. 2016; Fisher et al. 2016; Lindqvist et al. 2017; Mahfouda et al. 2019; Nobili et al. 2018; White Hughto and Reisner 2016).

Gender-Affirming Hormone Therapy

Although access to GAHT can positively affect recovery, some hormones are administered with needles, which can trigger those who have a history of injecting substances. Using a different formulation of hormone (e.g., gel, foam, patch, or pill), if available, may be preferable. Alternatively, a family member or support person can also hold on to the needles or lock them in a safe to minimize risk of relapse.

Gender-Affirming Surgery

There are no specific guidelines for assessing readiness for GAS in those with an SUD. Different surgeons have different requirements for how long one should remain abstinent from substances before being considered an appropriate candidate for GAS. Most list tobacco use as an absolute contraindication to surgery because of its potential to cause surgical complications (Grønkjær et al. 2014). It is helpful to check with the surgeon for clarification beforehand. A history of having an SUD should not automatically disqualify surgical candidates from GAS. Some research suggests that active substance use can lead to poor surgical outcomes or prevent people from fully participating in postsurgical aftercare. However, TNG people who actively engage with SUD treatment may be excellent surgical candidates. A history of good attendance or active engagement may show that the surgical candidate has the ability to follow through with aftercare and postsurgical recovery; this can be mentioned in a letter of support for gender-affirming care. It is preferable for the patient to not be actively engaged in at-risk substance use and to demonstrate the ability to achieve sustained recovery.

Surgery can be a challenging experience for anyone in recovery. The stress of the surgery itself, possible complications, and inadequate pain control can increase the risk of relapse. Because of their addictive potential, opioid pain medications can trigger relapse in patients with any SUD. But it is completely possible for someone in recovery to successfully undergo GAS. Additional support for the patient is essential; this may include having someone stay with them in the postoperative phase or increasing the frequency of recovery meetings and appointments with mental health clinicians. A family member or close friend may hold their opioid medications to minimize risk of misuse. Those on methadone, buprenorphine, disulfiram, or naltrexone may need special arrangements with the surgical team to avoid drug-drug interactions and ensure adequate pain control. Despite the risks, the benefits of GAS may reduce the risk of relapse through improvements in mental health and quality of life.

CONCLUSION

There are numerous gaps in our research, particularly when it comes to gathering epidemiologic information. Numerous TNG-specific studies have provided invaluable insights into addiction in our communities, but we need mainstream studies to collect demographic data on gender identity and gender assigned at birth.

Each year, the Substance Abuse and Mental Health Services Administration conducts a National Survey on Drug Use and Health, which estimates the prevalence and incidence of drug use in civilians >12 years old. The survey now collects data on lesbian, gay, and bisexual respondents, but gender is coded binarily (man or woman), and the survey does not collect data about respondents' gender modality (Rosner et al. 2021). These disparities in addressing gender identity are unfortunate, as there are clear differences among TNG people regarding how addiction develops, specific dangers, and best forms of treatment (Polak et al. 2015). There are also notable gaps regarding any specialized needs from an intervention for TNG individuals (Glynn and van den Berg 2017). Such work has implications for all mental health clinicians, regardless of specialization, owing to the widespread nature and prevalence of addiction.

REFERENCES

Alcoholics Anonymous World Services, Inc.: Twelve steps and twelve traditions. Alcoholics Anonymous World Services, 1982

Allen LR, Watson LB, Egan AM, Moser CN: Well-being and suicidality among transgender youth after gender-affirming hormones. Clin Pract Pediatr Psychol 7(3):302–311, 2019

American Psychiatric Association: Diagnostic and Statistical Manual of Mental Disorders, 5th Edition, Text Revision. Washington, DC, American Psychiatric Association, 2022

Babor TF, Hall W: Standardizing terminology in addiction science: to achieve the impossible dream. Addiction 102(7):1015–1018, 2007 17567379

Bawor M, Dennis BB, Samaan MC, et al: Methadone induces testosterone suppression in patients with opioid addiction. Sci Rep 4:6189, 2014 25155550

Benotsch EG, Zimmerman R, Cathers L, et al: Non-medical use of prescription drugs, polysubstance use, and mental health in transgender adults. Drug Alcohol Depend 132(1-2):391–394, 2013 23510637

Bjartveit K, Tverdal A: Health consequences of sustained smoking cessation. Tob Control 18(3):197–205, 2009 19228666

Botticelli MP, Koh HK: Changing the language of addiction. JAMA 316(13):1361–1362, 2016 27701667

Broyles LM, Binswanger IA, Jenkins JA, et al: Confronting inadvertent stigma and pejorative language in addiction scholarship: a recognition and response. Subst Abus 35(3):217–221, 2014 24911031

Buchting FO, Emory KT, Scout, et al: Transgender use of cigarettes, cigars, and e-cigarettes in a national study. Am J Prev Med 53(1):e1–e7, 2017 28094133

Center for Drug Evaluation and Research: Assessment of Abuse Potential of Drugs: Guidance for Industry. Silver Spring, MD, U.S. Food and Drug Administration, 2017. Available at: https://www.fda.gov/media/116739/download. Accessed June 24, 2023.

Centers for Disease Control and Prevention: Annual smoking-attributable mortality, years of potential life lost, and productivity losses—United States, 1997–2001. MMWR Morb Mortal Wkly Rep 54(25):625–628, 2005 15988406

Cochran BN, Peavy KM, Santa AF: Differentiating LGBT individuals in substance abuse treatment: analyses based on sexuality and drug preference. J LGBT Health Res 3(2):63–75, 2007 19835042

Connolly D, Gilchrist G: Prevalence and correlates of substance use among transgender adults: a systematic review. Addict Behav 111:106544, 2020 32717497

Cotaina M, Peraire M, Boscá M, et al: Substance use in the transgender population: a meta-analysis. Brain Sci 12(3):366, 2022 35326322

Day JK, Fish JN, Perez-Brumer A, et al: Transgender youth substance use disparities: results from a population-based sample. J Adolesc Health 61(6):729–735, 2017 28942238

de Freitas LD, Léda-Rêgo G, Bezerra-Filho S, Miranda-Scippa Å: Psychiatric disorders in individuals diagnosed with gender dysphoria: a systematic review. Psychiatry Clin Neurosci 74(2):99–104, 2020 31642568

De Pedro KT, Gilreath TD, Jackson C, Esqueda MC: Substance use among transgender students in California public middle and high schools. J Sch Health 87(5):303–309, 2017 28382667

Derbyshire KL, Grant JE: Compulsive sexual behavior: a review of the literature. J Behav Addict 4(2):37–43, 2015 26014671

Dhejne C, Van Vlerken R, Heylens G, Arcelus J: Mental health and gender dysphoria: a review of the literature. Int Rev Psychiatry 28(1):44–57, 2016 26835611

Drabble L: Alcohol, tobacco, and pharmaceutical industry funding: considerations for organizations serving lesbian, gay, bisexual, and transgender communities. J Gay Lesbian Soc Serv 11(1):1–26, 2000

Fisher AD, Castellini G, Ristori J, et al: Cross-sex hormone treatment and psychobiological changes in transsexual persons: two-year follow-up data. J Clin Endocrinol Metab 101(11):4260–4269, 2016 27700538

Flentje A, Heck NC, Sorensen JL: Characteristics of transgender individuals entering substance abuse treatment. Addict Behav 39(5):969–975, 2014 24561017

Frost MC, Blosnich JR, Lehavot K, et al: Disparities in documented drug use disorders between transgender and cisgender U.S. Veterans Health Administration patients. J Addict Med 15(4):334–340, 2021 33252409

Fullerton CA, Kim M, Thomas CP, et al: Medication-assisted treatment with methadone: assessing the evidence. Psychiatr Serv 65(2):146–157, 2014 24248468

Galanter M, Kleber HD, Brady K (eds): The American Psychiatric Publishing Textbook of Substance Abuse Treatment, 6th Edition. Washington, DC, American Psychiatric Publishing, 2015

Gerke DR, Call J, Atteberry-Ash B, et al: Alcohol use at the intersection of sexual orientation and gender identity in a representative sample of youth in Colorado. Am J Addict 31(1):61–68, 2022 34873759

Gibbons RD, Mann JJ: Varenicline, smoking cessation, and neuropsychiatric adverse events. Am J Psychiatry 170(12):1460–1467, 2013 24030388

Glynn TR, van den Berg JJ: A systematic review of interventions to reduce problematic substance use among transgender individuals: a call to action. Transgend Health 2(1):45–59, 2017 28861547

Gómez-Gil E, Simulionyte E, Balcells-Oliveró M, et al: Patrones de consumo de alcohol, tabaco y drogas ilegales en personas transexuales. Adicciones 31(3):201, 2018

Grønkjær M, Eliasen M, Skov-Ettrup LS, et al: Preoperative smoking status and postoperative complications: a systematic review and meta-analysis. Ann Surg 259(1):52–71, 2014 23799418

Guss CE, Williams DN, Reisner SL, et al: Disordered weight management behaviors, nonprescription steroid use, and weight perception in transgender youth. J Adolesc Health 60(1):17–22, 2017 28029539

Hembree WC, Cohen-Kettenis PT, Gooren L, et al: Endocrine treatment of gender-dysphoric/gender-incongruent persons: an Endocrine Society clinical practice guideline. J Clin Endocrinol Metab 102(11):3869–3903, 2017 28945902

Hendricks ML, Testa RJ: A conceptual framework for clinical work with transgender and gender nonconforming clients: an adaptation of the minority stress model. Prof Psychol Res Pr 43(5):460–467, 2012

Horgos B: Women and non-binary folks are changing the sobriety narrative: women in recovery are redefining rock bottom and taking the patriarchy out of sobriety. The Temper, September 3, 2019. Available at: https://www.thetemper.com/women-in-sobriety/. Accessed June 24, 2023.

Hughto JMW, Quinn EK, Dunbar MS, et al: Prevalence and co-occurrence of alcohol, nicotine, and other substance use disorder diagnoses among US transgender and cisgender adults. JAMA Netw Open 4(2):e2036512, 2021 33538824

Hunt J: Why the gay and transgender population experiences higher rates of substance use: many use to cope with discrimination and prejudice. Center for American Progress, March 9, 2012. Available at: https://www.americanprogress.org/article/why-the-gay-and-transgender-population-experiences-higher-rates-of-substance-use/. Accessed June 24, 2023.

Ip EJ, Barnett MJ, Tenerowicz MJ, Perry PJ: The Anabolic 500 survey: characteristics of male users versus nonusers of anabolic-androgenic steroids for strength training. Pharmacotherapy 31(8):757–766, 2011 21923602

James SE, Herman J, Rankin S, et al: The Report of the 2015 U.S. Transgender Survey. Washington, DC, National Center for Transgender Equality, 2016. Available at: https://transequality.org/sites/default/files/docs/usts/USTS-Full-Report-Dec17.pdf. Accessed June 24, 2023.

Jane E: The transgender alcoholic in AA. The Link, May 2019

Johnson EL, Kaplan PW: Caring for transgender patients with epilepsy. Epilepsia 58(10):1667–1672, 2017 28771690

Johnson K, Weissman-Ward A: Addiction treatment and recovery in an affirming environment, in Trans Bodies, Trans Selves: A Resource by and for Transgender Communities, 2nd Edition. Edited by Erickson-Schroth L. New York, Oxford University Press, 2022

Kanayama G, Brower KJ, Wood RI, et al: Treatment of anabolic-androgenic steroid dependence: emerging evidence and its implications. Drug Alcohol Depend 109(1-3):6–13, 2010 20188494

Kanayama G, Pope HG Jr: Illicit use of androgens and other hormones: recent advances. Curr Opin Endocrinol Diabetes Obes 19(3):211–219, 2012 22450858

Kcomt L, Evans-Polce RJ, Veliz PT, et al: Use of cigarettes and e-cigarettes/vaping among transgender people: results from the 2015 U.S. Transgender Survey. Am J Prev Med 59(4):538–547, 2020 32826126

Kelly JF, Westerhoff CM: Does it matter how we refer to individuals with substance-related conditions? A randomized study of two commonly used terms. Int J Drug Policy 21(3):202–207, 2010 20005692

Keuroghlian AS, Reisner SL, White JM, Weiss RD: Substance use and treatment of substance use disorders in a community sample of transgender adults. Drug Alcohol Depend 152:139–146, 2015 25953644

Kidd JD, Jackman KB, Barucco R, et al: Understanding the impact of the COVID-19 pandemic on the mental health of transgender and gender nonbinary individuals engaged in a longitudinal cohort study. J Homosex 68(4):592–611, 2021 33502286

Lindqvist EK, Sigurjonsson H, Möllermark C, et al: Quality of life improves early after gender reassignment surgery in transgender women. Eur J Plast Surg 40(3):223–226, 2017 28603386

Lombardi EL, van Servellen G: Building culturally sensitive substance use prevention and treatment programs for transgendered populations. J Subst Abuse Treat 19(3):291–296, 2000 11027900

Lucky M: Breaking down barriers: ensuring AA is accessible. The Link, May 2019

Lyons T, Shannon K, Pierre L, et al: A qualitative study of transgender individuals' experiences in residential addiction treatment settings: stigma and inclusivity. Subst Abuse Treat Prev Policy 10(1):17, 2015 25948286

Mahfouda S, Moore JK, Siafarikas A, et al: Gender-affirming hormones and surgery in transgender children and adolescents. Lancet Diabetes Endocrinol 7(6):484–498, 2019 30528161

Mathy RM: Transgender identity and suicidality in a nonclinical sample: sexual orientation, psychiatric history, and compulsive behaviors. J Psychol Human Sex 14(4):47–65, 2003

Matsuzaka S: Transgressing gender norms in addiction treatment: transgender rights to access within gender-segregated facilities. J Ethn Subst Abuse 17(4):420–433, 2018 28632095

McLellan AT, Lewis DC, O'Brien CP, Kleber HD: Drug dependence, a chronic medical illness: implications for treatment, insurance, and outcomes evaluation. JAMA 284(13):1689–1695, 2000 11015800

Meyer JS, Quenzer LF: Psychopharmacology: Drugs, the Brain, and Behavior. Sunderland, MA, Sinauer Associates, 2005

Miller SC, Fiellin DA, Rosenthal RN, et al: The ASAM Principles of Addiction Medicine, 6th Edition. Philadelphia, PA, Wolters Kluwer, 2019

Mooney AJ, Dold C: My recovery: Carla: Transgender and alcoholic, in The Recovery Book. New York, Workman Publishing, 1992

Myers SC, Safer JD: Increased rates of smoking cessation observed among transgender women receiving hormone treatment. Endocr Pract 23(1):32–36, 2017 27682351

Nagata JM, Murray SB, Compte EJ, et al: Community norms for the Eating Disorder Examination Questionnaire (EDE-Q) among transgender men and women. Eat Behav 37:101381, 2020 32416588

National LGBT Health Education Center: Addressing Opioid Use Disorder Among LGBTQ Populations. Boston, MA, Fenway Institute, 2018

Nemoto T, Operario D, Keatley J, et al: Promoting health for transgender women: Transgender Resources and Neighborhood Space (TRANS) program in San Francisco. Am J Public Health 95(3):382–384, 2005 15727962

Newcomb ME, Hill R, Buehler K, et al: High burden of mental health problems, substance use, violence, and related psychosocial factors in transgender, non-binary, and gender diverse youth and young adults. Arch Sex Behav 49(2):645–659, 2020 31485801

Nobili A, Glazebrook C, Arcelus J: Quality of life of treatment-seeking transgender adults: a systematic review and meta-analysis. Rev Endocr Metab Disord 19(3):199–220, 2018 30121881

Nuttbrock L, Bockting W, Rosenblum A, et al: Gender abuse, depressive symptoms, and substance use among transgender women: a 3-year prospective study. Am J Public Health 104(11):2199–2206, 2014 25211716

Pachankis JE: A transdiagnostic minority stress treatment approach for gay and bisexual men's syndemic health conditions. Arch Sex Behav 44(7):1843–1860, 2015 26123065

PDR Network: Methadone, in Prescriber's Digital Reference. Whippany, NJ, ConnectiveRx, 2022a

PDR Network: Spironolactone, in Prescriber's Digital Reference. Whippany, NJ, ConnectiveRx, 2022b

Peacock E, Andrinopoulos K, Hembling J: Binge drinking among men who have sex with men and transgender women in San Salvador: correlates and sexual health implications. J Urban Health 92(4):701–716, 2015 25591660

Polak K, Haug NA, Drachenberg HE, Svikis DS: Gender considerations in addiction: implications for treatment. Curr Treat Options Psychiatry 2(3):326–338, 2015 26413454

Reddy DS: Testosterone modulation of seizure susceptibility is mediated by neurosteroids 3α-androstanediol and 17β-estradiol. Neuroscience 129(1):195–207, 2004 15489042

Rider GN, McMorris BJ, Gower AL, et al: Gambling behaviors and problem gambling: a population-based comparison of transgender/gender diverse and cisgender adolescents. J Gambl Stud 35(1):79–92, 2019 30343416

Rosner B, Neicun J, Yang JC, Roman-Urrestarazu A: Substance use among sexual minorities in the US: linked to inequalities and unmet need for mental health treatment? Results from the National Survey on Drug Use and Health (NSDUH). J Psychiatr Res 135:107–118, 2021 33472121

Ruppert R, Kattari SK, Sussman S: Review: prevalence of addictions among transgender and gender diverse subgroups. Int J Environ Res Public Health 18(16):8843, 2021 34444595

Senreich E: The substance abuse treatment experiences of a small sample of transgender clients. J Soc Work Pract Addict 11(3):295–299, 2011

Shires DA, Jaffee KD: Structural discrimination is associated with smoking status among a national sample of transgender individuals. Nicotine Tob Res 18(6):1502–1508, 2016 26438646

Substance Abuse and Mental Health Services Administration: Medications for Opioid Use Disorder (Pub No PEP21-02-01-002; TIP Series 63). Bethesda, MD, Substance Abuse and Mental Health Services Administration, 2021. Available at: https://store.samhsa.gov/sites/default/files/pep21-02-01-002.pdf. Accessed June 24, 2023.

Sussman S, Lisha N, Griffiths M: Prevalence of the addictions: a problem of the majority or the minority? Eval Health Prof 34(1):3–56, 2011 20876085

Thombs DL: Introduction to Addictive Behaviors, 2nd Edition. New York, Guilford, 1999

University of Wisconsin Hospitals and Clinics Authority: Perioperative Medication Management, Adult/Pediatric: Inpatient/Ambulatory Clinical Practice Guideline. Madison, WI, UW Health, 2020. Available at: https://www.uwhealth.org/cckm/cpg/medications/Perioperative-Medication-Management-Clinical-Pratice-Guideline---August-2022.pdf. Accessed June 24, 2023.

U.S. Department of Health and Human Services: Office of the Surgeon General: Facing Addiction in America: The Surgeon General's Report on Alcohol, Drugs, and Health. Washington, DC, U.S. Department of Health and Human Services, 2016

White Hughto JM, Reisner SL: A systematic review of the effects of hormone therapy on psychological functioning and quality of life in transgender individuals. Transgender Health 1(1):21–31, 2016

World Health Organization: International Statistical Classification of Diseases and Related Health Problems, 11th Revision. Geneva, World Health Organization, 2019

Xavier J: Final Report of the Washington, DC Transgender Needs Assessment Survey (WTNAS). Washington, DC, Us Helping Us, 2000

CHAPTER 17

Perinatal Psychiatry and Affirming Gender Identity in the Setting of Pregnancy

Sarah Noble, D.O.

> The pregnant transgender man is radical, because he chooses,
> on the one hand, to mold his body to fit the image he identifies with
> and at the same time pragmatically uses the physical properties
> he decides to keep, his female reproductive organs,
> leading to a designification of the pregnancy as an exclusive
> determining sign of femaleness.
>
> *Verlinden 2012, p. 123*

GENDER TROUBLE
Trans, Nonbinary, and Gender-Expansive Pregnant Bodies Through the Theoretical Lens of Judith Butler and Erving Goffman

It is difficult to begin a conversation about transgender, nonbinary, and/or gender-expansive (TNG) pregnancy without a reference to Thomas Beatie, who is purported to be the first trans man in the United States to give birth to a child. Likely there have been many others throughout history, but Beatie's pregnancy made national headlines and was brought to the attention of the average American when he was a guest on *The Oprah Winfrey Show* in 2008 (Rakieten 2008). Jasper Verlinden, a professor of English and American Studies, states,

> The first shock occurs at the very beginning of the episode when Oprah tells them that "Thomas, not Nancy, is the one who is pregnant," and shows them a picture of "the pregnant man" ("First TV Interview"). The second shock comes when Oprah announces that Thomas used to be Tracy, a statement that is once again followed by photographic material, this time showing a very feminine Tracy as a model and Miss Hawaii Teen USA pageant finalist. (Verlinden 2012, p. 109)

Here, Verlinden highlighted the gender confusion—not of Thomas, but of the audience, who have been socialized to expect sex and gender to be the same and not be complicated by gender presentations that do not match expectations. This is the result of centuries of the Western world viewing gender as binary (woman/man) and as following directly from sex.

The 1990s birthed the field of transgender studies, with works by Judith Butler, Sandy Stone, Leslie Feinberg, and Jack Halberstam. Primarily created as a critique of the way transgender lives were discussed in feminist or gay/lesbian studies, transgender studies shifts TNG people from the objects of study to active subjects. TNG people existed in spaces well before the 1990s, but since that time, the language and ideas developed by academia have begun to permeate popular culture, enabling lay participation in the discourse regarding gender and sex.

Judith Butler's text *Gender Trouble* (1990) and Erving Goffman's earlier work (1956) *The Presentation of Self in Everyday Life* discussed gender performativity, asserting that gender/sex is something that is "done" in front of an audience, rather than an inherent biologic quality. Based on these seminal works, in particular, we deduce that a) gender is not a binary, b) sex is not a binary, c) gender does not follow from sex, d) the distinction between gender and sex is not always useful, and e) the gender/sex binary is harmful (Morgenroth and Ryan 2021). In their article, "The Effects of Gender Trouble," psychologists Thekla Morgenroth and Michelle Ryan explained,

> The ubiquity of the binary performance of gender/sex masks its performative nature and makes it appear natural. These processes are further reinforced by social sanctions faced by those who disrupt the gender/sex binary. (Morgenroth and Ryan 2021, p. 1121)

Butler (2020) argued that Western culture closely intertwines sex, gender, and sexual orientation in what she calls the *heterosexual matrix*. This matrix asserts that biological sex is binary (female/male) and forms the basis for gender, which is also binary (woman/man) and the basis for (hetero)sexual attraction. If we return to Thomas Beatie and Oprah's audience, we can immediately see the *gender trouble* Beatie presents: he does not fit Butler's heterosexual matrix. Butler argued that those who do not fit the heterosexual matrix are punished because the gender/sex roles are reinforced by social sanctions. Appearing on the *The Oprah Winfrey Show* may have catapulted Mr. Beatie and his family to fame, but his pregnancy was not universally accepted. Verlinden (2012) quoted conservative Minneapolis radio host Chris Barker as saying things such as, "I don't believe you're a guy. Can you stand up to pee?" As well as, "how can you say, 'I'm a guy,' and you had a baby and it wasn't even by cesarean?" (p. 114).

Goffman's exploration of the performativity of gender in *The Presentation of Self in Everyday Life* offered another way of analyzing TNG pregnancy. Using the metaphor of theater and the stage, Goffman explained that when we engage with others we are in fact "performing ourselves" and thus every interaction is actually a negotiation of the meaning and the roles of the people in it. In this way, society is constantly creating means to classify people, and when there are undesirable traits that contradict our stereotypes in relation to expectation, the individual with whom we are engaging will be stigmatized. When the audience is meeting Beatie, they are engaging with him using their stereotypes of what a man should be, of what a pregnant person should be, or what a beauty queen should be.

Costume is both body and presentation of the body, and a central part of any performance. Embodied changes of pregnancy, like clothes, are part of a costume. When a costume defies stereotypes—as is often with pregnant TNG people—that clear contradiction draws stigma. Per psychologist Damien Riggs, "Many transgender people are able to live their lives without other people knowing their transgender status. Transgender men who bear children, by contrast, are a priori treated as bodies requiring an explanation" (Riggs 2013, p. 63).

When we see Beatie on stage with Oprah, it is easy to forget that he would have also had to navigate the obstetrician's office, birthing center, and possibly a lactation center during his pregnancy. These traditionally "women's" spaces may not welcome him, despite his pregnancy.

Morgenroth and Ryan (2021) took Goffman's dramaturgical theory and Butler's gender trouble and created a strategy for generating change. They described broadly two categories of gender trouble: *category-based* (playing a different character, putting on a different costume, or deviating from the script) and *context-based* (dismantling the stage).

> Performance-based gender trouble can take a range of forms: switching character, costume, or script in a way that leads to misalignment; playing a character, putting on a costume, or enacting a script that is neither clearly

male/masculine nor clearly female/feminine; or switching characters, costumes, and scripts in a way that is still aligned but questions the immutability and innateness of gender/sex. (p. 1121)

Beatie engaged in performance-based gender trouble in character, costume, and script. He challenged the heteronormative matrix and the stereotypes of social interaction by being a pregnant trans man. He asked the audience, both literally and metaphorically, to challenge their assumptions in engaging with him.

Yet, as mentioned above, a TNG pregnant person still has to navigate "stages" that have been set up to reinforce the gender/sex binary. This is why the more powerful gender trouble is context-based: dismantling the stage. Rather than challenging the stereotypes one person at a time, it is much more effective to change the zeitgeist. Much as the advent of transgender studies in the 1990s brought into common parlance the terms trans and nonbinary, dismantling the stage suggests that the next phase is to dismantle the gender binary.

Before we discuss how clinicians can facilitate context-based gender trouble or dismantle the stage, we explore the ways in which gender trouble affects a pregnant TNG person.

MINORITY STRESS MODEL

Environmental Stressors: Medicolegal

The *minority stress model*, developed by Ilan H. Meyer in 2003, theorizes that proximal as well as distal factors contribute to the poor health outcomes of Two-Spirit, lesbian, gay, bisexual, queer, intersex, asexual, and more (2SLGBTQIA+) people (Meyer 2003). (Please see Chapter 2, "Stigma and Mental Health Inequities," for further discussion.) TNG people come into pregnancy having already experienced minority stress; this is compounded among those who are subject to additional minority stress for intersectional identities, for example, Black and Indigenous people of color (BIPOC), neurodivergent people, and disabled people (see chapters 5, 6, 7, 8, and 9). They may anticipate negative interactions with the medical or legal institutions that are inherently biased toward white, cis men (Institute of Medicine 2003).

It can be a struggle to deal with regulations and systems committed to upholding neat categories like female or male, woman or man. To pursue changing a birth certificate or to seek certain gender-affirming medical interventions, TNG people often need to first receive clearance from a therapist or psychiatrist; if they are lucky, their medical procedures might be covered by insurance. However, as Verlinden (2012) stated, "The therapists and medical professionals whom Thomas Beatie…and other trans men depend on for their physical and legal transitions would often see their wish to become pregnant as a 'contradiction of the diagnosis of transsexuality'" (p. 115). In addition, once a gender marker has been changed, there is an added complication that insurance might not cover a procedure such as childbirth for a person who is not female. For example, the following story from *Time* magazine called "My Brother's Pregnancy" describes the logistical challenges trans men face at the obstetrics office.

> When Evan arrived at the midwifery center for his first appointment, he filled out an intake form, but the receptionist had trouble entering his information: if she checked the "male" box, she couldn't open an obstetric record for him. This was a problem throughout the pregnancy—medical forms and insurance claims are not set up to allow people like Evan to be honest about their medical needs (Hempel 2016).

In addition to the systems and regulations struggling to recognize trans men as pregnant people, clinicians themselves often receive inadequate training. In one case, a transgender man whose boyfriend brought him to an emergency room for abdominal pain was triaged as "nonurgent" because a nurse failed to take the possibility of pregnancy seriously, despite being informed the patient was a transgender man who received a positive result on a home pregnancy test (Clarke 2019, p. 181). After several hours of delay, a physician realized the man's condition was urgent and he needed an emergency cesarean delivery. The baby was stillborn. Medical institutions use cisheteronormative standards, which often bias clinicians to not consider the possibility of TNG pregnancy. This is also seen in low rates of fertility preservation among TNG people: studies suggest a rate of 5%–15%, "in direct contrast to the 24%–58% of TNG patients who report the desire to have children" (Patel and Sweeney 2021, p. 254). This finding could indicate that TNG people do not feel comfortable discussing fertility preservation with their clinicians or do not believe it is an option for them. Further, there is misinformation among both clinicians and TNG people that testosterone can effectively prevent pregnancy. Testosterone does generally cause amenorrhea, but it does not always prevent ovulation.

The minority stress model shows us that TNG people face discrimination from the many systems that they need to engage with throughout the process of becoming pregnant and having a child, including assisted reproductive services, pregnancy and birthing services, and legal services related to child custody and access (Ross and Goldberg 2016). BIPOC are 300% more likely to be involved in the child welfare system than white peers (Harp and Oser 2016), resulting in extensive minority stress among BIPOC TNG parents.

Because of the expectation of stressful events and often viewing the medical system as unsafe for trans bodies, if TNG people do not avoid pregnancy altogether, they may choose home birth. One participant in a qualitative study on trans men's experiences with pregnancy said, "I never really wanted to do a home birth....I was only going to have a home birth just out of fear of how a hospital wouldn't be able to deal with me" (Hoffkling et al. 2017, p. 13). Another participant recalled, "the doctor asked me some weird questions that didn't have to do with [the reason I was there], but with my [genitals]" (p. 12). TNG people also may decide not to disclose their gender if they do not feel safe with a particular clinician, especially if disclosure has previously resulted in inappropriate or awkward care interactions.

Biologic Stressors: Hormonal and Physical Changes of Pregnancy

Once pregnant, TNG people may struggle with the embodied changes. The literature suggests that "some transgender men reconcile their pregnancies through the notion of simply being a 'host' for the child" (Riggs 2013, p. 64). For others, rather than exacerbating dissociation from their bodies, pregnancy can "paradoxically contribut[e] to, rather than undermin[e], a stable transmasculine identity" (p. 68). Interviewee Alex, in the documentary *Transparent* by Jules Rosskam (2005), offers an example: "During the pregnancy was the only time I felt right being in a female body." Individual comfort with bodily changes of pregnancy often fluctuates during pregnancy, and discrepancies between one's internal sense of gendered embodiment and (in)congruence should be considered separately from one's (dis)comfort interacting with others in society.

The hormonal shift of stopping testosterone is a major challenge for many TNG people initiating pregnancy. Hormonal shifts can bring significant mood and physical changes during pregnancy; this is robustly evident among cis women. Needing to cease testosterone therapy before conception adds an additional layer of hormonal complexity. One trans man told journalist Jessi Hempel, "When I went off the hormones [to get pregnant], all the mental-health stuff I had as a teenager came back" (Hempel 2016). Some patients maintain secondary sex characteristics (e.g., facial hair), but it is important for clinicians to anticipate increased dysphoria in pregnant TNG patients as masculinization decreases, particularly regarding enlarged breasts and hips during normal gestation.

In addition to dysphoria, elevated estrogen and progesterone can cause hormonal mood and physical changes. As with any pregnant person, it is important to be alert to peripartum depression, OCD, and other mood disorders. In cis women, the rates of peripartum depression and peripartum

OCD are 10%–20% and 4%, respectively (Sharma and Sommerdyk 2015; Van Niel and Payne 2020). Half of cis women with bipolar disorder suffer from postpartum depression (Clark and Wisner 2018). Suicide is the second leading cause of death for cis women postpartum (Van Niel and Payne 2020). As TNG people are already at increased risk for depression and suicidality, clinicians must diligently screen for worsening mood. "To date, no research into trans men's experiences of giving birth has focused on mental health, and none of the research has included their partners' experiences" (Darwin and Greenfield 2019, p. 341). In addition, pregnancy medication safety studies have all been conducted with cis women. Thus, we are left to extrapolate from the treatment protocols for pregnant cis women and non-pregnant TNG people.

The American College of Obstetricians and Gynecologists recommends that pregnant cis women with a history of major depressive disorder remain on their medication during pregnancy. In one study, 68% of pregnant [cis] women who discontinued antidepressants during pregnancy suffered a relapse of their illness, and in another study, 85% of study participants—pregnant [cis] women with a history of bipolar disorder who discontinued their use of mood stabilizers—experienced a relapse of their illness during pregnancy (Kalfoglou 2016). Kalfoglou continued:

> Two decades of experience have demonstrated that SSRIs are not a major teratogen like thalidomide or even cigarette smoking. Reviews of observational studies have argued that observed risks to the fetus may be due to detection bias and confounding factors including maternal depression; in all cases, the absolute risk is very small. (p. 616)

An article in the *Journal of Clinical Psychiatry* extended the conclusions:

> Reported associations between in utero exposure to antidepressants and physical, neurodevelopmental, and psychiatric outcomes, in large part, seem to be driven by the underlying maternal disorder. When limiting confounding by indication, prenatal exposure to antidepressants was significantly associated only with offspring BMI and affective disorders. (Rommel et al. 2020, p. 12965)

We can see how important it is to screen for and treat pregnant patients who might have peripartum anxiety or depression. The Edinburgh Postnatal Depression Scale is a simple tool validated for anxiety and depression. A cutoff value of 11 has good combined sensitivity and specificity; 13 is less sensitive but more specific (Levis et al. 2020, p. m4022).

When managing bipolar disorder, generally, clinicians ought to limit prescribing valproic acid, oxcarbazepine, and carbamazepine in pregnancy, as these have all been associated with significant teratogenicity. If at all possible, clinicians ought to avoid using such medications in all patients who are of reproductive age and not using some form of long-acting contraceptive. This includes TNG people who, as mentioned above, can still ovulate, even if amenorrheic.

Antipsychotics remain a viable option for mood stabilization. In a large cohort study from Hong Kong with >700,000 mother-child pairs, the findings "did not suggest that prenatal antipsychotic exposure increased the risk of [ADHD] or autism spectrum disorder (ASD) or small for gestational age" (Wang et al. 2021, p. 1332). Lithium and lamotrigine are good options for pregnancy, too, but they are not safe when chestfeeding, as levels can be high in milk and thus cause side effects for the infant such as Stevens-Johnson syndrome (in the case of lamotrigine) or lithium toxicity (Poels et al. 2018).

The topic of medication in pregnancy is rapidly evolving and can feel fraught. Two trusted sources of information on medication in pregnancy include the MGH Women's Center for Mental Health and MotherToBaby. After delivery, some TNG people will choose to chestfeed. Although many will have had chest masculinization surgery, such procedures differ from mastectomies in that some mammary tissue is left to prevent the appearance of a sunken chest. Depending on the surgical approach, there are "variable degrees of mammary gland/milk duct preservation" (Patel and Sweeney 2021, p. 257). Those who wish to lactate without gestation can pursue the same protocols as cis women. Domperidone is sometimes used in Canada and Europe to induce lactation (it is not approved by the U.S. Food and Drug Administration). Risks to the parent include arrhythmia, cardiac arrest, and sudden death; risks to the infant are unknown (Patel and Sweeney 2021).

Some TNG people may experience increased dysphoria with chestfeeding and may wish to resume gender-affirming hormone therapy. Little research speaks to the safety of testosterone, but owing to its "low oral availability and limited secretion into the breast milk, it is not likely to affect the baby adversely" (Patel and Sweeney 2021, p. 257). It is recommended that testosterone be held until lactation has been initiated, as it can suppress lactation, but once the parent has established a good chestfeeding routine, testosterone could be resumed. For patients on spironolactone, continuing the anti-androgen while chestfeeding is "potentially safe for the infant" due to "low secretion rate into breast milk (0.02% of the parental daily dose)" (p. 257).

Coping and Social Supports

The most important aspect of the minority stress and resilience model is that despite the toxic effects of both environmental and internal stressors, strength may be garnered from minority status. The source of this support is community. Some researchers have identified "a correlation between the social isolation and loneliness transgender men face during pregnancy and early parenthood and perinatal depression" (MacLean 2021, p. 133). Connecting patients to in-person or online groups where they can network with other trans and nonbinary parents can decrease isolation and increase a sense of shared experience. A good example is Postpartum Support International, which has expanded its online support groups to include a trans and queer support group. There are also two helpful Facebook groups: Birthing Beyond the Binary; and Birthing and Breast or Chestfeeding Trans People and Allies.

SUPPORTING TNG PEOPLE THROUGH THE PERIPARTUM PERIOD

TNG people who desire to become pregnant face many challenges. As behavioral health clinicians, we have the power to enable safer passage for our patients as they navigate medical systems. As stated in *The AMA Journal of Ethics*, we can "advocate for social, economic, educational, and political changes that ameliorate suffering and contribute to human well-being" (Freeman 2014, p. 722). This is how we begin to dismantle the stage of the heterosexual matrix that contributes to disparities of care for patients.

We need to advocate for equal insurance coverage for our TNG patients who, in the United States, are more likely "to be uninsured, to experience discrimination and mistreatment in health care settings, and to be adversely affected by limited clinician knowledge or refusal to provide care" (Moseson et al. 2020, p. 1060). Thankfully, federal law currently mandates covering gender-affirming care. For updates, refer to the National Center for Transgender Equality.

At the direct care level, it is essential that sexual and reproductive health care no longer be gendered. Rather than dubbing reproductive care "women's health"—which marginalizes transgender women, who cannot currently carry a pregnancy; cis women who either cannot or do not want to carry a pregnancy; and TNG people—these services can rather be known as sexual and reproductive health care. Along with this degendering of services and clinical spaces, all staff and clinicians should be trained to understand that not all people who visit clinical practices for sexual and reproductive health care are cis women. TNG patients are often misgendered by clinicians or staff, and distress, dysphoria, and shame accompany these experiences. For recommendations on how to degender clinical practices and make them more welcoming for TNG patients, see Moseson et al. 2020, pp. 1063–1064.

Electronic health records (EHRs) can be highly problematic for TNG patients (see Chapter 23, "Collecting and Analyzing Gender Identity Data"). EHRs often do not distinguish sex from gender and, for billing, may require that the patient's EHR gender match that listed on their insurance; this causes errors in care delivery when algorithms are built assuming correlations between gender and anatomy. For instance, "a clinician may find that the [EHR] does not display the appropriate checkboxes to document a prostate examination on a transgender woman who is registered as a woman, or that they are unable to complete charges for a man of transgender experience who is undergoing intrauterine device placement" (Moseson et al. 2020, p. 1061).

We should also ask TNG patients about fertility and family planning desires as part of our standard care considerations and, as needed, help connect patients to appropriate care. As stated earlier, we should screen patients for peripartum mood disorders and treat appropriately.

These changes require buy-in from hospital and clinical practice administrators, who can set the standard for each office to require training for all staff and clinicians. One incentive for administrators can be the Healthcare Equality Index, which categorizes hospitals and health care practices that have met standards for 2SLGBTQIA+ inclusion. In their own clinical offices, clinicians can make it a practice to have gender-inclusive intake forms. Our job as clinicians is to dismantle the stage and provide a multigendered or degendered space for all patients to receive care.

CONCLUSION

As we conclude our discussion of the peripartum period for TNG people, it is paramount to highlight that this is an area with limited research—not because TNG people do not have children, but rather because of bias in medicine and research. "Queer people's experiences of conception, pregnancy, birth and parenting are under-recorded, under-researched, and under-heard" (Darwin and Greenfield 2019, p. 341). As discussed at the beginning of this chapter, in a culture that is standardized to a heteronormative binary, it is easy for research to erase or ignore the possibility of those living outside the norm. Moseson et al. (2020) have excellent recommendations for researchers to more inclusively and responsively define gender identity and sex assigned at birth.

The most dangerous unique element of TNG pregnancies is exposure to discrimination and lack of culturally responsive care. No published data yet address the effects of testosterone exposure in unplanned TNG pregnancies; extrapolating from the pregnancies of cis women with high levels of androgen, only low birth weight is a potential complication (Patel and Sweeney 2021). Although little research has explored the mental health of children delivered by trans parents, what there is shows no differences in developmental trajectory for these children, unless there is a sudden loss of contact with the trans parent (Ross and Goldberg 2016).

Patients may avoid hospital births or prenatal care, anticipating discrimination and lack of skills serving TNG people in medical care settings. This is why gender-affirming care in the perinatal period must become the norm, with proper training for the entire team, not just clinicians. Patients interact with everyone: security guards, receptionists, phlebotomists. It is essential that each team member be fully gender affirming.

Clinicians should screen for and treat mental health concerns before, during, and after pregnancy. The Edinburgh Postnatal Depression Scale can assist with screening and treatment monitoring. Patients already on psychiatric medication should remain on their medication during pregnancy.

Most importantly, recognizing that we have all been socialized in a society that normalizes the heterosexual matrix and gender binary, we must constantly check our own unconscious biases. We can only become the best possible clinicians for all patients by being exquisitely aware of how unconscious bias is playing out in our interactions with people and the world around us.

ACKNOWLEDGMENTS

Thank you to all clinicians who are doing the work of caring for TNG patients as well as researching, writing, and educating our peers. I have learned much from you and hope that this chapter contributes to the ongoing improvement of care.

REFERENCES

Butler J: Gender Trouble: Feminism and the Subversion of Identity. Abingdon, UK, Rutledge, 1990

Clark CT, Wisner KL: Treatment of peripartum bipolar disorder. Obstet Gynecol Clin North Am 45(3):403–417, 2018 30092918

Clarke J: Pregnant people? Columbia Law Rev 119(6):173–199, 2019

Darwin Z, Greenfield M: Mothers and others: the invisibility of LGBTQ people in reproductive and infant psychology. J Reprod Infant Psychol 37(4):341–343, 2019 31387370

Freeman J: Advocacy by physicians for patients and for social change. Virtual Mentor 16(9):722–725, 2014

Goffman E: The Presentation of Self in Everyday Life. New York, Doubleday, 1956

Harp KLH, Oser CB: Factors associated with two types of child custody loss among a sample of African American mothers: a novel approach. Soc Sci Res 60:283–296, 2016 27712685

Hempel J: My Brother's Pregnancy and the Making of a New American Family. Time magazine, 2016. Available at: https://time.com/4475634/trans-man-pregnancy-evan/. Accessed August 20, 2021.

Hoffkling A, Obedin-Maliver J, Sevelius J: From erasure to opportunity: a qualitative study of the experiences of transgender men around pregnancy and recommendations for providers. BMC Pregnancy Childbirth 17(332 Suppl 2):332, 2017 29143629

Institute of Medicine: Unequal Treatment: Confronting Racial and Ethnic Disparities in Healthcare. Washington, DC, The National Academies Press, 2003

Kalfoglou AL: Ethical and clinical dilemmas in using psychotropic medications during pregnancy. AMA J Ethics 18(6):614–623, 2016 27322995

Levis B, Negeri Z, Sun Y, et al: Accuracy of the Edinburgh Postnatal Depression Scale (EPDS) for screening to detect major depression among pregnant and postpartum women: systematic review and meta-analysis of individual participant data. BMJ 371:m4022, 2020

MacLean LRD: Preconception, pregnancy, birthing, and lactation needs of transgender men. Nurs Womens Health 25(2):129–138, 2021 33651985

Meyer IH: Prejudice, social stress, and mental health in lesbian, gay, and bisexual populations: conceptual issues and research evidence. Psychol Bull 129(5):674–697, 2003 12956539

Morgenroth T, Ryan M: The effects of gender trouble: an integrative theoretical framework of the perpetuation and disruption of the gender/sex binary. Perspect Psychol Sci 16:1113–1142, 2021 32375012

Moseson H, Zazanis N, Goldberg E, et al: The imperative for transgender and gender nonbinary inclusion: beyond women's health. Obstet Gynecol 135(5):1059–1068, 2020 32282602

Patel S, Sweeney LB: Maternal health in the transgender population. J Womens Health (Larchmt) 30(2):253–259, 2021 33275854

Poels EMP, Bijma HH, Galbally M, Bergink V: Lithium during pregnancy and after delivery: a review. Int J Bipolar Disord 6(1):26, 2018 30506447

Rakieten E: First TV interview: The pregnant man. Chicago, IL, Harpo, 2008

Riggs D: Transgender men's self-representations of bearing children post-transition, in Chasing Rainbows: Exploring Gender Fluid Parenting Practices. Edited by Green FJ, Friedman M. Ontario, Canada, Demeter Press, 2013, pp 62–71

Rommel A, Bergink V, Liu X, et al: Long-term effects of intrauterine exposure to antidepressants on physical, neurodevelopmental, and psychiatric outcomes: a systematic review. J Clin Psychiatry 81(3):19r12965, 2020

Ross LE, Goldberg AE: Perinatal experiences of lesbian, gay, bisexual, and transgender people, in The Oxford Handbook of Perinatal Psychology. Edited by Wenzel A. New York,Oxford University Press, 2016, pp 618–630

Rosskam J (director): Transparent (film). San Francisco, CA, Frameline, 2005

Sharma V, Sommerdyk C: Obsessive-compulsive disorder in the postpartum period: diagnosis, differential diagnosis and management. Womens Health (Lond Engl) 11(4):543–552, 2015 26246310

Van Niel MS, Payne JL: Perinatal depression: a review. Cleve Clin J Med 87(5):273–277, 2020 32357982

Verlinden J: Transgender bodies and male pregnancy: the ethics of radical self-refashioning, in Machine: Bodies, Genders, Technologies. Edited by Hampf MM, Snyder-Körber M. New York, Winter Press, 2012, pp 107–136

Wang Z, Chan AYL, Coghill D, et al: Association between prenatal exposure to antipsychotics and attention-deficit/hyperactivity disorder, autism spectrum disorder, preterm birth, and small for gestational age. JAMA Intern Med 181(10):1332–1340, 2021 34398171

Affirming Gender Identity in the Setting of Serious Mental Illness

Michelle Joy, M.D.
Stephanie Bi, M.D.
Madeleine Lipshie-Williams, M.D.

ESTIMATES indicate that *serious mental illness* (SMI) affects >11 million adults in the United States (4%–6%) (Evans et al. 2016; Wang et al. 2002). According to federal legislation, SMI consists of one or more mental conditions that substantially impact one's life activities and ability to function (Wang et al. 2002). Typically, SMI refers to disorders with a significant psychotic component, such as schizophrenia and bipolar disorder (particularly Type I).

Treatment-resistant and psychotic depression are often included in this category, as can be anxiety disorder, personality disorder, and others, if severe. By definition, SMI is persistent, enduring, and functionally impairing, tending to affect a person's ability to work, form meaningful social relationships, and obtain stable housing (although this is not true for all those with such diagnoses). It is often associated with multiple psychiatric hospitalizations, incarceration, and co-occurring substance use disorders. The distinction is important, because SMI is frequently undertreated despite the need for an increased level of services. Although comprehensive evidence-based treatments do exist, those who do not receive them tend to face increased symptom burden and increased social isolation and stigma (Smith et al. 2019).

Undertreatment of SMI is common; one study found that only 15% of patients received minimally adequate treatment within the previous year (Wang et al. 2002). This undertreatment constitutes a serious public health problem, requiring increased access to care and improved quality of care (Wang et al. 2002).

Access barriers for SMI treatment are further compounded by other prognosticators of disparity, including racial minoritization, living in the rural United States, speaking English as a second language, older age, and lesbian, gay, bisexual, transgender, queer, intersex, asexual, and any sexual and gender minority (LGBTQIA+) identity (Evans et al. 2016). As of this writing, considerations for improving treatment access for those who are LGBTQIA+ and have SMI, outside of cultural competency, have been "left out completely" from research (Evans et al. 2016, p. 56). Individuals with SMI are often left out of research on sexuality and gender as well (Kidd et al. 2011). This neglect is notable, as estimates suggest that ~500,000 LGBTQIA+ individuals with SMI live in the United States (Kidd et al. 2016).

Illness-related stigma may have a large role in the lives of all those with SMI, but it has a specific presence for transgender, nonbinary, and/or gender-expansive (TNG) individuals with SMI (Chapter 2, "Stigma and Mental Health Inequities"). For much of the history of psychiatry, transness itself has been conceptualized as pathologic. More specifically, it was long understood to be a psychotic conception of the self, likened to a delusion, or other frameworks that posited being TNG as SMI. Today, being TNG remains conflated with gender dysphoria and is a diagnosable condition in DSM, albeit with the caveat of causing distress rather than being an inherently pathological state (American Psychiatric Association 2022). No world in which being TNG is itself a diagnosis will be free of the burdens of stigma for TNG people with actual mental health concerns. For TNG people who also experience SMI, particularly psychotic illness, the shadow of psychiatric failures to understand gender can notably impair care. Having a marginalized identity is itself a moderator of schizophrenia risk, as are related factors of childhood abuse and lower socioeconomic status (Barr et al. 2021). Relatedly, discrimination is associated with severity of mental illness among LGBTQIA+ populations (Smith et al. 2019). It is important to recognize that TNG individuals with SMI are resilient, but there remains a crucial role for mental health clinicians to disrupt stigma, rather than reinforce it. Current mental health practitioners and systems are often discriminatory; yet when clinicians are validating, accepting, and understanding, more positive clinical engagement is possible.

These trends underscore the need for evidence-based, community-informed mental health (and affiliated) services for TNG people with SMI. Such an endeavor requires first identifying the needs of this multiply stigmatized and undertreated population, then investing accordingly in education, systems improvements, and advocacy. In this chapter, we aim to guide clinicians in taking an active, inquisitive, and compassionate approach to the care needs of TNG persons with SMI. We call for a system that refuses to tolerate discrimination or to accept lack of awareness or experience as an adequate excuse. We examine diagnostic considerations, gender affirmation questions, and pharmacological factors relevant to TNG people with SMI.

PSYCHOTIC DISORDERS

Schizophrenia-spectrum diagnoses are reflective of the typical presentation of SMI. Symptoms include delusions, hallucinations, disorganization, bizarre behavior, and negative symptoms (loss of interest, lack of concentration) (American Psychiatric Association 2022). Schizophrenia and *schizoaffective disorder* tend to be chronic and substantially impairing and have been characterized as particularly difficult to treat (Peta 2020). Current epidemiological literature provides wildly disparate estimates of the rates of SMI among TNG individuals, reflecting the lack of high-quality data (Barr et al. 2021). Substance-induced psychotic disorders may further confound these data (Barr et al. 2021). Nonbinary populations are largely omitted from this literature. Clinical bias and misdiagnosis may contribute to variation in estimates of SMI prevalence among TNG people, given the controversial legacy of mental health clinicians pathologizing minoritized gender identities and expressions, including a tendency toward frank labeling of TNG identities as delusional and psychotic (Barr et al. 2021).

General access barriers for TNG persons with psychosis seeking health care also apply to gender-affirming care. In addition to financial, geographic, and other impediments, misattribution of symptoms might prevent a TNG person with a psychotic disorder from receiving gender affirmation; this is also seen for neurodivergent TNG people (see Chapter 8, "DoubleQueer"). Mental health clinicians can be reluctant to sign off on gender-affirming treatments for a person with a history of psychosis, despite such obstruction flying in the face of best practices (Barr et al. 2021; Smith et al. 2019). Psychosis alone is not a contraindication to gender-affirming services; in fact, gender-affirming care has been characterized as positive and protective for mental health, including for those with schizophrenia spectrum disorders and psychotic symptoms (Barr et al. 2021).

A commonly voiced concern among clinicians is "ensuring" that someone's experience of their gender is not part of a delusion in the setting of psychosis. We assert that this question is inherently reliant on continued conceptualizations of transness itself as pathology. This potential confusion exists as a result of ongoing belief that an internally held gender identity that is TNG may reflect an experience of reality that is pervasively different from the reality experienced by most others—that is, a delusion. Clinicians ought to be able generally to distinguish information about an individual's internal sense of self from beliefs about the external world (Smith et al. 2019).

This ability is at the crux of believing someone when they tell you their gender while recognizing that some statements (such as "the government is making me into a woman through a chip in my phone") may not reflect reality. We further suggest that determining the veracity of statements related to a person's gender is generally not productive. An associated common concern is what to do if someone with psychosis seeks referrals to medical or surgical gender-affirming treatment. The prevalence of this concern demonstrates "whataboutism" with regard to TNG care: most clinicians will never (or rarely) be in a situation in which someone with acutely impairing psychosis is actually in a position to access medical or surgical affirming care. Yet this question is often used to prevent TNG people from easily receiving referrals. Generally speaking, if a person who experiences psychosis is able to draw on their organizational and executive functioning as needed to establish care with a medical provider, seek a referral letter from a health care provider with relevant competencies, obtain medications or surgical dates, and so on, that person's psychotic symptoms are adequately managed to engage in informed consent discussions.

BORDERLINE PERSONALITY DISORDER

Borderline personality disorder (BPD) tends to be a common diagnosis in clinical settings that can qualify as SMI (Le et al. 2020). A personality disorder is an enduring and pervasive problem with cognition, emotions, relationships, and impulsivity and can lead to impairment and distress. BPD is characterized by unstable relationships, self-image, and emotion, as well as impulsivity (American Psychiatric Association 2022). BPD is associated with functional impairment, poor general health, and short life expectancy (Le et al. 2020). A few studies have reported higher prevalence of personality disorders, particularly BPD, in transgender populations, but the data remain inconclusive and subject to several confounding factors (Anzani et al. 2020; Goldhammer et al. 2019). For example, trauma (which is disproportionately experienced by TNG people) may be a mediating factor for BPD in this population (Anzani et al. 2020), and there may be a misattribution of identity diffusion of BPD with fluid gender expressions or vice versa (Goldhammer et al. 2019). Notably, BPD is highly stigmatized among patients and clinicians (Aviram et al. 2006), which compounds the stigmatization of TNG people with BPD, further alienating them from care.

BPD should not be considered an exclusion criterion for gender-affirming care. By nature, BPD can be difficult to treat and involve self-destructive behavior. This may have implications for gender-affirming care, including the possibility for inadequate treatment adherence and poor satisfaction with interventions (Anzani et al. 2020). Given the chronic and enduring nature of BPD, individuals must have access to quality, evidence-based care. This includes access to specialized psychotherapies such as dialectical behavioral therapy, distilled versions of these therapies by general mental health practitioners (Choi-Kain et al. 2017), and consideration of symptom-based psychopharmacology (American Psychiatric Association 2001).

SUICIDE

Suicidal thoughts and behaviors are a feature of numerous mental illnesses, particularly in instances of SMI. Suicide is a major TNG health disparity and public health crisis, as 40% of TNG individuals have engaged in suicidal behavior at least once (dickey and Budge 2020). Of note, the presence of suicidality may or may not reflect the presence of SMI and should not be used to conflate having a TNG identity with having SMI. Risk of suicidality among TNG people has one of the strongest associations for any marginalized group (dickey and Budge 2020). It often stems from experiences of oppression, discrimination, and violence, which can be exacerbated by additional marginalization related to intersecting factors, such as SMI and race (see Chapters 5–7 on Two-Spirit, Black, and Asian American and Pacific Islander experiences). Suicidality should not be used as a barrier to gender-affirming care when individuals maintain capacity for informed consent. In fact, numerous studies show the positive impact that affirmation can have on reducing suicidality in TNG individuals, including youth, nonbinary people, and veterans (Green et al. 2022; Lelutiu-Weinberger et al. 2020; Tucker et al. 2018). Paradoxically, the beginning of a gender affirmation process can be associated with increased suicidality, perhaps as a result of new experiences of rejection and discrimination related to asserting a gender that lacks societal acceptance, as well as initiating interactions with the health care system when seeking gender-affirming care (Rood et al. 2015). Overall, gender affirmation is a profound protective factor against suicide, and instances of transient increased distress do not justify withholding gender-affirming care.

TREATMENT ENVIRONMENTS

Inpatient mental health treatment, which often occurs for SMI, requires particular attention to be effective and meaningful for TNG patients (Saw

2017). Outpatient clinicians may need to advocate for patients and their needs when referring them to an inpatient or residential treatment setting. For TNG people, inpatient stays often include discrimination and violence and thus impede the very mental health goals they are intended to achieve (Peta 2020). Inpatients should have roommates based on their gender identity, not sex assigned at birth; if that is not feasible (and if desired by patients), private rooms should be considered, although this may further stigmatize TNG people or inadvertently out them to other inpatients. Private rooming should not be enforced against patient wishes, as private rooms are often associated with punishment in the behavioral health setting. Gender-affirming medications prescribed in the outpatient setting should be continued if there are no clear indications for altering the regimen. Access to prosthetics and tools for nonmedical gender affirmation, such as chest binders, should be allowed. Basic social affirmation, such as correct name and pronouns and clothing of choice, is crucial at all times and may require orientation and education for inpatient staff and other patients.

Of note, TNG communities may require specific consideration to adequately attend to housing, financial, and social support needs. Planning for times of increased medically associated stress and postoperative recuperation is particularly important. Because of widespread experiences of familial rejection, TNG patients may require coordination with support systems that are not based on biological or married family when planning discharge from an inpatient psychiatric admission or from the hospital after surgical affirmation. Acute inpatient care or surgery can be a stressful time for anyone, and particular attention should be paid to assessing, supporting, and developing support resources for TNG people. This might include leveraging TNG patients' *chosen family* as support, as well as providing access to TNG peer mentors, hospital navigators, or support groups with people who have shared marginalized gender identities. Advocating for the availability and access to such resources is well within any mental health clinician's ability, and recognition of such needs is important in establishing trust and rapport with patients.

PSYCHOPHARMACOLOGY

Psychopharmacological prescribing must consider some nuances in common treatments for SMI in a TNG population. One domain is potential side effects from SMI treatments and how these can impact TNG patients. Sexual side effects of psychiatric medications, in particular antipsychotic medications, are notable. Risperidone, paliperidone, and the first-generation antipsychotic medications can elevate prolactin levels, resulting in changes in menstruation, vaginal dryness, galactorrhea, loss or gain of body hair, erectile dysfunction, and gynecomastia. This is particularly relevant for patients taking cyproterone acetate—which can also cause hyperprolactinemia—as a component of gender-affirming hormone therapy (Sofer et al. 2020). Patients may not voice these changes for various reasons, ranging from desiring or lacking concern about these effects to discomfort discussing such topics with a mental health clinician. It is the responsibility of the prescribing practitioner to assess for and educate patients about these side effects, as well as the possibility of libido decrease, infertility, and mood symptoms. Options to address these issues include switching medications, adding low-dose aripiprazole, or adding other medications to target specific symptoms (e.g., erectile dysfunction). Given widespread discomfort discussing sexual health topics with patients—and the compounding effect of gender minority stigma—psychiatric prescribers should be particularly comfortable with discussing side effects and their implications. We must remain hypervigilant to biases that affect our care and not assume or avoid essential components of evaluation just because a patient with SMI is also TNG.

Antipsychotic medications increase the risk of metabolic side effects, including elevated blood sugar, lipids, and blood pressure. Although screening for and education about these effects has improved over time, they are still often neglected. There is a well-known mortality gap for individuals with SMI, who die earlier than those without SMI; while this phenomenon is multifactorial—including contributions from cigarette smoking, poor nutritional status, and lack of exercise—atypical antipsychotic medications appear to contribute as well (Riordan et al. 2011). This is not specific to TNG patients, but the compounding effects of inadequate access to care and stigma further increase the risk of metabolic complications. Further, body changes and weight gain that are also common side effects may induce increased severity of bodily or social dysphoria in TNG patients (Nagata et al. 2020a, 2020b). Discomfort with body changes can lead to further isolation and stigma. Conversations about weight gain should not stigmatize large bodies or equate health with size, while inviting TNG patients to discuss any concerns they may have (see Chapter 15, "Eating Disorders and Body Image Dissatisfaction in TNG People").

Extrapyramidal symptoms (EPSs), including parkinsonism and tardive dyskinesia, also require particular care with TNG patients. The risk of tardive dyskinesia increases with cumulative exposure, age, and concurrent substance use disorders. The physical impairment associated with tardive dyskinesia can limit activities and behaviors (Jackson et al. 2021) and is associated with concordant psychological distress (Jackson et al. 2021). As a marker of SMI, EPSs are associated with stigma and with demonstrated adverse impacts on employment, friendship, and romantic opportunities

(Ayyagari et al. 2020). Given the preexisting vulnerability of TNG populations to stigma, discrimination, and distress, the risk of isolation and impairment secondary to potential medication side effects warrants significant consideration and discussion with patients.

Clinicians tend to be unaware of and to underdiagnose tardive dyskinesia (Jackson et al. 2021). Those who recommend antipsychotic medications should be adept at discussing, monitoring, and adjusting treatment for EPSs. It is also worth noting that the habit of routinely prescribing anticholinergic medication for modulating such symptoms is not considered best practice (given the high side effect burden, particularly in older adults) and may in fact worsen tardive dyskinesia symptoms (Citrome et al. 2021). Clinicians can nonetheless seek to reduce or eliminate offending medications, prescribe a reversible inhibitor of vesicular monoamine transporter 2 (VMAT-2), or refer for management with botulinum toxin (Niemann and Jankovic 2018).

An evidence-based perspective is also helpful when considering the side effects of gender-affirming therapies. There is a general tendency to blame hormones for psychological decompensation, but that is rare, and careful interview and health history review are needed before making such an assumption. For instance, there are no known adverse psychiatric effects of estrogen used for gender affirmation, whereas testosterone's potential to affect manic or psychotic symptoms is conceivable only with excessive or supraphysiologic doses (Saw 2017).

Antiretroviral medications for prevention or treatment of HIV bear mentioning with regard to TNG populations with SMI, given both the higher prevalence of HIV and the higher incidence of sexual assault and sex work. HIV and SMI are both (independently) linked to higher cardiovascular risk (Edwards et al. 2011). Studies have shown that adding an antipsychotic medication to the regimen of a patient with HIV may worsen levels of total cholesterol, LDL, and non-LDL cholesterol (Edwards et al. 2011). Simultaneously, people with HIV can be more sensitive to first-generation antipsychotics owing to impact of the virus on certain areas of the brain (the hypothalamic-pituitary-adrenal axis and basal ganglia), which can worsen hyperprolactinemia as well as movement disorders (Vergara-Rodriguez et al. 2009). Notably, many HIV medications are metabolized by the liver's P450 CYP3A4 pathway, for which "lipid-friendly" second-generation antipsychotics (e.g., aripiprazole and ziprasidone) are substrates (Vergara-Rodriguez et al. 2009). These drug-drug interactions may exacerbate side effects, including sedation, priapism, and akathisia (Geraci et al. 2010).

Along with knowledgeable and careful management of the complicated pharmacology and education of patients about these risks, clinicians should incorporate behavioral interventions for TNG people with SMI. Smoking reduction/cessation, healthy diet, and aerobic exercise can be important avenues toward reducing cardiovascular risk (Saha et al. 2021). Reducing the use of illicit drugs (which can induce or perpetuate psychosis) may facilitate symptom control at lower antipsychotic medication doses, and accordingly mitigate side effects.

Of particular interest for this subpopulation, a few studies have considered a potential role for estrogen (Chua et al. 2005; Kulkarni et al. 2019) and testosterone (Brzezinski-Sinai and Brzezinski 2020; Misiak et al. 2018) in SMI treatment. Such work remains extremely preliminary and is not included in current practice guidelines. Future research on pharmacological interventions for SMI, including hormonal therapies, should consider TNG populations.

CONCLUSION

People who have SMI and those who are TNG independently experience discrimination and mistreatment in society at large and specifically within mental health care systems. Special attention should be paid to those who are at the intersection of these experiences and may be subjected to multiple minority stresses that have a profound impact on their health and lived experiences. In this chapter, we review pertinent psychosocial factors, diagnostic considerations, and potential interactions between gender-affirming care and psychopharmacology that all mental health clinicians should take into account to help achieve more equitable mental health care for TNG patients.

REFERENCES

American Psychiatric Association: Diagnostic and Statistical Manual of Mental Disorders, 5th Edition, Text Revision. Washington, DC, American Psychiatric Association, 2022

American Psychiatric Association: Practice Guideline for the Treatment of Patients With Borderline Personality Disorder. Washington, DC, American Psychiatric Association, 2001

Anzani A, Panfilis C, Scandurra C, Prunas A: Personality disorders and personality profiles in a sample of transgender individuals requesting gender-affirming treatments. Int J Environ Res Public Health 17(5):1521, 2020 32120872

Aviram RB, Brodsky BS, Stanley B: Borderline personality disorder, stigma, and treatment implications. Harv Rev Psychiatry 14(5):249–256, 2006 16990170

Ayyagari R, Goldschmidt D, Mu F, et al: An experimental study to assess the professional and social consequences of tardive dyskinesia. CNS Spectr 25(2):275–276, 2020 35078958

Barr SM, Roberts D, Thakkar KN: Psychosis in transgender and gender non-conforming individuals: a review of the literature and a call for more research. Psychiatry Res 306:114272, 2021 34808496

Brzezinski-Sinai NA, Brzezinski A: Schizophrenia and sex hormones: what is the link? Front Psychiatry 11:693, 2020 32760302

Choi-Kain LW, Finch EF, Masland SR, et al: What works in the treatment of borderline personality disorder. Curr Behav Neurosci Rep 4(1):21–30, 2017 28331780

Chua WLL, de Izquierdo SA, Kulkarni J, Mortimer A: Estrogen for schizophrenia. Cochrane Database Syst Rev (4):CD004719, 2005 16235377

Citrome L, Isaacson SH, Larson D, Kremens D: Tardive dyskinesia in older persons taking antipsychotics. Neuropsychiatr Dis Treat 17:3127–3134, 2021 34703232

dickey lm, Budge SL: Suicide and the transgender experience: a public health crisis. Am Psychol 75(3):380–390, 2020 32250142

Edwards KL, Chastain LM, Snodgrass L, et al: Effects of combined use of antiretroviral agents and atypical antipsychotics on lipid parameters. J Antivir Antiretrovir 3(3):34–39, 2011

Evans TS, Berkman N, Brown C, et al: Disparities Within Serious Mental Illness. Report No 16-EHC027-EF. Rockville, MD, Agency for Healthcare Research and Quality, 2016

Geraci MJ, McCoy SL, Crum PM, Patel RA: Antipsychotic-induced priapism in an HIV patient: a cytochrome P450-mediated drug interaction. Int J Emerg Med 3(2):81–84, 2010 20606815

Goldhammer H, Crall C, Keuroghlian AS: Distinguishing and addressing gender minority stress and borderline personality symptoms. Harv Rev Psychiatry 27(5):317–325, 2019 31490187

Green AE, DeChants JP, Price MN, et al: Association of gender-affirming hormone therapy with depression, thoughts of suicide, and attempted suicide among transgender and nonbinary youth. J Adolesc Health 70(4):643–649, 2022 34920935

Jackson R, Brams MN, Citrome L, et al: Assessment of the impact of tardive dyskinesia in clinical practice: consensus panel recommendations. Neuropsychiatr Dis Treat 17:1589–1597, 2021 34079257

Kidd SA, Veltman A, Gately C, et al: Lesbian, gay, and transgender persons with severe mental illness: negotiating wellness in the context of multiple sources of stigma. Am J Psychiatr Rehabil 14(1):13–39, 2011

Kidd SA, Howison M, Pilling M, et al: Severe mental illness in LGBT populations: a scoping review. Psychiatr Serv 67(7):779–783, 2016 26927576

Kulkarni J, Butler S, Riecher-Rössler A: Estrogens and SERMS as adjunctive treatments for schizophrenia. Front Neuroendocrinol 53:100743, 2019 30922675

Le H, Hashmi A, Czelusta K-L, et al: Is borderline personality disorder a serious mental illness? Psychiatr Ann 50(1):8–13, 2020

Lelutiu-Weinberger C, English D, Sandanapitchai P: The roles of gender affirmation and discrimination in the resilience of transgender individuals in the US. Behav Med 46(3-4):175–188, 2020 32787726

Misiak B, Frydecka D, Loska O, et al: Testosterone, DHEA and DHEA-S in patients with schizophrenia: a systematic review and meta-analysis. Psychoneuroendocrinology 89:92–102, 2018 29334627

Nagata JM, Compte EJ, Cattle CJ, et al: Community norms for the Eating Disorder Examination Questionnaire (EDE-Q) among gender-expansive populations. J Eat Disord 8(1):74, 2020a 33292636

Nagata JM, Murray SB, Compte EJ, et al: Community norms for the Eating Disorder Examination Questionnaire (EDE-Q) among transgender men and women. Eat Behav 37:101381, 2020b 32416588

Niemann N, Jankovic J: Treatment of tardive dyskinesia: a general overview with focus on the vesicular monoamine transporter 2 inhibitors. Drugs 78(5):525–541, 2018 29484607

Peta JL: Schizophrenia spectrum and other psychotic disorders among sexual and gender minority populations, in The Oxford Handbook of Sexual and Gender Minority Mental Health. Edited by Rothblum ED. New York, Oxford University Press, 2020, pp 125–134

Riordan HJ, Antonini P, Murphy MF: Atypical antipsychotics and metabolic syndrome in patients with schizophrenia: risk factors, monitoring, and healthcare implications. Am Health Drug Benefits 4(5):292–302, 2011 25126357

Rood BA, Puckett JA, Pantalone DW, Bradford JB: Predictors of suicidal ideation in a statewide sample of transgender individuals. LGBT Health 2(3):270–275, 2015 26788676

Saha SP, Banks MA, Whayne TF: Managing cardiovascular risk factors without medications: what is the evidence? Cardiovasc Hematol Agents Med Chem 19(1):8–16, 2021 32418531

Saw C: Transgender patient care on the inpatient psychiatric unit. AJP Residents J 12(11):7–8, 2017

Smith WB, Goldhammer H, Keuroghlian AS: Affirming gender identity of patients with serious mental illness. Psychiatr Serv 70(1):65–67, 2019

Sofer Y, Yaish I, Yaron M, et al: Differential endocrine and metabolic effects of testosterone suppressive agents in transgender women. Endocr Pract 26(8):883–890, 2020 33471679

Tucker RP, Testa RJ, Simpson TL, et al: Hormone therapy, gender affirmation surgery, and their association with recent suicidal ideation and depression symptoms in transgender veterans. Psychol Med 48(14):2329–2336, 2018 29331161

Vergara-Rodriguez P, Vibhakar S, Watts J: Metabolic syndrome and associated cardiovascular risk factors in the treatment of persons with human immunodeficiency virus and severe mental illness. Pharmacol Ther 124(3):269–278, 2009 19647020

Wang PS, Demler O, Kessler RC: Adequacy of treatment for serious mental illness in the United States. Am J Public Health 92(1):92–98, 2002 11772769

Affirming Gender Identity in the Setting of Incarceration

Michelle Joy, M.D.
Madeleine Lipshie-Williams, M.D.

FOR most of the 20th century, being lesbian, gay, bisexual, transgender, queer, intersex, asexual, or sexually and gender expansive (LGBTQIA+) was associated with criminal perversion (Stotzer 2014). The legal, law enforcement, and correctional systems have long used their state-given power to enforce normality and punish perceived deviance of gender and sexuality (Miles-Johnson 2020). Early in United States history, British-derived sodomy laws targeted sexual minorities. Later, so-called cross-dressing laws allowed officers to target people based on appearance, which particularly affected transgender people. It was not until 2003 that same-sex contact became legal with the Supreme Court's ruling in *Lawrence v. Texas*. And although far fewer laws specifically allow for state-sanctioned targeting of sexual and gender minorities, discrimination remains. In fact, in 2011, the United Nations issued a report highlighting laws discriminating against minority sexual orientations and gender identities around the world (Brown and Jenness 2020). In the United States, transgender people face staggering discrimination in arrest, case handling, and sentencing; violence in the carceral system; and a lack of legal remedies to address these issues (Buist and Lenning 2016; Redcay et al. 2020; Stotzer 2014).

ARREST

Internationally, bias in policing has been well established (Miles-Johnson 2020). Unjustified profiling, stops, arrests, and entrapment are common

(Mallory et al. 2015; Stotzer 2014). Unequal treatment by law enforcement is reported by 26%–47% of transgender, non-binary, and/or gender-expansive (TNG) people interacting with police (Stotzer 2014). TNG people tend to be wary of police independent of victimization status or personal experience with police (Miles-Johnson 2020). Police bias and victimization stem from transphobia and the expectation that gender follows a cisnormative binary pattern. This is compounded by a culture of "machismo" and hegemonic masculinity among law enforcement professionals (Miles-Johnson 2020). In the United States, the field tends to be dominated by white, working class, cisgender men (Miles-Johnson 2020). Stigma is perpetrated through police culture, attitudes, and training that perceive TNG identities as immoral sexual deviancy.

These practices are particularly significant for intersectionally disadvantaged LGBTQIA+ people, including racially minoritized people and people experiencing homelessness. Police disproportionately monitor these communities by targeting low-level crimes, such as sleeping or urinating in public, panhandling, loitering, or violating curfew. Most arrests of TNG persons are, in fact, for minor crimes and misdemeanors (Hughto et al. 2022). In essence, this is a carceral response to social problems (such as poverty) intersecting with racism and transphobia (Yarbrough 2021). These practices then create further poverty through downstream effects of contact with the criminal justice system (Yarbrough 2021).

With reduced access to stable employment, finances, and housing compared with cisgender peers, many TNG individuals engage in survival economies, such as sex work and the drug trade, placing them at increased risk of arrest and incarceration (Brömdal et al. 2019; Redcay et al. 2020; Yarbrough 2021). Transgender women—particularly TNG women of color—who engage in sex work have one of the highest arrest and incarceration rates of any population (Stotzer 2014; Yarbrough 2021). Some studies have shown that these arrests often occur under weak pretenses, such as portraying possession of a condom as evidence of engaging in sex work (Carpenter and Marshall 2017; Goldberg et al. 2019; Poteat et al. 2018). Further, TNG people are often profiled—and targeted, harassed, and victimized—as sex workers merely for being visible, a phenomenon known as *walking while trans* (Redcay et al. 2020; Stotzer 2014). Research has accordingly shown that the elevated risk of arrest for TNG people disproportionately surpasses rates that would be explained by increased engagement in survival crimes (Stotzer 2014).

There is widespread discrimination, harassment, and abuse of TNG communities by police (Mallory et al. 2015). Almost half of LGBTQIA+ victims of violence report experiencing police misconduct, as does more than half of the victimized TNG population (Goldberg et al. 2019). Harassment and verbal abuse are particularly common (Stotzer 2014). Many TNG people report ridicule and embarrassment by police (Miles-Johnson 2020). Police may "frisk" genitalia in attempts to verify someone's gender (Stotzer 2014). Police interactions represent the second most discriminatory venue (after retail stores) for transgender people, with 29% harassed and 6% physically abused by police (Grant et al. 2011). Of TNG people who interact with police, 22% report harassment; 6%, physical assault; and 2%, sexual assault (Grant et al. 2011). Almost 5% of sexual violence against TNG people is said to have been perpetrated by police (Munson and Cook-Daniels 2002); for sex work–related violence, this increases to >17% (Cohan et al. 2006). Transgender people of color are at particularly high risk of police violence. Of note, having been exposed to police violence was associated with later avoidance of health care in a study of Argentinian TNG women (Socías et al. 2014).

Paradoxically, while TNG people are often the targets of overpolicing as noted above, they are simultaneously underpoliced. They do not receive the same attention or response when victimized, despite being at elevated lifetime risk for multiple incidents and types of aggression (Goldberg et al. 2019; Stotzer 2009). TNG people asking for help may be perceived as liars about their gender identity and/or encounter disbelief about their reported crime (Stotzer 2014). About 50%–70% of large survey respondents were uncomfortable with and/or did not seek police assistance when victimized (Grant et al. 2011; Stotzer 2009); international studies show similar trends (Miles-Johnson 2020). When they do report, a vast majority of TNG people are not happy with their experience (Stotzer 2009); the reasons for this discontent vary from not being taken seriously to being revictimized. It is not uncommon for police to disregard the presence of a hate crime, for example.

INCARCERATION

Rates of incarceration in the United States are remarkably high: five times the global average, higher than any other country (Baćak et al. 2018; Joy 2020), and 40 times that of the country with the next lowest rates (Mauer 2017). Between 1982 and 2007, the number of incarcerated people in the United States quadrupled (Joy 2020). In 2010, ~2.3 million individuals were incarcerated, and many more were under community supervision (probation or parole). The expansion of the number of incarcerated people has been characterized as a confluence of changes in crime rates, the economy, political processes, policies, the law, and social conflicts (Campbell and Vogel 2019). International comparisons look at incarceration rates in terms of societal inequalities, racial implications, cultural values, and crime control (Mauer 2017).

Incarceration has many untoward effects on the individual, community, and society at large. These include increased physical and mental morbidity and mortality, decreased civic engagement, limited employment, family disruption, trauma, and homelessness (Bhuller et al. 2018; Mauer 2017; Weidner and Schultz 2019). Every year spent in prison translates into a 2-year reduction of life expectancy (Patterson 2013). Yet whether incarceration reduces crime or recidivism remains questionable.

Gender minorities are incarcerated at higher rates than the general population (Baćak et al. 2018). The criminal justice system has been described as one of queer injustice driven by criminalization of identity (Mogul et al. 2011). Estimates suggest that ~16% of TNG people experience incarceration during their lifetime; this corresponds to a 200%–570% greater risk of incarceration compared with cisgender peers (Brömdal et al. 2019; Clark et al. 2017; Grant et al. 2011; James et al. 2016). Global data, when available, show similar trends (Brömdal et al. 2019). The disparity is even more marked for transgender women (Sevelius and Jenness 2017), particularly for Black TNG women, whose lifetime incarceration risk is 47% (Grant et al. 2011). These stark disparities are largely driven by structural inequalities and stigma (Redcay et al. 2020).

Jails, prisons, and other carceral settings enforce a gender binary with "rigid heterosexist norms and hierarchies" (Baćak et al. 2018; Malkin and DeJong 2019). In particular, men's prisons are characterized by shows of traditional masculinity, heterosexuality, strength, dominance, and cisnormativity (Adorjan et al. 2021; Brown and McDuffie 2009; Buist and Lenning 2016). Incarceration has been characterized as a "terrifying" experience wherein institutional practices "erase" transgender lives (Edney 2004). TNG inmates are considered to be one of the most vulnerable and oppressed populations; they suffer misgendering, maltreatment, human rights violations, and abuse (Buist and Lenning 2016). Being a sexual or gender minority is one of the risk factors most closely linked to victimization behind bars (Baćak et al. 2018). Further associations include being gender non-binary or nonconforming, being a racial or ethnic minority, having been previously abused, and having HIV (Hughto et al. 2022). TNG inmates experience humiliation, verbal harassment, and physical and sexual assault from inmates and correctional staff alike (Clark et al. 2017; Grant et al. 2011; Hughto et al. 2022). Studies have found that 33%–56% of TNG inmates had been victimized (Beck et al. 2013; Hughto et al. 2022). In large surveys, 16%–43% of TNG inmates said that they were physically assaulted, and 15%–24% said that they were sexually assaulted (Caramico 2017; Grant et al. 2011; James et al. 2016). Another study found that 59% of TNG inmates in a male prison had been assaulted (Jenness et al. 2007). Around 15%–16% of transgender inmates report being sexually assaulted (Grant et al. 2011; Hughto et al. 2022).

TNG women housed with cisgender men are at particularly high risk of sexual assault given the tendency toward rape of vulnerable and/or feminine inmates in these settings (Baćak et al. 2018; Brömdal et al. 2019; Buist and Lenning 2016; Edney 2004). Black, Latina, and mixed-race TNG women are at highest risk (Reisner et al. 2014). Correctional officers have been characterized as "chronic and severe" perpetrators by failing to act on behalf of, humiliating, depriving the needs of, and physically, emotionally, and sexually abusing TNG inmates (Whitman 2017). Another report depicts correctional staff as requesting additional security checks for, humiliating, facilitating violence toward, and otherwise oppressing transgender inmates (Buist and Lenning 2016). Research has shown that correctional officers harass (38% of survey respondents), physically assault (9%), and sexually assault (7%) transgender inmates (Grant et al. 2011). At times victimization goes unreported, including by inmates themselves as well as health care providers aware of incidents (Brömdal et al. 2019; Ledesma and Ford 2020). Those inmates who report victimization are often assaulted multiple times, which may not be reflected in available data (James et al. 2016).

High rates of victimization of transgender inmates makes housing assignments particularly important, as they are related to physical, sexual, and other violence and have impacts on inmates' mental health (Brömdal et al. 2019; Ledesma and Ford 2020). In 2003, the Department of Justice issued the Prison Rape Elimination Act (PREA). It was intended to prevent sexual assault against vulnerable inmates. In 2009, PREA identified transgender inmates as being at highest risk and in 2012 developed further guidelines (Oberholtzer 2017). The act contains instructions for correctional administration and staff to understand and consider gender identity for inmate safety when deciding housing locations (Baćak et al. 2018; Kendig et al. 2019). However, its recommendations are not binding; many jurisdictions do not comply and may even have directly conflicting policies (Kendig et al. 2019; Malkin and DeJong 2019). For example, TNG inmates are often housed based on birth sex and genitalia (assessed by physical examination, itself a humiliation) (Bright 2018; Brömdal et al. 2019).

When TNG inmates are not housed with peers of their sex assigned at birth, they are often placed in protective custody (Hughto et al. 2022). This prioritizes physical safety but also creates social and emotional problems through forced isolation (Buist and Lenning 2016). Such segregation is considered a form of torture, with severe mental health consequences (Brömdal et al. 2019; Poteat et al. 2018). It also restricts transgender inmates from phone calls, work, and engagement in programming (Redcay et al. 2020); it worsens stigmatization; and it leaves TNG people vulnerable to abuse by correctional staff.

The best practice is for inmates to be housed based on gender identity and not sex assigned at birth (Buist and Lenning 2016; Ledesma and Ford

2020; Peek 2003). This approach should be flexible, however, and allow for assessment on a case-by-case basis (Brömdal et al. 2019; Hughto et al. 2022). Transgender inmates may be housed with cisgender or other transgender inmates, depending on institutional and individual factors. Some facilities have begun to implement appropriate policies (Sevelius and Jenness 2017). Whatever the case, segregation should be limited in duration and of a voluntary nature (Sevelius and Jenness 2017).

Inappropriate housing is tied to isolation, victimization, and psychological distress, including emotional dysregulation, self-esteem problems, and suicide (Baćak et al. 2018; Brömdal et al. 2019). Even at intake, TNG inmates have worse mental health than cisgender peers (Brown and McDuffie 2009) and often receive inadequate treatment because of barriers in accessing care. The transphobia and violence of incarceration environments compound these difficulties (Van Hout et al. 2020): these highly structured settings promote the gender binary and can in turn increase gender dysphoria (Kendig and Rosseau 2022). TNG inmates have more depression, anxiety, and self-harm than the general incarcerated population (Brömdal et al. 2019; Drakeford 2018). Their suicide rates are 900% that of the general U.S. population (Simopoulos and Khin Khin 2014).

In spite of more numerous medical needs, TNG inmates often receive inadequate health care (Brown 2014; Brown and McDuffie 2009). Gender-affirming care is difficult to access around the world (Petersen et al. 1996; Redcay et al. 2020). In one study, 55% of TNG inmates in the United States reported difficulty accessing appropriate health care (Wanta and Unger 2017). Transgender women have identified access to health care as their primary concern while incarcerated (Brown 2014). Clinicians may believe that being transgender is a form of mental illness; they often misgender, disrespect, harass, and mistreat TNG inmates; they also restrict access to gender-affirming medical, psychiatric, and psychological care (Brömdal et al. 2019; Clark et al. 2017; Hughto et al. 2022; White Hughto and Clark 2019). This behavior may be due to stigma as well as lack of knowledge (White Hughto and Clark 2019).

Even competent and well-meaning health care providers face barriers in providing adequate care. Many correctional institutions have policies restricting access to medical and psychological affirmation services (Baćak et al. 2018). In general, gender-affirming medications may be continued behind bars, but they often are not started (Brown and McDuffie 2009), although this practice is improving. Studies have found that 37%–44% of transgender people previously prescribed hormones did not receive them once incarcerated (Bright 2018; James et al. 2016). Inmate access to prescriptions may be significantly delayed (Hughto et al. 2022), and a diagnosis of gender dysphoria and proof of previous hormone use are often required. Always a barrier, this may create a particular difficulty for people with carceral histories, who may be more likely to have acquired medications without a prescription (owing to poverty and lack of access to care) (Clark et al. 2017; Van Hout et al. 2020). Correctional clinicians may even stop hormonal treatment as a form of punishment or behavioral control (Clark et al. 2017). Abrupt discontinuation of hormones—prescribed or not—can lead to mental and physical withdrawal symptoms, including distress and suicidality (Sevelius and Jenness 2017; Van Hout et al. 2020). Gender-affirming surgery is rarely provided (Brown and McDuffie 2009), and TNG inmates may attempt to perform procedures such as self-castrating (Brown and McDuffie 2009). There is a lack of relevant programming, such as support groups or therapy, tailored to the needs of transgender inmates (Trimble 2019); some states even prohibit it. Overall, lack of access to gender-affirming treatment is associated with depression, suicidality, and death (Brown and Jenness 2020; Clark et al. 2017; Drakeford 2018).

In recent years, courts have generally agreed that access to gender-affirming care is a legal requirement because gender dysphoria is a serious medical condition that cannot go untreated under the 8th and 14th Amendments (Brown and McDuffie 2009). Although this logic continues to inappropriately treat being TNG as an illness, it does establish clear legal precedent for continuing gender-affirming medical care. Courts have found both gender-affirming hormones and surgery to be medically necessary for TNG inmates (Van Hout et al. 2020), although surgery has also been denied by some courts (Kendig and Rosseau 2022). The Department of Justice issued a statement characterizing as unconstitutional the restriction of hormone prescription to persons previously prescribed them (Miller et al. 2020).

It is imperative that correctional clinicians understand the mental health and other needs of TNG inmates and, if lacking competence, engage in conferences, readings, and other methods of lifelong learning. TNG correctional health trainings have been found to be acceptable, feasible, worthwhile, and effective (White Hughto and Clark 2019; Kendig and Rosseau 2022; White Hughto et al. 2017). Competent clinicians must provide accessible, respectful gender-affirming care; furthermore, they should be involved in the creation of policies to ensure its delivery. The position statement of the National Commission on Correctional Health Care (NCCHC; 2020) on TNG health care in correctional settings can be used to introduce gender-affirming care to providers and systems. The NCCHC points to the World Professional Association for Transgender Health (WPATH) Standards of Care as appropriate to inform correctional TNG care, which should be equivalent to that in the community (NCCHC 2020). The American Psychological Association (2008) has also publicly recognized the importance of ensuring gender-affirming care in correctional settings.

As in all settings, best practices for gender-affirming care are based on an informed consent model and should not require a diagnosis of gender dysphoria to access care. Clinicians should let informed consent guide the prescription of hormones, whether continued or initiated (Brown and McDuffie 2009). This approach may involve advocacy for and involvement in the updating of institutional policies. If there are correctional budgetary concerns, clinicians can discuss the cost-saving nature of hormone prescriptions compared with the expenses associated with suicide, auto-castration, and severe mental distress that accompany lack of access (Brown and McDuffie 2009). Mental health clinicians should also support access to gender-affirming surgery and implementation of nonpharmacological mental health treatment that addresses the impact of discrimination and abuse. Potential interventions include Trauma Affect Regulation: Guide for Education and Therapy (TARGET), trauma and grief components therapy, cognitive processing therapy (CPT), or cognitive-behavioral therapy (CBT) (Tadros et al. 2020). Psychotherapy should explore relationships and identities (von Dresner et al. 2013). If competent mental health clinicians are not available on site, the institution needs to provide other access, such as through consultations or community appointments.

The entire correctional system, not just health care providers, needs to provide humane gender affirmation. Despite conflict between health care and security needs, correctional institutions may rely on the medical community in relevant policy decisions (Redcay et al. 2020). Adept clinicians can help to create institutional changes, such as promoting cultural competency of staff. Best practice recommendations exist for training correctional staff to provide a safe and respectful environment (Kendig and Rosseau 2022). Education can use existing resources. For example, the Los Angeles Police Department released information and guidelines on interactions between correctional officers and TNG inmates (Redcay et al. 2020). The National Center for Transgender Equality (NCTE) also published guidance for correctional organizations to improve the safety and well-being of TNG inmates (NCTE 2018). The document discusses community engagement, housing, screening, pronouns and names, searches, commissary, and undergarments. While there is no such thing as a humane prison, minimal basic standards can mitigate some harm.

REENTRY

Reentry to the community is a difficult time for anyone released from a correctional facility. Reentry may be associated with emergency room visits and hospitalizations; contracting sexually transmitted diseases, including HIV; drug overdose; and death (Kendig and Rosseau 2022).

Recent incarceration impedes access to resources and supports (Scheidell et al. 2021), a condition that is exacerbated for TNG individuals (Feingold 2021; Uggen et al. 2013) who, because of discrimination, frequently lack family and other support that could otherwise assist them during the transition (Kendig et al. 2019; Tadros et al. 2020). Recent incarceration has been shown to specifically decrease social support for Black transgender women (Scheidell et al. 2021). Housing and employment resources contain discriminatory policies based on biological sex, with effects compounded by the existence of a criminal record. Mental and physical health resources, in particular for HIV and substance use disorders, are important yet can be difficult to secure. Following release, TNG people face increased family betrayal, poverty, lack of insurance, homelessness, and unemployment (Kendig and Rosseau 2022; Tadros et al. 2020).

Correctional clinicians should prescribe sufficient quantities of psychopharmacologic, HIV/PrEP, and other medications to allow for continuity of care while awaiting treatment linkages in the community; referrals are important. Linking TNG inmates to community substance use disorder programming can reduce drug overdose and protect from communicable diseases (Kendig and Rosseau 2022). Correctional settings should also support connections to safe housing, identity documents, and employment opportunities. Unfortunately, adequate reentry support is often lacking (Kendig and Rosseau 2022).

TNG people are at high risk of recidivism (Kendig and Rosseau 2022). A primary predictor of incarceration in TNG and other populations is previous incarceration. Many steps toward preventing reincarceration begin behind bars, such as decreasing exposure to violence, increasing access to health care, and other programs that aim to address underlying causes of crime. Increased psychological distress might impede successful community reentry and increase recidivism, whereas adequate correctional treatment and continuity of care into the community have the opposite effects (Clark et al. 2017).

Most reentry services have historically focused on the needs of cisgender men and fail to adequately address community resource needs of TNG individuals (Clark et al. 2017; Zettler 2020). In addition to competency working with TNG individuals, clinicians should be aware of the mental health impact of a carceral history. In the general population, a history of incarceration is tied to subsequent major depressive disorder, bipolar disorder, dysthymia, and mental distress (Porter and DeMarco 2019; Schnittker et al. 2012; Turney et al. 2013), which may persist or even worsen over time (Steigerwald et al. 2021). Previously incarcerated transgender women have more polysubstance use, somatic symptoms of distress, homelessness, victimization, and intimate partner violence, as well as lower self-esteem (Anderson-

Carpenter et al. 2017; Brennan et al. 2012; Hughto et al. 2019). They are more likely to smoke, cope by using drugs, have HIV, engage in sex work, and experience physical and sexual assault; victimization during incarceration increases these odds (Reisner et al. 2014). Thus, a further recommendation for clinicians already working with TNG populations is to become more competent in post-incarceration care.

In addition to health care, social services must address other needs of previously incarcerated TNG populations. These services might be TNG competent or TNG focused. Homeless and intimate partner violence shelters, halfway houses, employment resources, rape crisis centers, case management, legal services, and peer supports can all play a role. Probation and parole programs should be similarly attentive to the needs of TNG supervisees.

Unfortunately, these settings are currently often characterized by transphobia, the effects of which are compounded by racism (Cicero et al. 2019; Kattari et al. 2017). The psychological consequences of encountering such discrimination include depression, anxiety, somatization, substance use disorders, and mental distress (Kattari et al. 2016). Research into the discriminatory practices of social services organizations calls for mental health clinicians to advocate against such practices on behalf of individual patients and in the system at large.

REFERENCES

Adorjan M, Ricciardelli R, Gacek J: 'We're both here to do a job and that's all that matters': cisgender correctional officer recruit reflections within an unsettled correctional prison culture. Br J Criminol 61(5):1372–1389, 2021 34489617

American Psychological Association: Transgender, Gender Identity, and Gender Expression Non-Discrimination. Washington, DC, American Psychological Association, 2008

Anderson-Carpenter KD, Fletcher JB, Reback CJ: Associations between methamphetamine use, housing status, and incarceration rates among men who have sex with men and transgender women. J Drug Issues 47(3):383–395, 2017 28670005

Baćak V, Thurman K, Eyer K, et al: Incarceration as a health determinant for sexual orientation and gender minority persons. Am J Public Health 108(8):994–999, 2018 29927654

Beck A, Berzofsky M, Caspar R, Krebs C: Sexual Victimization in Prisons and Jails Reported by Inmates, 2011–12. Washington, DC, U.S. Department of Justice, 2013

Bhuller M, Dahl GB, Loken KV, Mogstad M: Intergenerational effects of incarceration. AEA Pap Proc 108:234–240, 2018

Brennan J, Kuhns LM, Johnson AK, et al; Adolescent Medicine Trials Network for HIV/AIDS Interventions: Syndemic theory and HIV-related risk among young transgender women: the role of multiple, co-occurring health problems and social marginalization. Am J Public Health 102(9):1751–1757, 2012 22873480

Bright L: Now you see me: problems and strategies for introducing gender self-determination into the eighth amendment for gender nonconforming prisoners. J Crim Law Criminol 108:137, 2018

Brömdal A, Clark KA, Hughto JMW, et al: Whole-incarceration-setting approaches to supporting and upholding the rights and health of incarcerated transgender people. Int J Transgend 20(4):341–350, 2019 32999621

Brown GR: Qualitative analysis of transgender inmates' correspondence: implications for departments of correction. J Correct Health Care 20(4):334–342, 2014 25038142

Brown GR, McDuffie E: Health care policies addressing transgender inmates in prison systems in the United States. J Correct Health Care 15(4):280–291, 2009 19635927

Brown JA, Jenness V: LGBT people in prison: management strategies, human rights violations, and political mobilization, in Oxford Research Encyclopedia of Criminology and Criminal Justice. New York, Oxford University Press, 2020

Buist CL, Lenning E: Gender issues in corrections, in Issues in Corrections: Research, Policy, and Future Prospects. Edited by Hilinski-Rosick CM, Walsh JP. Blue Ridge Summit, PA, Lexington Books, 2016, pp 57–79

Campbell MC, Vogel M: The demographic divide: population dynamics, race and the rise of mass incarceration in the United States. Punishment and Society 21(1):47–69, 2019

Caramico G: Thank you Sophia Burset: a call on the federal bureau of prisons to break free of the chains of tradition in order to protect transgender inmates. Georget J Gend Law 18(1):81–102, 2017

Carpenter LF, Marshall RB: Walking while trans: profiling of transgender women by law enforcement, and the problem of proof. William Mary J Women Law 24(1):5, 2017

Cicero EC, Reisner SL, Silva SG, et al: Health care experiences of transgender adults: an integrated mixed research literature review. ANS Adv Nurs Sci 42(2):123–138, 2019 30839332

Clark KA, White Hughto JM, Pachankis JE: "What's the right thing to do?" Correctional healthcare providers' knowledge, attitudes and experiences caring for transgender inmates. Soc Sci Med 193:80–89, 2017 29028559

Cohan D, Lutnick A, Davidson P, et al: Sex worker health: San Francisco style. Sex Transm Infect 82(5):418–422, 2006 16854996

Drakeford L: Correctional policy and attempted suicide among transgender individuals. J Correct Health Care 24(2):171–182, 2018 29609484

Edney R: To keep me safe from harm? Transgender prisoners and the experience of imprisonment. Deakin L Rev 9(2):327–338, 2004

Feingold ZR: The stigma of incarceration experience: a systematic review. Psychol Public Policy Law 27(4):550, 2021

Goldberg NG, Mallory C, Hasenbush A, et al: Police and the Criminalization of LGBT People. New York, Cambridge University Press, 2019

Grant JM, Mottet LA, Tanis J, et al: Injustice at Every Turn: A Report of the National Transgender Discrimination Survey. Washington, DC, National Center for Transgender Equality, 2011

Hughto JMW, Reisner SL, Kershaw TS, et al: A multisite, longitudinal study of risk factors for incarceration and impact on mental health and substance use among young transgender women in the USA. J Public Health (Oxf) 41(1):100–109, 2019 29474682

Hughto JMW, Clark KA, Daken K, et al: Victimization within and beyond the prison walls: a latent profile analysis of transgender and gender diverse adults. J Interpers Violence 37(23-24):NP23075–NP23106, 2022 35195466

James S, Herman J, Rankin S, et al: The Report of the 2015 U.S. Transgender Survey. Washington, DC, National Center for Transgender Equality, 2016

Jenness V, Maxson CL, Matsuda KN, Sumner JM: Violence in California Correctional Facilities: An Empirical Examination of Sexual Assault. Irvine, CA, University of California Department of Criminology, Law and Society, 2007

Joy M: Incarceration reform, in Seeking Value: Balancing Cost and Quality in Psychiatric Care. Edited by Sowers WE, Ranz JM. Washington, DC, American Psychiatric Association Publishing, 2020, pp 491–518

Kattari SK, Whitfield DL, Walls NE, et al: Policing gender through housing and employment discrimination: comparison of discrimination experiences of transgender and cisgender LGBQ individuals. J Soc Social Work Res 7(3):427–447, 2016

Kattari SK, Walls NE, Whitfield DL, Langenderfer Magruder L: Racial and ethnic differences in experiences of discrimination in accessing social services among transgender/gender-nonconforming people. J Ethn Cult Divers Soc Work 26(3):217–235, 2017

Kendig NE, Cubitt A, Moss A, Sevelius J: Developing correctional policy, practice, and clinical care considerations for incarcerated transgender patients through collaborative stakeholder engagement. J Correct Health Care 25(3):277–286, 2019 31242806

Kendig NE, Rosseau NA: Advancing the care of transgender patients, in Public Health Behind Bars: From Prisons to Communities, 2nd Edition. Edited by Greifinger RB. Berlin, Springer, 2022, pp 383–394

Ledesma E, Ford CL: Health implications of housing assignments for incarcerated transgender women. Am J Public Health 110(5):650–654, 2020 32191518

Malkin ML, DeJong C: Protections for transgender inmates under PREA: a comparison of state correctional policies in the United States. Sex Res Soc Policy 16(4):393–407, 2019

Mallory C, Hasenbush A, Sears B: Discrimination and Harassment by Law Enforcement Officers in the LGBT Community. Los Angeles, CA, Williams Institute, 2015

Mauer M: Incarceration rates in an international perspective, in Oxford Research Encyclopedia of Criminology and Criminal Justice. New York, Oxford University Press, 2017

Miles-Johnson T: Policing transgender people and intimate partner violence (IPV), in Intimate Partner Violence and the LGBT+ Community: Understanding Power Dynamics. Edited by Russell B. Berlin, Springer, 2020, pp 281–304

Miller SL, Hodges RM, Wilner LL: Transgender inmates: a systems-based model for assessment and treatment planning. Psychol Serv 17(4):384–392, 2020 30550315

Mogul JL, Ritchie AJ, Whitlock K: Queer (In)Justice: The Criminalization of LGBT People in the United States, Vol 5. Boston, MA, Beacon Press, 2011

Munson M, Cook-Daniels L: Transgender Sexual Violence Project. Milwaukee, WI, Forge, 2002

National Center for Transgender Equality: Policies to Increase Safety and Respect for Transgender Prisoners: A Guide for Agencies and Advocates. Washington, DC, National Center for Transgender Equality, 2018

National Commission on Correctional Health Care: Transgender and Gender Diverse Health Care in Correctional Settings. Resource Document. Chicago, IL, National Commission on Correctional Health Care, 2020

Oberholtzer E: The dismal state of transgender incarceration policies. Prison Policy Initiative, November 8, 2017

Patterson EJ: The dose-response of time served in prison on mortality: New York State, 1989–2003. Am J Public Health 103(3):523–528, 2013 23327272

Peek C: Breaking out of the prison hierarchy: transgender prisoners, rape, and the Eighth Amendment. Santa Clara Law Rev 44:1211, 2003

Petersen M, Stephens J, Dickey R, Lewis W: Transsexuals within the prison system: an international survey of correctional services policies. Behav Sci Law 14(2):219–229, 1996

Porter LC, DeMarco LM: Beyond the dichotomy: incarceration dosage and mental health. Criminology 57(1):136–156, 2019

Poteat TC, Malik M, Beyrer C: Epidemiology of HIV, sexually transmitted infections, viral hepatitis, and tuberculosis among incarcerated transgender people: a case of limited data. Epidemiol Rev 40(1):27–39, 2018 29554240

Redcay A, Luquet W, Phillips L, Huggin M: Legal battles: transgender inmates' rights. Prison J 100(5):662–682, 2020

Reisner SL, Bailey Z, Sevelius J: Racial/ethnic disparities in history of incarceration, experiences of victimization, and associated health indicators among transgender women in the U.S. Women Health 54(8):750–767, 2014 25190135

Scheidell JD, Dyer TV, Hucks-Ortiz C, et al: Characterisation of social support following incarceration among black sexual minority men and transgender women in the HPTN 061 cohort study. BMJ Open 11(9):e053334, 2021 34588263

Schnittker J, Massoglia M, Uggen C: Out and down: incarceration and psychiatric disorders. J Health Soc Behav 53(4):448–464, 2012 23197484

Sevelius J, Jenness V: Challenges and opportunities for gender-affirming healthcare for transgender women in prison. Int J Prison Health 13(1):32–40, 2017 28299969

Simopoulos EF, Khin Khin E: Fundamental principles inherent in the comprehensive care of transgender inmates. J Am Acad Psychiatry Law 42(1):26–36, 2014 24618516

Socías ME, Marshall BD, Arístegui I, et al: Factors associated with healthcare avoidance among transgender women in Argentina. Int J Equity Health 13(1):81, 2014 25261275

Steigerwald VL, Rozek DC, Paulson D: Depressive symptoms in older adults with and without a history of incarceration: a matched pairs comparison. Aging Ment Health 26:2179–2185, 2021 34596476

Stotzer RL: Violence against transgender people: a review of United States data. Aggress Violent Behav 14(3):170–179, 2009

Stotzer RL: Law enforcement and criminal justice personnel interactions with transgender people in the United States: a literature review. Aggress Violent Behav 19(3):263–277, 2014

Tadros E, Ribera E, Campbell O, et al: A call for mental health treatment in incarcerated settings with transgender individuals. Am J Fam Ther 48(5):495–508, 2020

Trimble PE: Ignored LGBTQ prisoners: discrimination, rehabilitation, and mental health services during incarceration. LGBTQ Policy J 9:31–37, 2019

Turney K, Lee H, Comfort M: Discrimination and psychological distress among recently released male prisoners. Am J Men Health 7(6):482–493, 2013 23553444

Uggen C, Manza J, Behrens A: "Less than the average citizen": stigma, role transition and the civic reintegration of convicted felons, in After Crime and Punishment. Edited by Maruna S, Immarigeon R. London, Willan, 2013, pp 279–311

Van Hout MC, Kewley S, Hillis A: Contemporary transgender health experience and health situation in prisons: a scoping review of extant published literature, 2000–2019. Int J Transgender Health 21(3):258–306, 2020

von Dresner KS, Underwood LA, Suarez E, Franklin T: Providing counseling for transgendered inmates: a survey of correctional services. Int J Behav Consult Ther 7(4):38, 2013

Wanta JW, Unger CA: Review of the transgender literature: where do we go from here? Transgend Health 2(1):119–128, 2017 29082332

Weidner RR, Schultz J: Examining the relationship between U.S. incarceration rates and population health at the county level. SSM Popul Health 9:100466, 2019 31485477

White Hughto JM, Clark KA: Designing a transgender health training for correctional health care providers: a feasibility study. Prison J 99(3):329–342, 2019 31198227

White Hughto JM, Clark KA, Altice FL, et al: Improving correctional healthcare providers' ability to care for transgender patients: development and evaluation of a theory-driven cultural and clinical competence intervention. Soc Sci Med 195:159–169, 2017 29096945

Whitman CN: Transgender criminal justice: ethical and constitutional perspectives. Ethics Behav 27(6):445–457, 2017

Yarbrough D: The carceral production of transgender poverty: how racialized gender policing deprives transgender women of housing and safety. Punishment and Society 25:141–161, 2021

Zettler H: The gendered challenges of prisoner reentry, in Prisoner Reentry in the 21st Century: Critical Perspectives of Returning Home. Edited by Middlemass KM, Smiley C. New York, Routledge, 2020, pp 157–171

CHAPTER 20

Addressing the Adverse Impacts of Gender Identity Conversion Efforts

Talen Wright, M.Sc., B.Sc.

A BRIEF HISTORY OF GENDER IDENTITY CONVERSION EFFORTS

Overview

Gender identity conversion efforts (GICE) are known by many names. You may recognize them as *conversion therapy* or *reparative therapy*. GICE is the broad term that denotes any practice that seeks to suppress or change a person's gender identity, specifically from transgender, non-binary, and/or gender expansive (TNG) to cisgender. The central goal is to make someone cisgender, because being cisgender is seen as the only natural state of being, and thus a successful outcome of this approach (Wright et al. 2018).

GICE is in stark contrast to affirmative approaches. An affirmative clinical approach recognizes the importance of meeting patients where they are in their exploration of gender identity and expression. It neither encourages nor disparages a person's unique experience. An affirmative approach seeks to help the individual understand themselves more and gives them a holistic space to express their gender, thoughts, and feelings that is free from judgment, stigma, and pathologization (Hidalgo et al. 2013).

There have been legal movements toward the banning of GICE, and indeed other forms of conversion efforts such as sexual orientation change efforts (SOCE). At the time of writing, the practice of GICE and SOCE is still legal in the United Kingdom, with pressures on the government to outlaw its practice. In the United States, 18 states have banned the practice of conversion therapy, with further pressure in the remaining states to follow suit (Taglienti 2021). Argentina, Uruguay, Samoa, Fiji, and Nauru have also produced indirect bans on GICE and SOCE, whereas Brazil, Ecuador, Germany, and Malta have banned the practice altogether (Chatterjee and Mukherjee 2021). In their writing on conversion practice, Ashley (2019) discussed model law that addresses conversion practices' methods and distinguishes what constitutes GICE—and indeed, what does not. In this respect, they highlighted that "services that are part of a person's social or medical transition" do not constitute GICE, whereas "treatments, practices, and sustained efforts that delay or impede a person's desired social or medical transition without reasonable and non-judgmental clinical justification" do constitute GICE. Actively working to delay access to timely care may constitute a form of enforced biological GICE among TNG youth particularly (Wright et al. 2018). Ongoing work in this area has highlighted the ticking-time-bomb nature of accessing gender identity development services. For those close to puberty, there can be fear of developing physically into a body that is not desired; therefore, access to pubertal suppressant medications is vital to stall those changes. Actively denying timely referral because of a clinician's moral and ethical objections has as much of an adverse impact on the TNG person's well-being as formalized therapy to attempt to alter their identity. Such discussions are very much still ongoing, without consensus on legal approaches.

With the legal ramifications in mind, and indeed the juxtaposition between affirmation and conversion, in this chapter I outline how GICE has come to high prevalence, how it has changed historically, its contemporary uses, and the mental health effects it has had on TNG communities over time. The chapter ends by positing how we can move forward and create affirmative mental health care spaces for TNG patients.

History of GICE

I begin with a historical perspective on the practice of GICE. GICE has been, and perhaps in many circumstances continues to be, conflated with SOCE. The central tenet of any conversion practice is to not see gender diversity as valid and worth celebrating; therefore, it is possible that sexual minorities and gender minorities are seen as one and the same, and some of the literature summarized and highlighted in this chapter does not differentiate these two types of conversion efforts.

GICE has been intrinsically linked with morality and religiosity. Religion has played a substantial role in guiding ethics and morality among various cultures and populations. It therefore is no surprise that many of the GICE and SOCE practices we have seen occur in the counsel chambers of religious community leaders: long sessions with religious counsellors intended to convince individuals that their lives would be better if they adopted heterosexuality or maintained a celibate lifestyle (Haldeman 2002a). Similarly, for TNG people, efforts are common to convince an individual that life would be better if they conformed to the gender they were assigned at birth. In a study by Tozer and Hayes (2004), the motivation for seeking GICE was examined. The authors hypothesized a simple mediation model that religious orientation leads to a propensity to seek GICE, and that this relationship is mediated by internalized heterosexism. In their sample of 206 men and women who were "gay identified," they found that *quest orientation* was significantly associated with the propensity to seek GICE. *Quest* in this case is defined as the search for truth and relates to an individual who realizes that they may never know the final truth about religion but continues to seek answers. The authors also found that *intrinsic orientation*, the phenomenon in which religion is a central guiding principle in a person's life, was associated with the same propensity to seek conversion therapies.

Medical institutions also contribute significantly to the practice of GICE, with early attempts to "cure" sexual orientation and atypical gender identity documented in the late 19th century, when Richard von Krafft-Ebing in 1888 used hypnotic suggestion to attempt to cure homosexuality (Dickinson 2015). Various medical, biological, and psychological tools have been used to induce changes in sexual orientation and gender identity, including, in one case in the 1800s, a bicycle. (The bicycle intervention was administered to a man who was ordered to ride it to the point of exhaustion, in the hopes that this would "eliminate his appetite for other men" [Tozer and McClanahan 1999].) *Electroconvulsive therapy* (ECT)—which is administered through an electrical charge that is delivered to the brain through scalp electrodes, under general anesthesia, pharmacologic muscle relaxation, and constant oxygen saturation monitoring (Espinoza and Kellner 2022)—has been used in the treatment of depression for several decades with relatively good efficacy (Espinoza and Kellner 2022). It has also been used as "treatment" of sexual orientation and atypical gender identity through administration of electric shocks without the use of anesthesia, with the goal to eradicate feelings of same-sex attraction (Haldeman 2002b). Other techniques, such as visits to sex workers, isolation with the "other" sex for 2 weeks, and deprivation of fluids, have been used in a bid to rid the patient of homosexual tendencies. It is worth noting here that many of the accounts used do not explicitly mention TNG people in the vernacular we are accustomed to today. Instead, they used language and terminology such as "effeminate" or "dressing in men's clothing," which actively emphasize the person's gender assigned at birth.

Contemporary Understanding of GICE; What's Happening Now

Shifting to a more contemporary focus, and as mentioned in the overview, there is growing pressure internationally to outlaw the practice of SOCE and GICE, but what exactly are we banning? When we ask those who are likely to experience such practices, the picture becomes clear. In the United Kingdom, a large governmental survey was disseminated to lesbian, gay, bisexual, transgender, queer, intersex, asexual, and more (LGBTQIA+) people. At the end was a simple question: "Have you experienced, or been offered, conversion therapy?" Of the 108,100 respondents, 2% had experienced GICE or SOCE, and 5% had been offered it (Mordaunt 2019). Turban and colleagues published on the prevalence of GICE in the United States, finding that of the 27,715 TNG adults in the study, 14%, or 3,869 individuals, had experienced GICE (Turban et al. 2020). Higbee and colleagues investigated the occurrence of GICE in the southern United States, finding that 16% of the participants who reported experiencing this ($n = 143$) had done so before the age of 18, and that the survivors of GICE were more likely to have received this intervention from a religious leader than a medical professional (Higbee et al. 2022). Higbee et al. also highlighted the prevalence by state, finding that Mississippi had the highest prevalence in the region at 17% and West Virginia the lowest at 4%. Of note, Turban et al. (2020) found no difference in adverse outcomes between religious advisers and secular-type professionals, suggesting that any effort to change someone's gender identity to cisgender was harmful.

Regarding contemporary approaches, it has been argued that the simple withholding of gender-affirming care, such as pubertal suppression or gender-affirming hormone therapy, constitutes a form of GICE, or "biological GICE." For TNG youth, withholding pubertal suppression (ensuring their pubertal development in line with their gender assigned at birth) can be highly damaging.

Enforcing undesired pubertal development results in physical changes to the body that can increase distress and—particularly for those without the financial means or health insurance to pursue gender-affirming medical care—may cause a number of irreversible physical changes that increase the risk of violence. The harm caused by withholding gender-affirming medical care is linked, unsurprisingly, to the lack of appropriate education and training among clinicians, and in the United Kingdom may be linked to the lengthy waitlists for assessment of gender dysphoria (Arora et al. 2019; Barrett 2016).

To be clear on this point, for those who express a desire for more time to explore their gender identity, the withholding of medication would not itself constitute GICE. Exploratory therapy, which indeed can be beneficial, must involve the therapist having no preconceived notion about what the patient's gender identity ought to be. Health Liberation Now, a free resistance resource led by TNG survivors of GICE, highlights the need to be wary of terms such as *gender exploration therapy*, which are becoming synonymous with GICE (Leveille 2022). Leveille highlights the overlap between gender exploration therapy proponents and actors involved in the promotion of GICE practices. Any exploratory work related to gender identity should be guided by the underlying principle that the refusal to aid in someone's physiologic or medical gender affirmation is harmful. This refusal includes moral objections and often prioritizes a clinician's beliefs over the patient's wellbeing (Wright et al. 2018).

MENTAL HEALTH OUTCOMES ASSOCIATED WITH GICE

The mental health impact of GICE has been difficult to ascertain historically, but recent research offers rich insights into outcomes. I summarize these findings under categories of depression, anxiety, and suicidality.

Depression

Depression is characterized by persistent low mood and behavioral changes and is a key risk factor for self-harm (including nonsuicidal self-injury) and suicidality (including suicidal ideation and suicide attempts). Depression can be caused by biochemical changes in the brain or social factors, such as discrimination, harassment, bullying, and stigma.

In the published literature on GICE, very little research has assessed mental health outcomes generally; this is especially true for depression. According to what literature there is, those who have been subjected to conversion therapy are at increased risk of depression (Higbee et al. 2022). (To examine depression following exposure to GICE, we have to extrapolate from research on SOCE.) Shared experiences of LGBTQIA+ communities suggest common marginalization and experiences with conversion efforts, although there is a tendency to conflate sexual orientation with gender identity in the relevant literature.

In a study of 38 ex-ex-gay individuals, conversion efforts were perceived as harmful to their mental health. Within the short-term period after conversion efforts, themes of depression emerged (Flentje et al. 2014). In another study of 245 LGBT people in the United States, participants were asked to reflect on whether their parents had tried to change their sexual orientation and whether their parents took them to religious leaders to "cure, treat, or change their sexual orientation" (Ryan et al. 2020). Such attempts were found to be associated with depression, suicidal thoughts, suicide attempts, and lower education and income.

Anxiety

Anxiety is characterized by restlessness, a sense of dread, feeling on edge, difficulty concentrating, and irritability. In the United Kingdom, anxiety is endemic in TNG communities: a large U.K. survey of TNG mental health found that 75% of the 1,054 participants were currently or previously diagnosed with anxiety. In another study, anxiety following GICE was explored in a sample of 6,418 Australians 14–21 years old. In this population, 4% had experienced GICE (Jones et al. 2022). For those who experienced GICE, there was an increase in anxiety symptoms.

There are multiple possible mechanisms for this increase in anxiety. The goal of GICE is to cause suppression of gender identity, and this can intensify feelings of internalized transphobia, which in turn can feel all-consuming and unmanageable. Also, it is widely acknowledged that concealment of gender identity, especially among youth, can increase anxiety symptoms, as concealment involves the need for complex calculations and cost-benefit analysis to determine the appropriate course for any given social environment (Bry et al. 2017). This concealment therefore may underpin a feeling of dread and being on edge.

Suicidality

Suicidality is an overarching term that encompasses a continuum, in which there is a progression in phenomena from suicidal ideation (i.e., thinking about suicide) to attempts to take one's life (Sveticic and De Leo 2012). Suicide disproportionately affects TNG communities, with recent figures suggesting that 88% of trans people in the United Kingdom have thought about suicide and ~40% have attempted suicide. In the United States, the numbers are equally high, with 82% of the 27,715 survey respondents to the 2015 U.S. Transgender Survey having thought about suicide at some point in their lives, and 40% having attempted suicide (Herman et al. 2019). Many underlying mechanisms are thought to increase TNG people's risk of suicidality: cisgenderism, discrimination, gender minority stress, stigma, and poor access to health care (Herman et al. 2019; Romanelli et al. 2018).

An association has been found between recalled exposure to GICE and subsequent suicidality (Turban et al. 2020). Turban et al. (2020) found that lifetime exposure to GICE increased the odds of lifetime suicide attempts by 2.27. Thus, exposure to GICE has a clear detrimental impact on mental health, particularly suicidality. When factoring in age of exposure, those who were < 10 years old when they experienced GICE had odds of attempting suicide that were doubled again, with an increase in odds of 4.15 compared with participants who had not been exposed to GICE. These findings show quite plainly that exposure to GICE is traumatic, and that youth are particularly susceptible to the damaging effects of GICE.

In the 2015 U.S. survey of TNG people, respondents who had been rejected by their religious communities or had undergone conversion efforts were more likely to have reported suicidal ideation and suicide attempts. In that report, 13% of those who reported religious rejection or GICE had attempted suicide in the previous year, compared with 6% of those who received religious acceptance (Herman et al. 2019). Furthermore, Herman et al. (2019) found that suicide attempts were more common among TNG people if a professional had tried to stop them from being TNG (12% vs. 6% of those who had not had that experience).

HOW TO MAKE PSYCHIATRIC CARE MORE AFFIRMATIVE

To make psychiatric care more affirming, we first must understand the numerous ways in which psychiatric care has hurt TNG people. In this chapter, I characterize some such harmful practices, and we also should apply an intersectional approach. *Intersectionality* is an analytical framework for understanding how different aspects of a person's social and political identities combine to result in unique experiences around discrimination and stigma (Atewologun 2018). Examples of intersecting identities are gender, race, ethnicity, disability, and sexual orientation, all of which have social and political meaning (Naples 2009). For Black, Indigenous, and people of color (BIPOC) communities, lack of health care access, broken patient-clinician trust, and race-related stigma associated with nonadherence to medication are just some of the barriers to accessing high-quality care (Price et al. 2022). For disabled people, ableism and a lack of accessible space are barriers to psychiatric care, especially for the young (Coomer 2013). These are just a few examples. Affirmative approaches must be intersectional to be truly affirmative.

Recognizing the traumas that the field of psychiatry has inflicted, mental health clinicians must actively aim to increase culturally responsive care for TNG communities. Affirmation in clinical care is not a practice that either encourages or disparages gender transition as the goal of a therapeutic relationship. Affirmation simply seeks to support an individual and address their needs holistically. Having preconceived negative beliefs about TNG lives and engaging in practices meant to hurt TNG people, such as willful deadnaming or misgendering, is incompatible with an affirmative approach to care. Affirmative approaches are nonjudgmental and allow for full exploration, following the process, pace, and path set by the patient.

REFERENCES

Arora M, Walker K, Luu J, et al: Education of the medical profession to facilitate delivery of transgender health care in an Australian health district. Aust J Prim Health 26(1):17–23, 2019 31738874

Ashley F: Model law—Prohibiting conversion practices. Social Science Research Network, 2019. Available at: https://ssrn.com/abstract=3398402. Accessed July 18, 2023.

Atewologun D: Intersectionality theory and practice, in Oxford Research Encyclopedia of Business and Management. New York, Oxford University Press, 2018

Barrett J: Doctors are failing to help people with gender dysphoria. BMJ Online 352, 2016

Bry LJ, Mustanski B, Garofalo R, Burns MN: Management of a concealable stigmatized identity: a qualitative study of concealment, disclosure, and role flexing among young, resilient sexual and gender minority individuals. J Homosex 64(6):745–769, 2017 27633070

Chatterjee A, Mukherjee T: On conversion talk in Indian clinical contexts: a pilot venture. J Psychosex Health 3(4):308–314, 2021

Coomer RA: The experiences of parents of children with mental disability regarding access to mental health care. Afr J Psychiatry (Johannesbg) 16(4):271–276, 2013 24051566

Dickinson T: 'Curing queers': mental nurses and their patients, 1935–74, in Curing Queers. Manchester, UK, Manchester University Press, 2015

Espinoza RT, Kellner CH: Electroconvulsive therapy. N Engl J Med 386(7):667–672, 2022 35172057

Flentje A, Heck NC, Cochran BN: Experiences of ex-ex-gay individuals in sexual reorientation therapy: reasons for seeking treatment, perceived helpfulness and harmfulness of treatment, and post-treatment identification. J Homosex 61(9):1242–1268, 2014 24960142

Haldeman DC: Gay rights, patient rights: the implications of sexual orientation conversion therapy. Prof Psychol Res Pr 33(3):260, 2002a

Haldeman DC: Therapeutic antidotes: helping gay and bisexual men recover from conversion therapies. J Gay Lesbian Psychother 5(3–4):117–130, 2002b

Herman JL, Brown TN, Haas AP: Suicide Thoughts and Attempts Among Transgender Adults: Findings From the 2015 U.S. Transgender Survey. Los Angeles, CA, Williams Institute, 2019

Hidalgo MA, Ehrensaft D, Tishelman AC, et al: The gender affirmative model. Hum Development 56(5):285–290, 2013

Higbee M, Wright ER, Roemerman RM: Conversion therapy in the southern United States: prevalence and experiences of the survivors. J Homosex 69(4):612-631, 2022 33206024

Jones T, Power J, Hill AO, et al: Religious conversion practices and LGBTQA+ youth. Sex Res Soc Policy 19:1155–1164, 2022

Leveille L: A new era: key actors behind anti-trans conversion therapy. Health Liberation Now!, June 1, 2022

Mordaunt P: LGBT Action Plan: Annual Progress Report 2018 to 2019. London, Government Equalities Office, 2019

Naples NA: Teaching intersectionality intersectionally. Int Fem J Polit 11(4):566–577, 2009

Price JL, Bruce MA, Adinoff B: Addressing structural racism in psychiatry with steps to improve psychophysiologic research. JAMA Psychiatry 79(1):70–74, 2022 34613345

Romanelli M, Lu W, Lindsey MA: Examining mechanisms and moderators of the relationship between discriminatory health care encounters and attempted suicide among U.S. transgender help-seekers. Adm Policy Ment Health 45(6):831–849, 2018 29574543

Ryan C, Toomey RB, Diaz RM, Russell ST: Parent-initiated sexual orientation change efforts with LGBT adolescents: implications for young adult mental health and adjustment. J Homosex 67(2):159–173, 2020 30403564

Sveticic J, De Leo D: The hypothesis of a continuum in suicidality: a discussion on its validity and practical implications. Ment Illn 4(2):e15, 2012 25478116

Taglienti J: Therapists behind bars: criminalizing gay-to-straight conversion therapy. Fam Court Rev 59(1):185–199, 2021

Tozer EE, Hayes JA: Why do individuals seek conversion therapy? The role of religiosity, internalized homonegativity, and identity development. Counsel Psychol 32(5):716–740, 2004

Tozer EE, McClanahan MK: Treating the purple menace: ethical considerations of conversion therapy and affirmative alternatives. Counsel Psychol 27(5):722–742, 1999

Turban JL, Beckwith N, Reisner SL, Keuroghlian AS: Association between recalled exposure to gender identity conversion efforts and psychological distress and suicide attempts among transgender adults. JAMA Psychiatry 77(1):68–76, 2020 31509158

Wright T, Candy B, King M: Conversion therapies and access to transition-related healthcare in transgender people: a narrative systematic review. BMJ Open 8(12):e022425, 2018 30580262

Psychiatric Evaluations in Support of Gender-Affirming Surgical Procedures

Morgan Faeder, M.D., Ph.D.

AN enduring frustration of transgender, non-binary, and/or gender-expansive (TNG) people is obtaining letters from mental health clinicians in support of gender-affirming surgery (GAS). Some version of this letter is required by surgeons and insurance companies—often separate letters written by two clinicians—in addition to whatever letters are needed from hormone prescribers. Surgeons and insurance carriers have related, but not identical, interests in establishing medical necessity and ensuring that the patient is able to consent to and tolerate the intended procedure. At first, the point was for a mental health clinician to establish the patient's identity within a narrow framework of what it means to be TNG, and thus certifying their eligibility for the procedure. Over time, the emphasis has expanded to include establishing medical necessity, preventing regret, documenting psychological "stability," and ensuring ability to tolerate the procedure and any complications.

This chapter reviews the historical context of the letter and discusses gatekeeping and the ethical role of the psychiatrist. We emphasize the impact of prior traumatic experiences on the patient and on the letter-writing process and conclude by describing the mechanics of letter-writing visits and what components the letter should contain.

HISTORICAL CONTEXT

For most of history, surgery for TNG people was not an option (or was available to very few). The first modern genital reconstruction surgeries ("lower surgery") were performed in the early to mid-20th century (Frey et al. 2017). The first documented transfeminine lower surgery was performed in 1931 at the Institute of Sexual Science in Berlin (Meyerowitz 2004), and the first transmasculine procedures, from 1946 to 1949 in Great Britain by Dr. Harold Gillies (Riverdale 2012). The first high-profile lower surgery, sensationalized in the American news media (Walsh 2012), was performed in Copenhagen for Christine Jorgensen in 1952. The case report of her treatment describes "very thorough continuous psychiatric assessment" over the 2 years between the initiation of estrogen and the time of her lower surgery (Hamburger et al. 1953). At that time, each surgeon or surgical center had extensive selection criteria, focusing on a narrow conceptualization of TNG identities and privileging straight white transgender women who were deemed by the evaluators as most likely to be perceived as cisgender. At the Johns Hopkins University School of Medicine Gender Identity Clinic, patients underwent a week of evaluation, including individual psychiatric evaluation, family interviews, and neuropsychological testing (Siotos et al. 2019).

The move toward standardization of health care for TNG people began with Harry Benjamin, who took a stance advocating for body modification to treat gender dysphoria by aligning the body with experienced gender, rather than what was then the standard of conversion therapy (psychological attempts to align gender identity with societal expectations based on sex assigned at birth) (Benjamin 1967). In 1979, the Harry Benjamin International Gender Dysphoria Association was founded (renamed the World Professional Association for Transgender Health [WPATH] in 2007), and the first Standards of Care (SOC) were released. The most current SOC, Version 8 (Coleman et al. 2022), continues to require assessment of individuals seeking GAS to establish a diagnosis of gender incongruence and identify any co-occurring mental health disorders. According to the SOC, this assessment can be done by any qualified health care professional, not limited to mental health clinicians, and without requiring a specific psychiatric assessment. The SOC define a qualified professional as one who holds a master's degree or equivalent in a relevant clinical field; is competent in using a diagnostic taxonomy such as the World Health Organization's ICD; is able to identify coexisting mental health concerns and distinguish them from gender dysphoria or incongruence; is able to assess capacity to consent for treatment; is qualified to assess clinical aspects of gender dysphoria, incongruence, and diversity; and undergoes continuing education related to gender dysphoria, incongruence, and diversity. These requirements of the assessor make it very likely that it will be mental health professionals that assess GAS candidates for the foreseeable future. In fact, recommendation 5.3.d, "Ensure that any mental health conditions that could negatively impact the outcome of gender-affirming medical treatments are assessed, with risks and benefits discussed, before a decision is made regarding treatment," all but ensures the frequent involvement of mental health professionals (Coleman et al. 2022).

Although it is no longer strictly necessary for the letter in support of GAS to be written by a mental health clinician, it is useful to examine the evolution of the psychiatric view of TNG identities to put the modern assessment in historical context. In parallel with societal recognition and changing attitudes toward TNG people, the American Psychiatric Association (APA) first included mention of transgender identity in DSM-III (American Psychiatric Association 1980), classifying *transsexualism* as a *psychosexual disorder*. In DSM-IV and DSM-IV-TR (American Psychiatric Association 1994, 2000), the diagnosis changed to *gender identity disorder*. In DSM-5 and DSM-5-TR, it became *gender dysphoria* (American Psychiatric Association 2013, 2022), in response to criticism that diverse gender identities are not, in themselves, pathological.

The inclusion of TNG identities in DSM marks the entry of TNG people into the mainstream consciousness. The evolution of diagnoses illustrates the shift from viewing TNG identities first as sexual deviance, then as character pathology (where the logical response is either societal shaming or psychotherapy to "cure" the mistaken view of self), and finally as a maladaptive response to a natural variation of human experience. The most recent shift in diagnostic classification comes from ICD-11 (World Health Organization 2020), which classifies the TNG experience as a "condition related to sexual health" rather than a mental health disorder, implicitly recognizing that the increased mental health difficulties TNG people face compared with the general population are caused by stigma and discrimination rather than any pathology inherent to being TNG.

GATEKEEPING

Access to medical and surgical gender affirmation has always been limited to those whom the medical establishment identifies as "appropriate." This initially was decided in a rather haphazard way, by the surgeon or clinic performing the surgery or the clinician referring for surgery. For example, the Johns Hopkins University Gender Identity Clinic performed GAS on only 24 patients in its first 2.5 years (Meyerowitz 2004). The introduction of the original WPATH SOC and subsequent revisions, along with better access to insurance coverage of GAS, has led to standardization of the process and has cemented mental health professionals as the gatekeepers of access to GAS. Before the Affordable Care Act (The Patient Protection and Affordable Care Act 2010) in the United States, most insurance health plans did not cover GAS, and surgeons established their own procedures, often using practice guidelines such as the WPATH SOC or similar references (Center of Excellence for Transgender Health 2016; Coleman et al. 2012; Lichtenstein et al. 2020), in determining suitable candidates. Thus, although most insurance carriers rely on WPATH SOC to determine eligibility for coverage, individual surgeons or surgical practices may require more documentation than the insurance carrier. The letter writer therefore must clarify with the surgical candidate what must be included to satisfy all parties. There have also been restrictions on who may write letters: although the policy is not stated in any practice guidelines, many insurance carriers and surgeons have insisted on at least one letter of support written by a doctoral-level clinician (M.D., D.O., Ph.D., or Psy.D.).

Inherent to the criteria for access to surgery is the assumption of *cisnormativity* (that cisgender identities are normal and TNG identities are not), thus implicitly framing GAS as removing healthy tissue from a mentally ill person (Strand and Jones 2021). This assumption has led to several problems. One is that an evaluation for GAS requires TNG people to prove their identities to a mental health professional and establish medical necessity for the procedure. Mental health evaluation for GAS is often compared to a transplant or bariatric surgery evaluation but differs in that a transplant or bariatric surgery candidate is not asked to prove the medical necessity of the procedure, only that they will be able to follow postoperative instructions and cope reasonably with both intended and unintended outcomes. Their identity is not called into question. The GAS evaluation puts the clinician and the TNG individual in an adversarial relationship, with the clinician requiring "proof" and the TNG person being challenged to produce it, thus increasing the power differential between clinician and patient. As a result, the TNG person seeking GAS is incentivized to produce a history that is consistent with what they think the clinician will require to give a diagnosis that, in turn, their insurance company will accept as a prerequisite for surgery (essentially, adjusting testimony to what they believe the insurance company wants to hear). This history also needs to establish medical necessity apart from the certification that the TNG person is who they say they are (the diagnosis), by establishing significant impairment that will be alleviated by surgery. The TNG person needs to walk a line between being impaired enough to require GAS but not so impaired that they are considered to possess insufficient psychological stability to tolerate it. This has been particularly difficult for non-binary people (whose identities are neither female/

woman nor male/man) because their stories have entered relatively late in mainstream consciousness, as well as the difficulty of many clinicians to conceptualize a body that is phenotypically neither female nor male (Lykens et al. 2018).

The clinician then has two conflicting roles: the accustomed role as patient advocate and support, and the assigned role as arbiter of the identity of the TNG person and certifier of their surgical needs. The task is to remain patient centered while still fulfilling the assigned duty. The TNG person is in a complementary, though significantly disadvantaged, position: needing documentation to be able to access their surgical goals, and also being a human in need of respect and support. The path of least resistance for both parties is to fulfill the insurance and surgical requirements and let the less tangible needs of the patient fall by the wayside, and thus losing an opportunity to help the patient achieve the best outcome possible, both surgically and in terms of mental health in general.

ROLE OF THE LETTER WRITER

A clinician may be asked to write a letter for GAS under two broad sets of circumstances: as a one-time consultation, or for an existing patient in longitudinal care with the clinician. The information in the letter itself will be essentially similar; however, the approach with the TNG person will likely be quite different, as the process of rapport and trust-building is truncated in a one-time consultation. In either case, trust is essential; if the clinician has not established themselves as trustworthy, the TNG person will tell a story that gives them the best chance of obtaining the letter they need and omit much that does not fit the current culturally acceptable narrative surrounding TNG identities and experiences. When writing a letter for an established patient with whom the clinician has a good working relationship, there need not be a heavy emphasis on establishing trust at the beginning of the process, particularly if gender dysphoria and associated mental health disorders have been the focus of treatment. Nevertheless, with patients for whom this has not been a primary focus in the past, establishing safety around these particular issues is still necessary. An appointment can be scheduled for the purpose of gathering information to be included in the letter, with appropriate explanation of why the information is necessary. The letter writer can also use this time to agree with the TNG person on any interventions to increase the likelihood of an optimal surgical outcome, including identifying supports or clarifying questions that the patient may have for their surgeon. This is also a good time to discuss what constitutes an optimal outcome for the patient and what concerns they have about complications.

When engaging with a TNG person as a limited consultant for a letter in support of gender-affirming care, it is necessary to consider explicitly the role of the letter writer. Given the history of psychiatric gatekeeping discussed earlier and the impact of trauma on the relationship-building process, discussed below, the letter writer must be clear with themselves and the TNG person about what exactly the letter-writing visit is meant to accomplish. It is important to frame the visit from the start as one that is person centered and focused on helping the TNG person succeed with their goals for gender affirmation without making any assumptions beforehand about what the goals are. To build trust and openness, the clinician should acknowledge personal and community medical trauma and the intention to establish a trauma-informed environment. Ideally, a letter-writing visit will end with the TNG person understanding that the clinician will be able to write a letter in support of their goals, and this is true most times in practice as well. At times, the visit will uncover areas where the TNG person needs more support to have an optimal outcome. In those cases, the emphasis must be on how to help them meet these needs and not on delaying support for the procedure. This may mean connecting them with community resources or helping them to access more information about the procedure so that they will be able to participate in granting informed consent to their surgeon. Whether the letter writer is a one-time consultant or an established care clinician, they may write the letter in collaboration with the TNG person during the office visit. If the letter writer decides to write the letter at another time, an additional visit should be scheduled to review the letter and confirm with the TNG person that it portrays their experiences accurately and respectfully. They can then collaboratively specify changes as needed before the letter is finalized.

TRAUMA

The impact of trauma on any interaction of a TNG person with the medical establishment is hard to overstate. Classically, clinicians consider a traumatic event one that fulfills diagnostic criterion A for PTSD, requiring "exposure to actual or threatened death, serious injury, or sexual violence" (American Psychiatric Association 1980). Nevertheless, "nontraumatic" events, those that have a marked negative impact but do not fulfill criterion A, may still evoke a trauma response (Alessi et al. 2013). These may include events such as familial rejection, losing access to stable housing, and discrimination in health care, among many others. So medical trauma, in this context, will include both criterion A events and non–criterion A events. The history of gatekeeping, denial of care (nontraumatic), and medical assault (traumatic) is ongoing, and most, if not all, TNG people will either have experienced one of these or know someone who has (James et al. 2016). Over the years 2018–2022, legislation targeting gender-affirming care gradually increased, with two bills proposed in 2018 and 35 in 2022. At the time of writing (June 2023), 168 bills have been introduced, many of them criminalizing or banning gender-affirming care for young people (up to age 26 in some cases) (Health care; prohibiting gender transition procedures for children; authorizing certain civil actions and relief; licensure; adding violations and penalties 2023) and others intending to make care inaccessible, if not strictly illegal, to adults (Gender Clinical Interventions, HB 1421, Florida House of Representatives 2023). While this chapter does not address the added complexities of writing a letter in support of gender affirmation for minors, these laws are manifestations of the stigma attached to TNG identities and a clear indication of the current climate TNG people face. The stress associated with institutionalized discrimination against some community members has an impact on the mental and physical well-being of the entire community and will affect interactions with health care clinicians (Institute of Medicine 2011).

Any interaction with a medical professional must be seen in the context of the stigma associated with TNG identities and the ongoing history of medical trauma experienced by TNG people. When a TNG person seeks a letter in support of gender-affirming care, they must engage with a system that has been a source of trauma for them and/or their community and may display reasonable and adaptive behaviors that are viewed as maladaptive by the clinician. Core posttraumatic symptoms such as avoidance, hypervigilance, and hyperarousal may be interpreted as hostility and lack of cooperation with the evaluation. This fundamental misunderstanding precludes a thorough understanding of the patient's experiences, goals, and challenges. In the best case under these circumstances, a TNG person will leave the encounter with a supporting letter; however, the opportunity will have been lost for identifying and increasing their natural supports and providing resources to assist with any challenges. The worst-case scenario leaves the patient further traumatized and without a letter.

Another aspect of trauma that the letter-writer must consider is the impact of prior trauma on a TNG person's ability to fulfill postoperative requirements and cope with complications. A history of medical trauma may make anything other than the most routine follow-up care difficult. Past sexual trauma may negatively impact a person's ability to adhere to a dilation schedule after vaginoplasty, for example. The role of the clinician in these cases is not to make resolution of prior traumas a condition of writing a letter in support of surgery, lest they get in the way of optimal surgical outcomes, but to identify and connect the TNG person with appropriate supports to allow them to succeed despite their experiences of trauma.

LETTER-WRITING VISIT

When working with a TNG person to support their surgical goals, the clinician should also be collaborating with the patient's other clinicians of gender-affirming care. Ideally, a one-time consultation will take place in an integrated care setting, where the mental health clinician works with either a gender-affirming medical clinician, a surgeon, or both (Manrique et al. 2021). Unfortunately, most patients do not have access to fully integrated services, and most clinicians do not work in an integrated center. If they are able to interface with the medical and surgical clinicians, even if they are not part of a multidisciplinary center, the clinician can help the TNG person navigate the process more easily, and less of the visit needs to be devoted to prior history of gender-affirming care or understanding the nuances of working with a particular surgeon. If possible, obtaining consent to communicate with other clinicians and requesting medical records can be done before the visit, to streamline the process and guide discussion of any points that may be less clear. Many surgeons and insurance companies have letter templates; obtaining these before the first visit will save time.

As noted earlier, establishing rapport is the first order of business and can be complicated by many factors, including personal or community history of medical trauma and the transactional nature of a limited-time consultation to obtain a surgical letter. On meeting the patient, one should give an introduction with both name and pronouns and ask for both from the patient. It is best then to open with a clear introduction of the purpose of the visit (to fulfill insurance and surgical requirements) and a statement acknowledging the pressures the TNG person may feel to tell a story that fits in with a "classic" narrative. This can be followed by a statement of acceptance of whatever their experiences have been that have brought them to this point and a commitment to helping them realize their goals in seeking care. These statements align the clinician's interests with the TNG person's and help to establish a safe and affirming environment. It is important, however, not to leave the TNG person with the impression that they will leave the first visit with a letter in hand. Although it will be possible in the vast majority of cases to write a letter of support after one or two visits, there will be times when the clinician may need to make recommendations for the TNG person to pursue before a supporting letter is provided.

After establishing the framework for the visit and clarifying the task ahead, the clinician and TNG person can explore the history of the patient's gender development as an affirming way to assess for gender dysphoria. The clinician will want to know when (approximately) they identified their gender as different from their sex assigned at birth, what steps they have taken

to affirm their gender thus far, and what the responses of the people important to them have been. It will be important to note a timeline for when the
TNG person started social transition (name change; changes in clothing,
hair, and other reversible external modifications of appearance); when they
started medical interventions for gender dysphoria; what kinds of treatments they have already pursued (puberty blockers, hormone treatment,
other surgeries); and what the effects of those have been. To establish medical necessity, clinicians may describe distress that has improved with prior
interventions but has not been fully relieved. Standard mental health assessment concludes the information-gathering portion of the session.

Part of the evaluation will be to help establish *capacity* to provide informed consent for the desired procedure. As capacity depends on other factors, it cannot definitively be assessed at a visit that is necessarily well in
advance of the procedure itself; therefore, the final capacity determination
falls to the surgeon at the time of the procedure. The clinician does not need
to know the details of each gender-affirming procedure to be able to help the
patient participate in an informed consent discussion with their surgeon.
Nevertheless, some attention must be paid to this issue in the letter, as surgeons and insurance companies want to know that, broadly speaking, the
TNG person is able to reason about the risks and benefits of the surgery and
is entering the process with knowledge of the important issues. During the
evaluation, the clinician can explore the patient's understanding of the details
of the procedure, the known risks, and the requirements for postoperative
care. If the TNG person needs to travel for the procedure, they will need to
consider housing and postoperative support away from home. Some insurance plans will pay for a stay in a skilled nursing facility; however, many TNG
people will need to arrange appropriate lodging and identify a caregiver who
can travel with them. In their discussion about the procedure, the clinician
and patient can explore what aspects of major surgery in general, and of their
surgery in particular, are of most concern and make a list of questions to ask
the surgeon. The clinician can assist with identifying supports and connecting the patient with resources. In this way, the clinician can document that
the patient is participating actively in the informed consent process and that
concern is low for lack of decisional capacity at the time of the procedure.

During the interview, the TNG person may discuss issues that could impede recovery, such as current smoking or heavy alcohol use. The clinician
can use the visit as an opportunity to offer education on smoking and wound
healing (including the likelihood that cessation of nicotine use for a time before and after the surgery will be required by the surgeon), or on the risk of
postoperative alcohol withdrawal, and offer appropriate treatment or referral to a more intensive treatment program. They can also use the evaluation
as an opportunity to identify areas in which the TNG person may need more

support and offer referrals to service coordination and other relevant programs. Likewise, the clinician and TNG person can strategize ways to limit the impact of prior trauma on the patient's ability to perform postoperative tasks, such as vaginal dilation or wound care.

Throughout the process, the clinician must remain centered on the needs of the TNG person. One can view the visit as a collaboration with the clinician to meet the needs of the person for access to surgical care and as an opportunity to identify ways in which to improve access and surgical outcomes. At the end of the visit, the TNG person should leave with the understanding that they will have a letter in support of their surgery or clear knowledge of what must be done to receive it. The clinician should never place barriers to surgery, only identify those that exist and assist with overcoming them. The clinician may write the letter and share it with the TNG person to solicit corrections to any misunderstanding of the patient's history and conceptualization of themselves. Alternatively, they may choose to schedule another visit to write the letter collaboratively with the patient. This is often easiest to accomplish when working with a defined format for the letter already in place that the two working together then populate with the details of the patient's experience. Insurance carriers or clinicians may provide their own format, and examples are available online (TransLine 2022); however, after starting to work with patients, the clinician may want to construct their own optimized template.

CONCLUSION

When writing a letter in support of GAS, the clinician must approach the TNG person with the historical context of the process in mind. Historically and currently, psychiatry has had a role in perpetuating stigma around TNG identities and in gatekeeping access to medically necessary care, and this needs to be addressed with every TNG patient seeking a surgical letter. The clinician must also factor in the role of trauma, both personal and that of TNG communities, in the evaluation and be alert for the potential to reinforce past trauma or, conversely, to provide a corrective experience. Despite the potential pitfalls, the clinician who is familiar with the history and culture of TNG communities and the basics of gender-affirming medical and surgical care has the potential to improve the TNG person's experience and outcomes. Taking a collaborative approach to both the mental health evaluation and the process of letter writing is one way to maximize the potential for this externally imposed and often unwelcome requirement to contribute to better surgical and mental health outcomes, and to minimize the probability of perpetuating harm.

REFERENCES

Alessi EJ, Meyer IH, Martin JI: PTSD and sexual orientation: an examination of Criterion A1 and non-Criterion A1 events. Psychol Trauma 5(2):149–157, 2013 26113955

American Psychiatric Association: Diagnostic and Statistical Manual of Mental Disorders, 3rd Edition. Washington, DC, American Psychiatric Association, 1980

American Psychiatric Association: Diagnostic and Statistical Manual of Mental Disorders, 4th Edition. Washington, DC, American Psychiatric Association, 1994

American Psychiatric Association: Diagnostic and Statistical Manual of Mental Disorders, 4th Edition, Text Revision. Washington, DC, American Psychiatric Association, 2000

American Psychiatric Association: Diagnostic and Statistical Manual of Mental Disorders, 5th Edition. Arlington, VA, American Psychiatric Association, 2013

American Psychiatric Association: Diagnostic and Statistical Manual of Mental Disorders, 5th Edition, Text Revision. Washington, DC, American Psychiatric Association, 2022

Benjamin H: The transsexual phenomenon*. Transact NY Acad Sci 29(4 Series II):428–430, 1967

Center of Excellence for Transgender Health: Guidelines for the Primary and Gender-Affirming Care of Transgender and Nonbinary People, 2nd Edition. Edited by Deutsch MB. San Francisco, CA, University of California, 2016. Available at: https://transcare.ucsf.edu/sites/transcare.ucsf.edu/files/Transgender-PGACG-6-17-16.pdf. Accessed December 15, 2022.

Coleman E, Bocking W, Botzer M, et al: Standards of care for the health of transsexual, transgender, and gender-nonconforming people, version 7. Int J Transgenderism 13(4):165–232, 2012

Coleman E, Radix AE, Bouman WP, et al: Standards of care for the health of transgender and gender diverse people, version 8. Int J Transgender Health 23(Suppl 1):S1–S259, 2022 36238954

Frey JD, Poudrier G, Thomson JE, Hazen A: A historical review of gender-affirming medicine: focus on genital reconstruction surgery. J Sex Med 14(8):991–1002, 2017 28760257

Gender Clinical Interventions, HB 1421, Florida House of Representatives, 2023

Hamburger C, Sturup GK, Dahl-Iversen E: Transvestism; hormonal, psychiatric, and surgical treatment. J Am Med Assoc 152(5):391–396, 1953 13044539

Health care; prohibiting gender transition procedures for children; authorizing certain civil actions and relief; licensure; adding violations and penalties. Emergency., SB 613, Oklahoma Senate, 2023

Institute of Medicine: The Health of Lesbian, Gay, Bisexual, and Transgender People: Building a Foundation for Better Understanding. Washington, DC, National Academies Press, 2011

James S, Herman J, Rankin S, et al: The Report of the 2015 U.S. Transgender Survey. Washington, DC, National Center for Transgender Equality, 2016

Lichtenstein M, Stein L, Connolly E, et al: The Mount Sinai patient-centered preoperative criteria meant to optimize outcomes are less of a barrier to care than WPATH SOC 7 criteria before transgender-specific surgery. Transgend Health 5(3):166–172, 2020 33644310

Lykens JE, LeBlanc AJ, Bockting WO: Healthcare experiences among young adults who identify as genderqueer or nonbinary. LGBT Health 5(3):191–196, 2018 29641314

Manrique OJ, Bustos SS, Bustos VP, et al: Building a multidisciplinary academic surgical gender-affirmation program: lessons learned. Plast Reconstr Surg Glob Open 9(3):e3478, 2021 33968551

Meyerowitz J: How Sex Changed: A History of Transsexuality in the United States. Boston, MA, Harvard University Press, 2004

The Patient Protection and Affordable Care Act, Pub. L. No. 111–148, 2010

Riverdale J: A brief history of FTM trans civilization. TransGuys, October 29, 2012

Siotos C, Neira PM, Lau BD, et al: Origins of gender affirmation surgery: the history of the first gender identity clinic in the United States at Johns Hopkins. Ann Plast Surg 83(2):132–136, 2019 30557186

Strand NK, Jones NL: Invisibility of "gender dysphoria." AMA J Ethics 23(7):E557–E562, 2021 34351266

TransLine: Surgery sample letter, in Gender Affirming Surgery. TransLine, 2022. Available at: https://transline.zendesk.com/hc/en-us/articles/229372788-Surgery-Sample-Letter. Accessed December 15, 2022.

Walsh M: It's been 60 years since the first he turned she: Bronx-born Christine Jorgensen's historic sexual reassignment surgery in Denmark. Daily News, November 30, 2012. Available at: https://www.nydailynews.com/news/world/60-years-christine-jorgensen-born-article-1.1211068, Accessed December 15, 2022.

World Health Organization: International Statistical Classification of Diseases and Related Health Problems, 11th Revision. World Health Organization, 2020

CHAPTER 22

Standardized Language and Nonstandard Identities

Sex and Gender Taxonomies and Data Collection, Storage, and Use

Clair Kronk, Ph.D.
Roz Queen, B.S.

ASPECTS OF GENDER AND SEX

Conceptualizations of gender and sex are considered in this chapter, including historical examinations of gender, cultural examples of gender diversity, and notes on effectively and respectfully communicating with transgender, non-binary, and/or gender-expansive (TNG) patients.

In the mid-20th century, sexologist John Money defined six sex variables in relation to human beings, and postulated a seventh: "Gender role and orientation as male or female, established while growing up" (Table 22–1) (Money et al. 1955). Anti-trans backlash in the 1970s overwrote such intricacies in favor of a purely biological/gender essentialist binary that actively disregarded variation as a possibility (Joffe 2017; Williams 2014). Today, our understanding has evolved beyond Money's variables and essentialism to include a complex intertwining of biological, psychological, sociological, cultural, and environmental factors and forces in the formation of sex and gender.

Electronic health records (EHRs) use rule-based systems to decide what types of care may be appropriate or inappropriate for a given patient in a given context. Historically, EHR rule systems were based on studies that assumed that sex was a steady, static, uniform variable. Recently, some EHRs

TABLE 22–1. Seven variables said to define sex and gender in 1955

Variable	Approximate contemporary equivalent
Assigned sex and sex of rearing	Assigned gender (at birth); gender of rearing
External genital morphology	External genitalia (primary sex characteristics)
Internal reproductive structures	Internal genitalia (primary sex characteristics)
Hormonal and secondary sex characteristics	Gonadocorticoid levels during key developmental stages; status of gonadocorticoid receptors; secondary sex characteristics
Gonadal sex	Type of gamete produced; status of gamete production
Chromosomal sex	Gonosomal karyotype; SRY gene inactivation, transfer, mutation, etc.
Gender role and orientation	Gender identity; gender expression; gender modality; gender role

Source.   Money et al. 1955.

have added gender identity and *assigned gender at birth* (AGAB) variables, as well as the ambiguous *legal sex* variable. The first two changes intended to replace a single proxy (the sex datum) with a two-step proxy, providing better estimations and predictions of structures relevant to medical care (such as hormone levels or organ inventories) (Figure 22–1).

AGAB, sometimes erroneously labeled as assigned sex at birth (ASAB), is typically the value indicated via a gender marker in birth-related documentation, such as a birth certificate or birth registry (Kronk et al. 2022). Formats vary by jurisdictions, and values other than F or M can be included, such as X in Canada and the United States, or D or blank in Germany (Holzer 2018; Jao 2018; Sweeney and LaCroix 2021).

Inclusion of gender identity and AGAB in a two-step proxy is essential to measuring *gender modality*: an individual's alignment or nonalignment between AGAB and gender identity (Ashley 2022). This provides a more consistent and reproducible definition of terms such as *cisgender* (alignment between gender identity and AGAB) and *transgender* (nonalignment between AGAB and gender identity) and allows for better comparison studies over time by avoiding terminology shift (Kronk et al. 2022).

Sex, like gender, has many nuances to consider. Often *sex* is used to refer to legal gender markers in documents (e.g., birth certificates or driver's licenses), where it supposedly represents biological sex. However, that is often not the case owing to a lack of clear guidance or verification in the collection and use of these data. *Sex Parameters for Clinical Use* (SPCU), or sex-related data specific to a given clinical context, is recommended to account for the

What is your gender identity? *Choose all that apply.*
To see how this information is used or to contact us with questions, please see [URL]

☐ Female; Woman; Girl

☐ Male; Man; Boy

☐ Non-binary

☐ Exploring; Questioning

☐ Prefer not to respond/disclose

☐ Gender identity not listed (please specify) [＿＿＿＿＿]

What is your assigned gender at birth, meaning the gender marker which appears on your original birth certificate?
Choose one.
Note that intersex status is covered in another section. To see how this information is used or to contact us with questions, please see [URL]

○ Female ('F')

○ Male ('M')

○ X

○ Unsure

○ Prefer not to respond/disclose

○ Assigned gender at birth not listed (please specify) [＿＿＿＿＿]

FIGURE 22–1. A mock-up of a two-step process to use when considering implementation.
Source. Adapted by Queen from Kronk et al. 2022.

diversity of human biology. SPCU should be used only when absolutely necessary for care, after discussion with a patient to ensure transparency in communication, and with consent (Kronk et al. 2022; McClure et al. 2022).

Gender and Sex Diversities

Please note that this section discusses only a small proportion of identities related to gender and sex diversities, which are more complicated than can be succinctly described here.

In this chapter, we use *gender and sex diversities* (GSDs) as an umbrella term viewed specifically within a Eurocentric or Anglocentric, binaristic framework. Therefore, when a given identity or role is viewed as an expression of diversity in this context, the view may not be universally applicable. That is to say, outside of a specific context, it rarely makes sense to refer to an individual person as diverse.

With medical colonialism, preexisting GSDs were, and continue to be, converted into inappropriate frameworks and classifications. By imposing Euro- or Anglocentric beliefs on ways of being, these structures redefine traditional roles as deviant or disruptive. It is difficult and counterproductive to separate translations from forces of globalization, imperialism, and colonialism. For instance, *hijra* have lived for centuries on the Indian subcontinent. In the late 20th and 21st centuries, however, in the American Psychiatric Association's DSM, hijra are referred to in research as "male transvestites" and "men with gender identity disorders" (Baqi et al. 1999; Kalra 2012). This trend follows from earlier anthropological and ethnographic research that examined GSD through a Eurocentric, binarizing lens and labeled GSDs as "third genders."

Some umbrella terms are coined within cultural communities as endonyms for the purposes of organizing; *Two Spirit* is one such term (Weedon 2019) (see Chapter 5, "Affirming and Intersectional Psychiatric Care for Two-Spirit People"). Of note, the conceptualization of an individual as having two spirits has been criticized by some Native American and First Nations peoples as a form of erasure of individual tribal identities, such as *lhamana, wik'ovat,* and *sipiniq* (Inuktitut: ᓯᐱᓂᖅ), among numerous others (O'Brien 2009).

Terminologies relating to diversities of sex characteristics are likewise diverse. The term *intersex* was coined in reference to moths by Richard Goldschmidt in 1917, although the term in common parlance at that time was *hermaphrodite* and its variants. In the 1990s, the term intersex surpassed hermaphrodite in usage, with the latter classified as a pathologizing and medicalizing slur. Concurrently, the phrase *disorders of sex development* (DSD) entered use among biomedical researchers and clinicians, reinforcing pathologization and medicalization. Although DSD has been redefined as differences or diversities of sex development, it retains its pathologizing history, making *intersex* the term preferred and used by most individuals and activist organizations, such as interACT, Organisation Intersex International, and the Intersex Campaign for Equality. There is no consensus definition of intersex. interACT (2021) defines intersex as "an umbrella term for unique variations in reproductive or sex anatomy," compared with the two usual paths of human sex development.

Taxonomies of Sex and Gender

By the late 19th century, sex-, sexual-, and gender-diverse people were grouped together by defects perceived to originate congenitally or from vice, leading to the umbrella label *sexual inversion* (American Psychiatric Association 1952). Use of this label pathologized and marginalized people systemically, shaping the trajectories of health information standards communities, such as Medical 203, an early classification system of mental disorders that was adopted by the U.S. Armed Forces. From it, DSM-I (American Psychiatric Association 1952) was derived, and such terminology continues to pathologize people today. Terminological standards can be slow moving and are influenced by significant bias and political forces. For instance, systems such as Systematized Nomenclature of Medicine, Clinical Terms (SNOMED CT) simply graduated terms from previous iterations of standards, rather than investigating terms individually and reflexively (Figure 22–2).

These standards have a long history in medical standards of care, including the World Professional Association for Transgender Health Standards of Care (WPATH SOC). Legislation has adopted these influential recommendations. In many jurisdictions, legal documents require specific codes and diagnoses, along with letters of support from health professionals, for name and gender marker changes. As depathologization and demedicalization movements gain momentum, it is important to keep in mind in what ways legal systems may make these changes difficult, and to support legislative changes. Of note, not all TNG people undergo surgical or hormonal procedures. Not all TNG people experience gender dysphoria, and gender euphoria has become a prioritized sensation for many TNG people. Some TNG people, when faced with significant barriers to care, may attempt do-it-yourself, or self-managed, hormone therapy, which can result in further complications.

Pronouns, Names, and Titles

Clinicians, in person and via EHR, should aim for respectful communication to build trust with patients—better communication leads to better health outcomes (Stewart 1995). Clinicians should use the terminology that makes patients most comfortable; when a mistake is made, apologize quickly, correct oneself, and move on. EHRs can potentially help alleviate some errors, by providing clinicians with layouts of pronoun usage, patient names, etc., before and during encounters, as a form of passive practice. Putting the patient's pronoun information in a prominent, consistent position on every screen within the EHR can help reinforce correct pronoun usage by increasing the number of times a clinician sees the information while interacting with the EHR.

Unfortunately, EHRs often list pronoun, name, and title entities as *preferred, chosen*, or *affirmed*, rather than what they really are: a person's name, pronouns, or title (without qualification). Cisgender people are awarded unconditional naming status, so why the need to qualify a TNG person's name and pronouns? Systems are beginning to add pronoun and name fields, but many EHRs do not yet capture this information, so seeking consent and recording these data in notes can be crucial to avoiding negative outcomes.

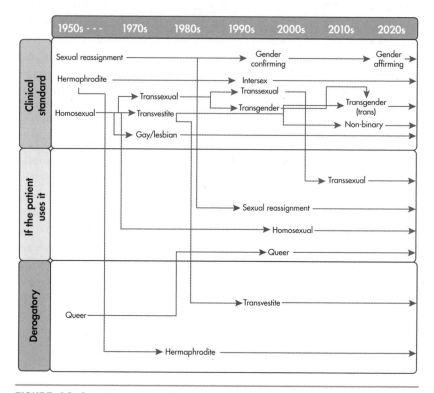

FIGURE 22–2. Summary of the etymology of some terms relevant to LGBTQIA+ people in medical settings.

Source. Adapted by Queen from Kloer et al. 2021.

Another language-related barrier between clinicians and TNG patients may be specific jargon, slang, or argots that TNG people use to avoid discrimination, marginalization, and persecution in various jurisdictions (T 2020). Clinicians should respect that although trust and understanding are important, aspects of TNG people's lived experiences may never be understood by people without those experiences.

DATA COLLECTION, STORAGE, AND USE

Please note that the information provided in this section does not, and is not intended to, constitute legal advice; instead, all information, content, and materials available in this chapter are for general informational purposes only and may not be the most up-to-date available.

Classically, the first thing that happens when an individual enters a clinical setting is they are handed a paper intake form with questions pertaining to the visit, their demographics, and their family history, among other things. Paper has transitioned with increasing velocity toward electronic forms of data collection, such as patient portals, but paper persists in many places, creating a digital divide (Bradford et al. 2015) (Figure 22–3).

Both of these methods form what is known as *patient-centered data collection*: trusting a patient to give answers that they believe are best for their own health. Conversely, a staff member may be positioned as more knowledgeable on health-related jargon and someone who could more efficiently help patients by translating their words into "medicalese." With this method, the danger is that staff members may make snap judgments based on appearance and their underlying biases, losing information and distorting the picture of what health care services are needed.

Data Representations

Given the previously discussed gender and sex diversities, it may seem nearly impossible to accurately represent those diversities in a database. However, paradigms such as using the two-step process mentioned earlier, asking for gender identity followed by AGAB, have been shown to be more effective than either category individually (Kronk et al. 2022).

It should be noted that these questions do not incorporate intersex status, as being intersex is almost never considered a gender identity or AGAB. For medical situations, interACT has published an extensive guide on suggestions for intersex data collection, also using a two-step process (interACT 2020). Step 1 captures intersex status after explaining the meaning of the term; in Step 2, the individual selects the specific intersex conditions. These could be easily integrated into other EHR workflows, such as karyotyping, surgical histories, or organ inventories.

Data Storage and Privacy

Despite the existence of legal data protections and advanced cybersecurity systems, maintaining security of health care systems has long been a struggle. Considerations of data storage and privacy in these contexts are important for all patients, but for TNG persons who choose to discuss their lives and experiences with medical professionals, these considerations may have unique repercussions. Outing a person can have legal and psychological affects, and inappropriate release of confidential information can fuel enactments of cisgenderism or gender/sex binarism, with severe adverse consequences.

Clinicians should be aware of their institution's data breach history and current approaches. Clinicians can judiciously select what information to record based on their assessment of the data's safety and the scale of potential negative outcomes if such information were to become public. Clini-

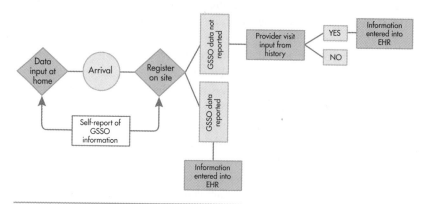

FIGURE 22–3. Generic workflow for collecting gender, sex, and sexual orientation (GSSO) data in a clinical setting using a patient portal or paper forms.. Data may be input from a patient from home via a patient portal, at the clinic during intake, or during the clinical visit.

Source. Adapted by Queen from Bradford et al. 2015.

cians should always discuss these possibilities with patients to determine whether significant safety concerns exist.

Data Usage

Usage of data regarding gender modality and identity, as well as intersex status, can take a number of different forms. This section analyzes primary usage of data in care settings, not secondary or tertiary use. For information on secondary and tertiary use of sex- and gender-related data, such as in research, see Chapter 23, "Collecting and Analyzing Gender Identity Data."

The SPCU concept discussed earlier allows for data to be used in tailored ways for the purposes of individualized care. In most EHRs (at least currently), the single "administrative gender" field is used for everything: insurance claims, patient matching, medication dosing, laboratory testing and reference ranges, and clinical decision-making algorithms (Lau et al. 2020b; McClure et al. 2022; Moscoe 2014). Thus care teams must switch data values for gender back and forth, which can cause challenges with regard to institutional compliance statutes, for instance asking a patient if they could be pregnant (SoRelle 2019). Toggling a single administrative gender field datum requires individuals to make trade-offs in terms of safety while within clinical settings. For example, changing the administrative gender field to align with one's gender identity can increase psychological safety and guard against misgendering but can also cause other clinical errors related to sex-based clinical reminders, medication dosages, and laboratory test values, compromising patient safety (Burgess et al. 2019). Forcing patients and their care teams to make these decisions and safety trade-offs is a direct result of the single administrative gender field being used to capture a complex, diverse phenomenon.

Finally, sex and gender data are used by health care professionals to communicate with patients and form interpersonal relationships. These applications of sex and gender data can function to make a patient either comfortable or uncomfortable in a given moment and affect patients' overall care experiences, perceptions, outcomes, and trust of health care professionals and institutions. Many TNG people avoid care until it becomes an emergency, so considering their overall well-being while accessing care can save lives (Lau et al. 2020a).

Cases in which these data are misrepresented may be subject to legal recourse. In 2015, the U.S. Department of Health and Human Services Office for Civil Rights noted that the nondiscrimination provision in the Affordable Care Act was applicable to TNG patients when data were used or entered in a manner that could be considered discriminatory. This ruling resulted from a "transgender female who presented as a female at the hospital [but was assigned] to a double occupancy patient room with a male occupant" (Atlantic Information Services 2015). In this case, it was likely that a health care worker entered the administrative sex field as "male" against the patient's wishes.

Data Sharing

Sharing of biomedical data, which is essential to research and clinical practice (Federer et al. 2015; Villanueva et al. 2019), introduces a number of challenges and uncertainties. Depending on the type and usage of patient-level biomedical data (and on a jurisdiction's laws), unauthorized disclosures of information can result in severe legal consequences. Clinicians should always be aware of their jurisdiction's laws and current ethical procedures regarding data sharing before proceeding.

Accordingly, deciding when and how to share patient data can be daunting. In general, the answer is "if, and only if, needed." In practice, we cannot necessarily predict all possible future data needs and requirements, especially for health surveillance and public health applications.

Data sharing can affect people's lives in a number of unintended ways. For instance, unauthorized disclosure of a person's status as TNG, intersex, gay, lesbian, or bisexual (known as *outing*) may adversely impact that person's social structures (e.g., leading to familial or social rejection), cause severe emotional/psychological distress, lead to loss of employment or housing, or indirectly or directly cause an individual's death.

In some jurisdictions, knowingly revealing an individual's status as TNG, intersex, gay, or otherwise may be a criminal offense. Many current mass health surveillance platforms, including EHRs, do not allow for, or incorporate, omissions of information by patients. In this sense, EHRs are inaccurate representations of actual public health status and represent only distorted pieces of a larger public health puzzle. Moreover, as EHRs incorporate sex- and gender-related data, discussions of privacy protections have rarely taken place. Because these protections are uncertain, it may be advisable in some situations to not record information about a person's status as transgender, intersex, or otherwise. Further confusing matters, clinicians are, in many jurisdictions, allowed to lie to their patients unless those lies themselves cause harm to the patient, including covering a clinician's mistake or disguising fraud (Palmieri and Stern 2009; Zolkefli 2018).

To omit information about status (TNG, intersex, or otherwise) is permitted in most jurisdictions and can be essential to patient safety in certain situations. Therefore, although no known case law exists on the subject, it may be permissible for one clinician to withhold information about such a status from another clinician, if harm is likely to occur should such a status be disclosed. For instance, if a TNG person has a cancer-related crisis that is urgent and the only available oncologist regularly denies care to transgender patients, it is theoretically advisable not to include information about that status when transmitting the EHR.

Some major concerns may arise if documentation of a particular diagnostic code is needed to change gender on documents or in other processes. Use of a particular diagnostic code may unintentionally out an individual, cause unnecessary distress, and complicate future access to other legal and medical needs. Additionally, some jurisdictions are subject to anti-TNG legislation, so audits of TNG-related information could result in legal consequences. For instance, if a law states that providing TNG youth with pubertal suppressants is a felony and allows that jurisdiction's governing body to ascertain medical records for the purpose of bringing felonious charges, application of felony charges would be made much easier with structured sex and gender data collection. For these reasons, some clinicians and patients have suggested or used diagnostic codes such as "endocrine disorder, unspecified" in lieu of "transsexualism" or "gender identity disorder." In such complex and sensitive situations, it may be beneficial to contact legal services within the health care organization or relevant civil liberties groups such as the American Civil Liberties Union (ACLU) or the National Center for Transgender Equality.

CONCLUSION

Structured collection of gender- and sex-related data has many patient-level and research benefits, such as patient safety, health outcomes, and visibility in datasets. However, it may also have unintended consequences, such as breaches of privacy and serious legal ramifications. Therefore, this collection must be done carefully, with special consideration given to privacy.

REFERENCES

American Psychiatric Association: Diagnostic and Statistical Manual of Mental Disorders. Washington, DC, American Psychiatric Association, 1952

Ashley F: 'Trans' is my gender modality: A modest terminological proposal, in Trans Bodies, Trans Selves: A Resource by and for Transgender Communities, 2nd Edition. New York, Oxford University Press, 2022

Atlantic Information Services: First-ever transgender settlement sets standards for privacy, better patient care. Report on Patient Privacy 15(8):1–4, 2015

Baqi S, Shah SA, Baig MA, et al: Seroprevalence of HIV, HBV, and syphilis and associated risk behaviours in male transvestites (Hijras) in Karachi, Pakistan. Int J STD AIDS 10(5):300–304, 1999 10361918

Bradford JB, Cahill S, Grasso C, Makadon HJ: How to Gather Data on Sexual Orientation and Gender Identity in Clinical Settings. Boston, MA, The Fenway Institute, 2015. Available at: https://fenwayhealth.org/wp-content/uploads/2015/09/Policy_Brief_HowtoGather..._v3_01.09.12.pdf. Accessed June 5, 2023.

Burgess C, Kauth MR, Klemt C, et al: Evolving sex and gender in electronic health records. Fed Pract 36(6):271–277, 2019 31258320

Federer LM, Lu Y-L, Joubert DJ, et al: Biomedical data sharing and reuse: attitudes and practices of clinical and scientific research staff. PLoS One 10(6):e0129506, 2015 26107811

Holzer L: Non-Binary Gender Registration Models in Europe: Report on Third Gender Marker or No Gender Marker Options. Brussels, ILGA-Europe, 2018. Available at: https://www.ilga-europe.org/sites/default/files/non-binary_gender_registration_models_in_europe_0.pdf. Accessed June 5, 2023.

interACT: Intersex Data Collection: Your Guide to Question Design. Sudbury, MA, interACT, 2020. Available at: https://interactadvocates.org/intersex-data-collection. Accessed May 5, 2021.

interACT: Intersex Definitions. Sudbury, MA, interACT, 2021. Available at: https://interactadvocates.org/intersex-definitions. Accessed December 9, 2021.

Jao A: Gender "X": Ontario issues its first "nonbinary" birth certificate. NBC News, May 9, 2018. Available at: https://www.nbcnews.com/feature/nbc-out/gender-x-ontario-issues-its-first-ever-non-binary-birth-n872676. Accessed June 5, 2023.

Joffe G: Profile on the right: Paul McHugh. Political Research Associates, 2017. Available at: https://politicalresearch.org/2017/04/27/profile-on-the-right-paul-mchugh. Accessed June 5, 2023.

Kalra S: The eunuchs of India: an endocrine eye opener. Indian J Endocrinol Metab 16(3):377–380, 2012 22629502

Kloer C, Blasdel G, Morris M, et al: Overview of gender affirming surgery for the gynecologic surgeon. J Gynecol Surg 37(4):269–274, 2021

Kronk CA, Everhart AR, Ashley F, et al: Transgender data collection in the electronic health record: current concepts and issues. J Am Med Inform Assoc 29(2):271–284, 2022 34486655

Lau F, Antonio M, Davison K, et al: An environmental scan of sex and gender in electronic health records: analysis of public information sources. J Med Internet Res 22(11):e20050, 2020a 33174858

Lau F, Antonio M, Davison K, et al: A rapid review of gender, sex, and sexual orientation documentation in electronic health records. J Am Med Inform Assoc 27(11):1774–1783, 2020b 32935124

McClure RC, Macumber CL, Kronk C, et al: Gender harmony: improved standards to support affirmative care of gender-marginalized people through inclusive gender and sex representation. J Am Med Inform Assoc 29(2):354–363, 2022

Money J, Hampson JG, Hampson JL: An examination of some basic sexual concepts: the evidence of human hermaphroditism. Bull Johns Hopkins Hosp 97(4):301–319, 1955 13260820

Moscoe GB: Beyond the Binary: A Proposal for Uniform Standards for Gender Identity and More Descriptive Sex Classifications in Electronic Health Records. Portland, OR, Oregon Health and Science University School of Medicine, 2014

O'Brien J (ed): Encyclopedia of Gender and Society. Thousand Oaks, CA, SAGE, 2009

Palmieri JJ, Stern TA: Lies in the doctor-patient relationship. Prim Care Companion J Clin Psychiatry 11(4):163–168, 2009 19750068

SoRelle J: When gender goes awry in electronic health records. Lablogatory, August 14, 2019. Available at: https://labmedicineblog.com/2019/08/14/when-gender-goes-awry-in-electronic-health-records/. Accessed June 5, 2023.

Stewart MA: Effective physician-patient communication and health outcomes: a review. CMAJ 152(9):1423–1433, 1995 7728691

Sweeney C, LaCroix R: Oklahoma issues first nonbinary birth certificate. KOSU, October 22, 2021. Available at: https://www.kosu.org/local-news/2021-10-22/oklahoma-issues-first-nonbinary-birth-certificate. Accessed June 5, 2023.

T A: Opacity—Minority—Improvisation: An Exploration of the Closet Through Queer Slangs and Postcolonial Theory. Bielefeld, Germany, transcript, 2020

Villanueva AG, Cook-Deegan R, Koenig BA, et al: Characterizing the biomedical data-sharing landscape. J Law Med Ethics 47(1):21–30, 2019 30994069

Weedon A: Understanding the Pacific's alternative genders. RNZ, August 31, 2019. Available at: https://www.rnz.co.nz/international/pacific-news/397872/understanding-the-pacific-s-alternative-genders. Accessed June 5, 2023.

Williams C: Fact checking Janice Raymond: the NCHCT Report. TransAdvocate, 2014. Available at: https://www.transadvocate.com/fact-checking-janice-raymond-the-nchct-report_n_14554.htm. Accessed December 8, 2021.

Zolkefli Y: The ethics of truth-telling in health-care settings. Malays J Med Sci 25(3):135–139, 2018 30899195

Collecting and Analyzing Gender Identity Data to Enhance Your Practice

Juwan Campbell, M.A.

Dan E. Ferrari Funk, M.A.

Chris Grasso, M.P.H.

THE health care sector captures a variety of data elements in patient health records, often electronic health records (EHRs). At minimum, this includes the patient's name, home address, insurance information, and details about the care they have received. It is also well documented that sociodemographic information and social determinants of health (e.g., race, ethnicity, primary language spoken, income, housing status, country of origin, immigration status, veteran status) are important data elements to capture in a health record, as these identities and factors are related to health outcomes. The previous chapter discussed considerations for collecting gender identity data, particularly with regard to transgender, non-binary, and/or gender-expansive (TNG) people. In this chapter, we discuss the collection and maintenance of important gender-related data elements and the use of these data to enhance clinical practice.

In addition to improving individual patient experiences, collecting gender identity data facilitates local analysis of disparities in care delivery. Data maintenance and quality assurance are major components of any clinical practice's data management plan; such plans must include gender identity data. Asking patients these important questions often ensures that we refer to them accurately (e.g., name, labels). All data should be reviewed for quality and completeness before analysis. As research robustly links gender identity (and other sociodemographic metrics) with psychiatric health, it is important to analyze access to services, outcomes related to services delivered, and disparities across an organization's patient population.

Here we outline best practices for collecting gender identity and other gender-related data, leveraging gender identity data for culturally responsive patient interactions, and guidelines for reporting, monitoring, and analyzing these data.

GENDER IDENTITY DATA COLLECTION, QUALITY, AND MAINTENANCE

Despite increasing protocolization guiding provision of gender-affirming medical care, TNG people remain largely invisible to their clinicians, experience delays in access to care, face stigma, and encounter barriers to accessing care, resulting in health disparities and poor outcomes compared with non-TNG peers. Numerous published articles have highlighted the negative health outcomes among TNG people attributed to the denial of care for basic treatment, which often contributes to a higher disease burden compared with the general population (Stroumsa 2014).

A key component to addressing these gaps is creating robust health information technology (HIT) systems to collect, store, and harness patient information. Culturally responsive patient-clinician interactions that involve sensitive and effective communication are critical to ensuring a positive therapeutic experience (Keuroghlian 2021). HIT can assist care teams in building and maintaining a culturally affirming environment. This process begins by ensuring the patient can provide important information about themselves, including name used, pronouns, gender identity, and gender assigned at birth (Grasso et al. 2019). Gender response categories should be expansive, to provide options that recognize the range in how people identify and allow for a self-defined field. While there has been an increase in research related to TNG health outcomes, evidence-based practice remains limited due to the paucity of available data. Expanding gender categories will allow for analysis of outcomes data that is inclusive of an invisible and too-often understudied patient population (Dragon et al. 2017). Dedicated structured EHR data fields to capture name used and pronouns signal to patients that the clinical practice is affirming. Many EHRs now support visibility of name used and pronouns throughout the patient's record from registration to clinical care; this helps ensure that patients are addressed respectfully.

Improved data capture supports clinical practice compliance with preventive screening and quality measures, such as the Electronic Clinical Quality Measures (Centers for Medicare and Medicaid Services n.d.). When gender categories are conflated with anatomy, care teams are unable to accurately determine whether TNG patients are receiving appropriate preventive care and screenings (Keuroghlian 2021). Although psychiatric teams may not conduct physical procedures (e.g., cervical cancer screening), understanding a patient's anatomy and the words they use to describe their anatomy remains critical to respectful mental health care interactions. This also presents an opportunity to practice trauma-informed care and advocate for any specific patient needs related to undergoing a procedure on a part of their anatomy that is associated with gender-related distress (Grasso et al. 2021).

Initial and ongoing training is essential. While clinical teams commonly receive training on collecting gender identity data and establishing a culturally affirming environment, it is equally important to develop similar training for nonclinical staff. Nonclinical staff often serve as the face of an organization and can have more frequent interactions with patients, including serving as the first interaction patients have with an organization—prior to receiving any clinical care or assessments. For instance, if a billing person calls a patient about a bill, then that billing person must be sensitive and effective in using the patient's name, pronouns, and gender correctly. The goal is to create a patient-centered experience that is neither differential nor fragmented, regardless of which staff members interact with the patient.

Patients may have privacy concerns about information in their EHR chart; many EHRs offer settings that limit who can view a patient's record. Clinicians can assure patients that their data will be kept private, confidential, and only accessible to staff involved in their care.

Clinicians can also ask patients their preferences for documentation of certain information and who has privileges to view their chart. Organizations should have a process where patients can request changes to privacy settings at any point during their care, as such wishes may change over time. Personal circumstances may impact a patient's comfort with information documented in their chart (e.g., a patient may be hesitant to have their gender identity documented for fear of repercussions: a minor with unsupportive parents, an undocumented immigrant). In many states, a parent or guardian may have limited access to view a minor's information over a patient portal but can request a copy of the minor's full records, which may include gender identity, name used, and pronouns (Goldhammer et al. 2022). For a minor, these conversations should occur without the parent or guardian in the room and include shared decision-making about which information should be documented. All staff (regardless of patient population) should be trained in the good clinical practice of viewing a patient's EHR record only when relevant to clinical care. The federal Health Insurance Portability and Accountability Act (HIPAA) Privacy Rule establishes that any patient is entitled to a report of staff who viewed their records (U.S. Department of Health and Human Services 2022). To maintain integrity and accountability over protecting patient data, organizations should prepare correction plans for addressing unprofessional behavior, such as reading a patient's visit note despite not being involved in their care. At a minimum, such a plan should require retraining, and disciplinary action may be appropriate in some cases.

Whether in person or via telehealth, clinical and administrative staff ought to avoid assumptions and have a process to discuss name and pronouns with each patient. Some organizations minimize the use of the wrong name or pronouns by using more generic terms like "Dear Patient" or removing the use of pronouns from EHR chart documents, letters, or emails. As more organizations move toward having "open notes" where patients can view office visit notes through a portal, the language in the documentation should reflect the patient's gender, name, and pronouns accurately. Reading notes with incorrect information can be traumatizing to a patient and negatively impact the patient-clinician relationship.

As part of a coordinated care plan, the psychiatric team may need to refer a patient to a specialist or consult with a patient's primary care team. Prior to external conversations, clinicians ought to confirm with the patient what information can be shared externally. Many privacy groups are taking the privacy controls one step further to restrict information that is transmitted to external organizations. National interest groups, such as the Protecting Privacy to Promote Interoperability Workgroup (Drummond Group n.d.), are developing standards and recommendations to retain privacy of data used in interoperability; this area will continue to develop over time.

Often, organizations implement processes for collecting gender identity and gender assigned at birth data fields without conducting quality checks or analysis to evaluate patient outcomes. Linking gender identity data to other clinical data can inform the quality of care provided, identify gaps, and point to systems to improve patient health outcomes (Grasso et al. 2021). This process begins by assessing opportunities for data collection by EHR vendors. The Office of the National Coordinator for Health Information Technology (ONC) certified EHR vendors will have designated fields to collect these data (Office of the National Coordinator for Health Information Technology 2022). If your organization is not using a certified product, then consult with your internal technical teams or vendor to identify fields to document these data.

Clinical practices may struggle to codify patients' responses and to analyze and report on the findings. In Tables 23–1 and 23–2, we offer brief guidance for this critical work

In the endeavor of leveraging data to address the health disparities observed among TNG people, do not neglect analyzing data completeness. Missing data can be as informative as those recorded. Evaluating data completeness for a given patient demographic variable against other demo-

TABLE 23–1. Data integrity categories.

Accurate/reliable: Numerators and denominators correct and based on the measure specifications; consistent results generated from the same reporting tool.

Documentation issues

Are each of the questions their own data field? (For instance, are GI and gender assigned at birth each mapped to their own field?)

Are data entered into proper EHR fields? (For instance, are staff documenting gender assigned at birth, as well as GI?)

Does the system differentiate between refused/missing and unknown values?

Are there response categories that do not belong in that field?

Logic issues

Is the report logic querying data from the proper EHR fields? (For instance, is it incorrectly extracting sexual orientation from the GI field?)

Are all eligible data fields being captured in the report logic? (For instance, is the query arbitrarily omitting certain ages?)

Are patients who are of a certain age relative to the measure specifications (e.g., older than the age limit) being included or excluded correctly?

Is the date the GI data were reported extractable?

Are patients able to update their GI information at subsequent visits?

Do updates to GI data overwrite previous entries?

Are the correct codes consistently associated with the field being measured (e.g., did mapping break due to a new EHR upgrade)?

Face validity checks

Does the number of distinct patients who had encounters closely match the number of aggregated GI data units collected?

Are numerators/denominators relatively consistent over time? If not, is there is a logical reason they are changing over time (e.g., new site opened)?

Retrievable: Desired data elements are in the EHR in a format possible to query.

Are data elements consistently documented in structured fields or using standardized free text, rather than as inconsistent free text, so that these appear consistently in query results?

Are data points (e.g., GI) in another place in the EHR that is not able to be queried?

Are patient responses extractable over time?

Complete: All data elements, including any repeat/re-analysis data, are included.

How does the collection of GI data compare to other data being collected at the same visit (e.g., rates of completeness for race or income)?

How does the completeness compare among GI questions (e.g., higher response rate for current GI vs. gender assigned at birth)?

Are select sites, providers, or patients missing from the data set?

Is the data capture being limited to certain sites, clinicians, or patients?

Note.   EHR = electronic health record; GI = gender identity.

TABLE 23–2. What is driving your data?

Is the parameter or test being measured correctly?

Are staff trained on GI questions and how to respond to patient questions?

Do certain staff have lower response rates?

Are patients properly supported to answer GI questions (e.g., through linguistic translations, clear terminology definitions, and patient handouts)?

Do staff have privileges to enter GI data into the EHR?

Are you able to combine the gender assigned at birth and current GI data to identify TNG patients?

Are patients given the opportunity to answer GI questions?

Are all patients given the opportunity to report GI (e.g., both new and existing patients vs. just new patients)?

Are staff giving the patients registration forms or other forms that contain the GI questions to complete?

Do patients have adequate time to complete the GI questions?

Have all forms been updated to include GI questions?

Is patient GI being reported in a way that eliminates it from being counted (e.g., in a clinical visit note)?

Are there specific common factors among patients who are not reporting GI data?

Are there trends in demographic factors (e.g., age, gender, race, ethnicity, location) among patients?

Are there trends by locations of care, encounters, departments, or clinicians?

Are there trends by new vs. existing patients?

Note. EHR = electronic health record; GI = gender identity; TNG = transgender, non-binary, and/or gender-expansive.

graphic fields facilitates comparing response rates. When a difference is observed, it is important to elucidate if this is a widespread issue or if certain staff or clinicians have lower rates of collection. In turn, this helps guide additional, focused patient outreach and/or staff trainings.

For example, consider stratifying screening data (e.g., depression screening) by gender identity. At a process level, such quality reports help identify gaps in screening and compare screening rates of different populations (e.g., cisgender vs. TNG) and indicate opportunities to evaluate and reform the internal processes that exacerbate that disparity. At an outcomes level, such reports also facilitate inter-demographic outcome comparisons and guide development of additional mechanisms to support the most vulnerable patients (Grasso et al. 2021).

Data monitoring and quality control is an ongoing process. Health care organizations that have been successful implementing and harnessing gender identity data collection have typically integrated these processes into existing workflows or workgroups.

MONITORING, REPORTING, AND ANALYZING GENDER IDENTITY DATA

The purpose of establishing data collection tools and implementing protocols for their utilization is to reliably access appropriate data when needed for reporting and analysis. These data must be readily accessible because every location of care has funding agencies, local public health authorities, and internal standards that will require routine reporting of patient experiences and outcomes. Being unable to meet the reporting needs of entities that support the operation of the clinical practice could have adverse ramifications on the ability to continue providing beneficial psychiatric care for patients (Grasso et al. 2021). Further, keeping updated and efficient data collection systems in place is a key part of ensuring that the practice can sustain providing care (Grasso et al. 2021).

Providing ethical psychiatric care requires committing to provide the highest quality services possible to all patients who come to the practice. To do so, a practice must routinely assess its performance according to patient needs and standards of care. Reviewing performance data holds the practice accountable to the promise of delivering optimal quality of care (Grasso et al. 2021).

The health care organization's performance should be compared against national standards, and the institution should adhere to current best practices within the field. Notably, such standards and practices are based on patient needs, which are not static. By monitoring patient experiences and outcomes, an organization can update its systems and practices to best serve its patients and identify opportunities to evolve to meet their changing needs (Grasso et al. 2021).

Having established that data reporting and analysis are important parts of meeting reporting requirements from funding entities, holding the practice accountable for providing the highest quality care, and maintaining a flexible practice that adapts to evolving needs of patients, the next step is to consider methods of reporting and analyzing data.

PREPARING TO ANALYZE SEX AND GENDER DATA

On a basic level, building reports to assess gender identity data will use similar methods to any other type of clinical data analysis. Before attempting advanced analyses, it is crucial to check data quality. We achieve this by monitoring factors such as accuracy, completeness, and stratification. Most organizations have existing reports to this end for other demographic data points. Such reports look at the completeness of insurance, contact information, race, and ethnicity data for active patients. The design of the report is simple and flexible, making it easy to monitor the completeness of additional fields. Gender identity and gender assigned at birth may be added without disrupting existing templates. This is often the best initial step the practice can take in analyzing gender identity data once sex and gender data collection processes are in place. First and foremost, how complete data are determines their usability. During the early stages of data collection, the practice may find that more data are missing than anticipated. In this case, the report may guide you to the conclusion that your practice needs to go back and look for flaws in the data collection tools and protocols before putting effort into more detailed usages of the data.

There are a few places it is important to check for completeness of sex and gender data. First, the data should be collected at the practice's initial touchpoint with patients. In comparing the collected data with the practice's database, any incongruence suggests that the technology is not working as intended, and it may be necessary to contact HIT staff for further assistance. If HIT staff confirm that the technology is working as intended, the next step is to investigate staff training. If the data collection protocol requires staff to administer forms to patients, all staff members responsible need the appropriate training. Perhaps front desk staff have been accidentally administering older versions of the patient registration form that are missing gender assigned at birth and gender identity questions. The solution is to dispose of the remaining copies of the old registration form, direct staff to the new version, and demonstrate how to confirm whether it is the correct version of the form as a final quality check. These two scenarios are common challenges to data completeness, and investigating them first may save staff time and effort.

If neither technology nor staff training affects the completeness of sex and gender data, reviewing additional data may be necessary. Stratifying sex and gender data according to other demographics may pinpoint which patient groups are less likely to include their sex and gender data. For example, sorting gender identity by language spoken among patients can identify whether patients who speak a language other than English are disproportionately missing gender identity data. This information is invaluable and provides a high-impact starting point for improving the completeness of gender identity data for the practice.

ANALYZING AND UNDERSTANDING YOUR DATA

Once the practice's sex and gender data are of adequate quality and integrity for analysis, the practice can develop a more nuanced understanding of its patients, including their gender assigned at birth and gender identity. Intersectionality principles inform our understanding that people's lives are not impacted solely by a single identity but rather by how all their identities interact with one another to create unique experiences (Crenshaw 1991). Any reports stratifying gender identity and gender assigned at birth according to other demographics will provide insight into the many distinct positionalities held by patients served at the practice.

Research has also demonstrated that gender identity is a key determinant of mental health. A review of ~60 million patients in the United States found that TNG patients are more likely than the general population to be diagnosed with mood disorders, anxiety disorders, psychotic disorders, PTSD, substance use disorders, and a myriad of other mental health concerns (Wanta et al. 2019). Therefore, monitoring psychiatric care delivery for TNG patients may require stratifying a practice's clinical quality measures by gender identity and gender assigned at birth. Adding gender identity and gender assigned at birth data to the reports of key clinical quality measures that are already being considered will help the practice monitor any psychiatric care needs (e.g., clinical services or interventions) specific to TNG patients. Accordingly, such reports help the practice remain accountable for providing the best psychiatric care possible for all patients.

The most common error in identifying TNG patients is using the gender identity field alone. If there are five gender identity options in the EHR (man, woman, trans man, trans woman, and non-binary), TNG patients may opt to mark their gender identity as man or woman. Accordingly, although aggregating the count of patients listed as trans man, trans woman, or non-binary will certainly capture many—if not most—of the practice's TNG patients, it will miss others. Instead, cross-tabulating gender assigned at birth with gender identity identifies all patients whose gender identity is not the societal expectation based on their gender assigned at birth, regardless of the specific gender identity marked in their EHR chart; this provides a more complete count of TNG patients than the gender identity field alone. If the EHR has other fields and protocols used to identify TNG patients (e.g., an ICD-10 code), then the practice should consider harnessing those fields to help account for missing, inaccurate, or outdated sex and gender data.

Often, there are several ways to structure analyses using these separate sex and gender data fields: for instance, comparing mental health outcomes among cisgender patients to those among their TNG counterparts; contrasting the different mental health outcomes between women and men, regardless of whether they are cisgender or TNG; or homing in on TNG patients by comparing the mental health outcomes of TNG patients with a binary gender identity (man or woman) to those of non-binary patients. There is no specific formula to follow for deciding how to structure an analysis using these data, but careful consideration should always be given to how to operationalize sex and gender.

Finally, language around sex and gender is rapidly evolving; thus, data must be clearly and accurately labeled. Careful labeling helps prevent misrepresentation of data and their meaning. For example, when presenting an analysis of 9-item Patient Health Questionnaire (PHQ-9) results of TNG patients assigned female gender at birth versus TNG patients assigned male gender at birth, miscategorizing patients as trans men or trans women mislabels and erases experiences of many non-binary, genderqueer, and gender-expansive patients.

TURNING DATA INTO IMPACT

As noted above, gender identity is a key determinant of mental health. A practice can improve its service delivery by identifying ways to address the disparities that analysis unveils. Working groups can engage staff in the practice to address problems identified in the data.

When a disparity is noted, the first step is to research effective strategies for reducing that disparity. Practices can cross-tabulate race/ethnicity and sexual orientation and gender identity (SOGI) data. The percentage values in a table can represent the rate at which a given group receives a service across a given row and down a given column (e.g., Asian cisgender sexual minority men; Black straight trans women; Latinx LGBQ trans men). The midpoint of the table's color gradient can be set to the rate for the overall population, and the color gradient makes obvious which groups are performing above and below the average.

Such a table can be applied to screenings for depression, for example, to help deduce whether TNG patients in the practice are screened for depression at lower rates than their cisgender counterparts, at a risk of underestimating depression prevalence. An intervention to address screening of TNG patients would be needed to rectify this disparity, possibly including a focus group to better understand the reasons that patients are not responding to screeners; training for staff to improve cultural responsiveness; or outreach methods that are specifically tailored to TNG people. A practice may also deduce that white/non-Latinx TNG people have higher screening rates than TNG patients of color. Deeper analysis is needed to better understand this disparity: Are there structural barriers or biases that affect access to appropriate screening, such as cultural responsiveness for TNG patients of color specifically? Do other demographic data offer more context, such as access to transportation or technologies needed for screening?

Data collection, quality, maintenance, monitoring, and analysis provide critical tools and information to improve gender-affirming mental health care. Collecting accurate sex and gender data metrics affords patients the opportunity to share the words that they use to describe themselves with their clinicians, which in turn allows clinicians to earn trust with patients by using these affirming names, pronouns, and terms. Monitoring and analyzing sex and gender data allows health care organizations to evaluate the effectiveness and equity of the services they offer. Assessing gender-related disparities in these data helps to identify areas in which a practice can improve its mental health services for TNG people.

REFERENCES

Crenshaw K: Race, gender, and sexual harassment. Calif Law Rev 65:1467, 1991

Dragon CN, Guerino P, Ewald E, Laffan AM: Transgender Medicare beneficiaries and chronic conditions: exploring fee-for-service claims data. LGBT Health 4(6):404–411, 2017 29125908

Drummond Group: Protecting Privacy to Promote Interoperability (PP2PI) Workgroup. Portsmouth, NH, Drummond Group, n.d. Available at: https://www.drummondgroup.com/shift/. Accessed June 22, 2023.

Goldhammer H, Grasso C, Katz-Wise SL, et al: Pediatric sexual orientation and gender identity data collection in the electronic health record. J Am Med Inform Assoc 29(7):1303–1309, 2022 35396995

Grasso C, Goldhammer H, Thompson J, Keuroghlian AS: Optimizing gender-affirming medical care through anatomical inventories, clinical decision support, and population health management in electronic health record systems. J Am Med Inform Assoc 28(11):2531–2535, 2021 34151934

Grasso C, McDowell MJ, Goldhammer H, Keuroghlian AS: Planning and implementing sexual orientation and gender identity data collection in electronic health records. J Am Med Inform Assoc 26(1):66–70, 2019 30445621

Keuroghlian AS: Electronic health records as an equity tool for LGBTQIA+ people. Nat Med 27(12):2071–2073, 2021 34811548

Office of the National Coordinator for Health Information Technology: About the ONC Health IT Certification Program. HealthIT.gov, n.d. Available at: https://www.healthit.gov/topic/certification-ehrs/about-onc-health-it-certification-program. Accessed November 7, 2022.

Stroumsa D: The state of transgender health care: policy, law, and medical frameworks. Am J Public Health 104(3):e31–e38, 2014 24432926

U.S. Department of Health and Human Services: Your Rights Under HIPAA. Health Information Privacy. Available at: https://www.hhs.gov/hipaa/for-individuals/guidance- materials-for-consumers/index.html.

Wanta JW, Niforatos JD, Durbak E, et al: Mental health diagnoses among transgender patients in the clinical setting: an all-payer electronic health record study. Transgend Health 4(1):313–315, 2019 31701012

CHAPTER 24

Cultivating Inclusive and Gender-Affirming Mental Health Care Environments

Mason Dunn, J.D.
Steph deNormand, M.A.

IN this chapter, we introduce the broad but critically important topic of building an inclusive and respectful environment for transgender, nonbinary, and/or gender-expansive (TNG) people seeking care. All people, including TNG people, deserve high-quality psychiatric care in which they feel valued, affirmed, and safe. Meeting these needs begins long before a TNG person enters a clinical setting or is seen by a clinician. Building a welcoming environment begins with considerations for an inclusive workforce, policies, visual affirmations, or cues and an organizational commitment to respect and affirmation for gender diversity.

WORKFORCE DEVELOPMENT

Although we here prioritize and focus on the needs of TNG patients, it is critical to understand that these communities also exist outside the realm of those served by clinicians; TNG people are colleagues, mentors, and supervisors and should have a place in every facet of the workplace. Building an inclusive practice includes providing a safe and welcoming workplace for TNG staff and colleagues. Through workforce development, clinicians not only invite diverse and talented perspectives into their practice, but also make the space more welcoming for TNG patients, who can see aspects of their identity reflected in the clinical and administrative staff.

Building an inclusive workforce environment is an ongoing, long-term investment. According to a recent publication by the National LGBTQIA+ Health Education Center, building an inclusive environment relies on leadership to "set the tone for the entire health center by clearly communicating that…the organization's commitment to diversity includes patients and staff of all sexual orientations and gender identities" (National LGBTQIA+ Health Education Center 2021). Those in leadership should develop plans and policies that are tailored to their practices or sites. Outlined here are some considerations in developing a TNG-inclusive workforce.

Policies and Documentation

A nondiscrimination policy or statement is an important beginning step for an inclusive practice. The statement should be publicly available, easy to find, and clear. Here is one example adapted from the policies of Fenway Health (2021):

> [Entity] is an Equal Opportunity and Affirmative Action Employer and encourages applications from all qualified individuals without regard to race, color, religion, sex, gender identity, national origin, sexual orientation or identification, age, marital status, disability or veteran status, or any other characteristic protected by law. [Entity] prohibits any such discrimination or harassment.

Although a nondiscrimination statement is an important place to start, it is not sufficient on its own to address the realities of discrimination in the workplace. The process of reporting and documenting discriminatory or harassing behavior must also be articulated. Here is one example (Fenway Health 2021):

> [Entity] encourages reporting of all perceived incidents of discrimination or harassment. It is the policy of [Entity] to promptly and thoroughly investigate such reports. [Entity] prohibits retaliation against any individual who reports discrimination or harassment or participates in an investigation of such reports. Incidents of harassment or discrimination should be reported to [HR staff or URL].

To make public such policies ensures that applicants may see and understand their rights as a potential clinician. Other important policies include insurance coverage of gender-affirming care; policies and procedures when an employee comes out as TNG (e.g., name change, time off, office notification); and requests for accommodations regarding mental health, disability, or gender affirmation.

Hiring Practices

The process of applying and interviewing for employment within organizations can be made unintentionally difficult for TNG candidates. Below are some areas to examine in a practice's hiring protocols:

- *Application forms:* Asking for an applicant's name on a standardized form may seem simple. For TNG applicants, however, this question can be ambiguous: is the form asking for legal name or common use name? If an applicant does not have space to clarify their common use name (if different from legal name), unintentionally stressful interactions may result. On any standardized form, common use name should be prioritized, and an option can be added to state "legal name, if different," if that information is necessary. It is helpful for hiring managers and human resources staff members to know which specific documentation should be referenced if an applicant has different names on various forms of legal documentation.
- *Pronouns:* Any interaction with new applicants (or patients) should be an opportunity for someone to introduce their pronouns. There are many ways this can be done, such as through documentation on a form or articulated in an introduction.
- *References:* If an applicant is asked to submit the names/contacts of references, it is important to ensure that the reference in question has all the same information about the applicant. Applicants should be provided with the opportunity to articulate any important information ahead of the reference calls, such as a change in name or pronouns.

Training and Continued Education

All clinicians and health care staff should receive training on the inclusion of TNG communities in the workplace. Inclusion training should be a part of onboarding for all new staff; training updates should occur annually. Language and practices may change over time; consequently, all training should be revisited regularly to ensure the information conveyed is accurate and up-to-date. In addition, practices should offer continuing education resources that build on foundational knowledge and awareness of TNG communities.

Employee Resources and Retention

Along with hiring a diverse workforce that includes TNG staff, clinicians in leadership should prioritize ensuring that the workplace is welcoming and inclusive for all staff. This includes examining internal policies, procedures, and benefits available to staff. For instance, health insurance policies should cover gender-affirming medical care, family planning, and assisted reproductive technology, and organizations should have clear, easy-to-understand protocols for communication when a staff member changes a name or pronouns.

Clinical and administrative staff may also benefit from peer-to-peer mentoring or support. Having channels dedicated to meeting such needs (e.g., employee resource groups, mentoring, reading groups) can foster a collaborative and welcoming workplace for TNG and allied staff.

SIGNS, SYMBOLS, AND CUES

When entering any kind of health care office or facility, many TNG people, particularly those seeking psychiatric care, will be keenly aware of visual cues or signs indicating the space is welcoming and affirming. Equally important is the proactive work necessary to live up to the expectations these signs indicate. A sign, flag, or poster may be an important visual indicator, but it is the work done to reinforce the sign that is most valuable for the patient and the provider.

Myths and Misconceptions About So-Called Safe Zone Images

Although the intentions of various "safe zone" images are laudable, too often they lack the training or infrastructure to live up to their communicated expectations. This is evidenced by the alarming statistics of TNG people having to educate their providers. Signs often feature rainbow flags with text and communicate that the person or place displaying them is supportive and open to discussing lesbian, gay, bisexual, transgender, queer, intersex, asexual, and more (LGBTQIA+) identities. However, without recent culturally responsive service training, the site may unknowingly still communicate anti-LGBTQIA+ biases, undermining the intention of the safe zone moniker. It is recommended that individuals or organizations interested in becoming a safe zone and displaying the corresponding notices should commit to baseline cultural responsiveness training, with regular updates.

Bathroom Signs

Anti-transgender activists have turned public bathrooms into a hot-button issue in the discussion of rights and equity for TNG people. Although bathrooms are by no means the most important aspects of TNG lives, they can be a point of pressure and concern when accessing services, including health care. Facilities that have restrooms available should be mindful of access and the signage involved.

Ideally, health care facilities should offer single-stall/single-room, gender-inclusive bathrooms (also called "gender neutral," "all gender," or "family" restrooms). Not all facilities have such spaces available, so some buildings may offer single-stall restrooms with gender designations, and others may have gender-segregated multistall restrooms.

Single-stall gender-designated restrooms represent an opportunity for advocacy by converting them into gender-inclusive restrooms. A simple sign change can facilitate access for TNG patients, clients, and staff on site. Turning one-room "women's" and "men's" facilities into two inclusive restrooms can also increase access for families with young children and people with disabilities and prevents disparities in availability according to gender.

Gender-segregated multistall restrooms make access for TNG people more complicated. In these cases, supplemental signage can be added, articulating a policy of affirmation for TNG patients and staff; for example: "you are welcome to use the restroom that best aligns with your gender identity." It may also be helpful to describe where the nearest inclusive restroom is for those who may not feel comfortable in segregated spaces.

As described earlier for safe zone images, it is important that these signs are accompanied by both staff training and written policy. Staff should understand how to handle questions or potential conflicts about restroom signs and usage. Simple examples of how to defuse moments of implicit bias can transform a complaint into an educational opportunity to align an organization's mission of welcome with action.

In recent years, some organizations have taken a more creative approach to restroom signage, intending to bring humor or levity to the discussion. In many cases, unfortunately, such efforts make light of the real anxiety or violence that TNG people have experienced in restrooms. Table 24–1 describes common signs to avoid, and Figure 24–1 is an example of inclusive signage.

Ideal restroom signage for gender-inclusive restrooms should be simple and easily convey that the facility is open to all people, genders, and needs. This can include "family" restrooms and disability access. These signs can also illustrate what facilities are available inside the restroom, such as a urinal, changing tables, or menstrual product dispensers or baskets.

Pronoun Pins and Other Personal Accessories

Along with organization-wide signage, clinicians may have the opportunity to convey inclusivity through personal accessories, such as pins, stickers, lanyards, or individual office signage. By no means are these individual accessories required to convey allyship, but they can make TNG patients feel more seen. Pronoun buttons can be an important tool not only to convey a person's pronoun usage but also help open conversations with TNG patients about their pronouns. They should not replace an affirmative introduction of pronouns, however.

Public-Facing Materials/Images

If a clinician or organization publishes printed materials, such as brochures, or if they have a digital presence (website, social media), it is import-

TABLE 24–1. Restroom signage language to avoid.

Description	Why It Shouldn't Be Used
A sign shows the traditional male figure, female figure, and a third figure that is half man, half woman, along with the wording "gender neutral restroom."	The "half man, half woman" figure wrongly communicates that TNG people are "half and half," rather than their affirmed gender as woman, man, or nonbinary.
A sign shows the transgender symbol, combining the symbols for Mars, Venus, and a third line that combines both symbols, followed by the word "Restroom." Below the restroom title, the sign says, "This restroom may be used by any person regardless of gender identity or expression."	The intentions of this sign are affirmative, but it leads many to assume that this is "the TNG restroom" and not actually accessible to everyone, particularly cisgender people.
A sign shows traditional and nontraditional bathroom figures (woman, man, wheelchair figure, alien, two-headed person, and Roman centurion). Text below reads, "Whatever, just wash your hands."	TNG people may feel this sign suggests that their gender identity or expression is "alien" or "bizarre." The "whatever" messaging is overly passive rather than affirmative.

ant to consider the messages conveyed. Advertisements and materials should include individuals and families with diverse gender expressions, ages, abilities, race and ethnicities, and other intersecting identities. When possible, consult community-created resources and educators about the use of different symbols, flags, and language. Such cues shift over time and across contexts, and the incorrect or inappropriate use of these indicators may express a wholly different message than intended.

Social media offers an opportunity to express allyship, particularly during LGBTQIA+ holidays or current events. However, it is important that public messages of support for LGBTQIA+ people are not limited to June (Pride Month); allyship should be expressed all year round. There are multiple opportunities throughout the year to convey solidarity with TNG communities, as well as mental health awareness. Some examples are included in Table 24–2.

Forms and Systems

In many care contexts, registration and intake processes are the first encounter someone has with policies, procedures, and structures in a health care setting. According to best practices in sexual orientation and gender

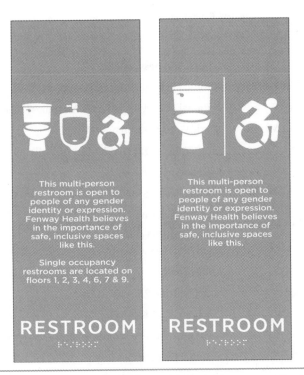

FIGURE 24–1. Fenway Health believes in the importance of safe, inclusive spaces.

identity (SOGI) data collection, sexual orientation, gender identity, and gender assigned at birth are essential data for health centers to collect (Kronk et al. 2022; Suen et al. 2022). Similarly important is collecting intersex status, but no published, peer-reviewed, validated questions are yet available (Baker et al. 2021). Information about partners, parents, siblings, children, and emergency contacts may also be solicited in the context of registration and intake, and such forms should not assume that anyone in a person's life is cisgender. Electronic health records (EHRs) pose a number of issues for TNG people and the clinicians who serve them. Establishing intentional and well-documented workflows to record, display, and reference the pronouns and common use names of all patients is essential, though it may require the creative use of preexisting fields within the EHR. Clinically relevant information may also be difficult to locate, as the sex that is listed on a patient's insurance is often most visible and by default used in clinical decision support tools. Please see Chapter 22, "Standardized Language and Nonstandard Identities," and Chapter 23, "Collecting and Analyzing Gender Identity Data," for more information about EHRs and SOGI data collection.

TABLE 24–2. Holiday calendar

Date/month	Event
January	Mental Wellness Month
Last week of February	National Eating Disorders Awareness Week
Late March	National LGBTQIA+ Health Awareness Week
Last week of March	World Autism Awareness Week
March 31	International Transgender Day of Visibility
April 26	Lesbian Visibility Day
May	Mental Health Month
May 3	International Family Equality Day
May 17	International Day Against Homophobia, Transphobia, and Biphobia
June	Pride Month
September 10	World Suicide Prevention Day
September 23	Celebrate Bisexuality Day
October	LGBTQIA History Month, ADHD Awareness Month
October 11	National Coming Out Day
October 26	Intersex Awareness Day
November 20	Transgender Day of Remembrance

When in interdisciplinary practices or when necessary and appropriate, the use of an anatomical inventory is a cohesive way to record a person's body parts. Data about gender identity and gender assigned at birth cannot accurately predict the body parts a person has at any point in time, so directly asking about specific body parts is an effective way to capture this information. These inventories are typically conducted to allow for more informed clinical decision-making, including supporting preventive health care needs through clinical decision support tool integration (Grasso et al. 2021). Data may additionally be leveraged for population health management and assessments of quality measures, allowing for greater oversight and ongoing assessment of social factors of health.

Community Accountability

Finally, continuous engagement with, responsiveness to, and accountability toward our communities is a cornerstone of cultural humility, especially for those historically marginalized and underserved. Clinical education still lacks adequate training about providing care to TNG communities, and clinician baseline skills of even asking about sexual orientation and gender identity are highly perishable (Newsom et al. 2022). The quickly growing body of knowledge in best care and practices may present additional barriers, even for clinicians regularly engaging in new literature and research. Continued education in the field is essential to the health and well-being of TNG clients and must include both clinical and nonclinical content on an ongoing basis.

Appropriate care for TNG communities goes far beyond clinical guidance and must include understanding the historical and social context of TNG communities. Lack of trust in health care systems has been earned, and it is the role of those within systems of institutional power to be overtly transparent and engaged with the communities they serve. Community advisory boards, community feedback sessions, and appropriate expedient responses to individual feedback can all contribute to a culture of community and trust, but only when these recommendations and feedback are acted on. Working for TNG communities almost universally requires advocacy within systems that were not constructed with consideration for TNG lived experiences. This engagement, advocacy, and accountability to the community facilitates trust-building and makes space for partnerships among TNG communities and clinicians to address these systems and create a better health care environment for all.

DEPATHOLOGIZATION

Western medical and academic institutions have long approached gender diversity as a matter of medical or behavioral diagnosis, including early medical literature, the first documented gender affirmation surgery, and the eventual inclusion in DSM in 1980 (Koh 2012). While this characterization has provided some limited benefits in access to affirming health care (such as insurance coverage), the pathologizing of gender identity has been repeatedly shown to correspond with stigmatization, social isolation, and anti-transgender violence (Castro-Peraza et al. 2019). Furthermore, equating TNG identities with psychological trauma ignores the reality that traumas or sufferings embodied by TNG people are not inherent to TNG identities, but more often result from social stigmatization (Puckett et al. 2020).

In building a space that conveys inclusion, clinicians should consider how an approach to TNG care can dismantle the pathologizing of gender identity. This is particularly relevant in mental and behavioral health care, which is often a "gatekeeper" to gender affirmation. Inclusive and affirming health care for TNG people should be built on models of informed decision-making, rather than models that create unnecessary barriers and propagate assumptions such as binaries or linear trajectories for transition (Cavanaugh et al. 2016).

Clinicians should work to affirmatively communicate with TNG patients about their rights to information, autonomy, and consent when accessing gender-affirming care (Suess Schwend 2020). Even if a clinician is bound by institutional policies (such as those established by health insurance providers), open and honest communication with TNG patients about these policies can reduce feelings of stigma or shame (Asquith et al. 2021).

Clinician choices when discussing gender identity or mental health can communicate stigmatizing pathology or break those biases down (Cavanaugh et al. 2016). For instance, clinicians should not use unrelated mental health diagnoses as barriers for gender-affirming care. In one study, TNG participants specifically cited their mental health being used as a rationale to deny access to gender-affirming care (such as hormones or surgery) (Puckett et al. 2018). Although some mental health considerations may be linked to the social stigma TNG people face, by no means is being TNG intrinsically linked to a diagnosis of depression or anxiety. In fact, multiple studies have shown that affirmation from family, friends, and health care professionals leads to better mental health outcomes for TNG people (Puckett et al. 2018).

In considering TNG youth, pathologizing is further amplified and creates even more alarming barriers to care (Kearns et al. 2021). Clinicians are often stymied by concerns that a young person may "change their mind" or that affirmative health care may somehow be "irreversible." In reality, gender affirmation for youth, particularly prepubertal children, lies predominantly in areas of social affirmation rather than clinical treatment. This pathologizing has led to stigmatization of TNG youth and attempts by anti-transgender activists to ban gender affirmation in health care, which could affect access to mental and behavioral health. More information about care for TNG youth can be found in Chapter 13, "Working With TNG Youth and Their Families."

Clinicians may be faced with institutions, policies, or procedures that force a pathologized view of TNG people. This is most commonly embodied by a triadic model of TNG health (gender dysphoria diagnosis, gender-affirming hormone treatment, surgery), which is further enforced by legal gender recognition and policies relating to affirming identity documents (Suess Schwend 2020) (see Chapter 25, "Legal and Policy Considerations," for more discussion of identity documents).

These interactions with institutionalized pathologizing can be an opportunity for clinicians to advocate for a more affirmative view of TNG lives and experiences. In any case, clinicians should work with their patients to discuss where advocacy could intertwine with care and always allow patients autonomy in their care. Although clinicians may be limited in their ability to change or challenge some policies, they can make space for patients to process the implications of institutionalized stigma embodied by pathologized views of TNG experiences.

CONCLUSION: BREAKING DOWN BARRIERS TO CARE

Despite the documented benefits of harm reduction models, much gender-affirming care has restrictive gatekeeping measures, resulting in significant barriers to lifesaving treatment. Many examples exist, but a particularly representative one is the requirement for documentation to access gender-affirming surgery. In the United States, when gender-affirming care is a covered service, insurance companies generally follow the recommendations of the WPATH Standards of Care, either version 7 (World Professional Association for Transgender Health 2012) or version 8 (Coleman et al. 2022). At the time of writing, these include requiring documentation of assessments from health care professionals, depending on the surgery pursued. This requirement can create a significant barrier to patients, and its benefits are not well documented (Yuan et al. 2021). In the context of a shortage of qualified and affirming providers, the barrier becomes insurmountable. In addition to advocating for evidence-based approaches to care, creating referral networks, expedited assessment processes, and low/no-cost assessment and documentation opportunities all play a part in reducing barriers, increasing access, and improving the health and well-being of TNG communities.

Given the broad diversity of potential goals and needs of TNG community members, a robust and well-connected network of referrals is paramount to providing adequate care. Even the most well-resourced clinicians cannot meet all the possible medical, surgical, behavioral, emotional, and social needs of all TNG community members. Of the many community-built referral databases available, no single one has the breadth and scope to address all patient needs in all regions. Those working within health care settings may have easier access to networking and relationship building with local providers and international experts compared with the lay community. Providing a warm handoff by a trusted provider can also make a difference in further access to and engagement in care.

Necessary resources go beyond just the clinical realm. Providing access to supplies, education, and support needed for daily living can have an even greater impact on a person's well-being than an appointment with a clinician, especially when these resources are provided in affirming spaces and ways. Food pantries and clothing closets with affirming policies for TNG people are essential resources, whether in-house or in the community. Similarly, creation of or knowledge of affirming resources to address and/or assist with housing, at-risk substance use, safer sex, discrimination, and other needs disproportionately impacting TNG communities are helpful ways to address the most current and pressing needs among the most marginalized members of our communities.

Facilitated connections to other forms of community-based support are similarly necessary in building a robust support network. One-time and re-curring programming can be another way to directly provide resources, ed-ucation, and support to address specific disparities in health and well-being of TNG communities, while simultaneously advertising other available ser-vices and supports. This may include informational presentations about a new local resource or frequently asked questions, or perhaps social events designed to build community and awareness of local offerings. Open access to no-cost, nonbilled one-on-one assistance is another valuable way to sup-port TNG communities. Insurance assistance, questions about individual care access, and more sensitive topics may be better addressed in more pri-vate individualized settings. While helpful in any capacity, these services within the context of a health care organization additionally allow for easy and direct referral between resource providers and care teams, closing the loop and ensuring patients receive the support they need.

To authentically engage and build trust with TNG communities, more is needed than just skilled clinical intervention delivery. The deeply political nature of gender-affirming care and working within transgender health care necessitate a community-engaged, politically active practice (Ashley and Domínguez 2021). Whether taking action toward political and social change at the governmental level or advocating for and supporting local TNG com-munity advisory boards, engaging in community builds rapport and con-nects clinicians to the people they serve, improving their ability to provide culturally responsive care.

REFERENCES

Ashley F, Domínguez S: Transgender healthcare does not stop at the doorstep of the clinic. Am J Med 134(2):158–160, 2021 33228952

Asquith A, Sava L, Harris AB, et al: Patient-centered practices for engaging transgen-der and gender diverse patients in clinical research studies. BMC Med Res Methodol 21(1):202, 2021 34598674

Baker KE, Streed CG Jr, Durso LE: Ensuring that LGBTQI+ people count: collecting data on sexual orientation, gender identity, and intersex status. N Engl J Med 384(13):1184–1186, 2021 33793150

Castro-Peraza ME, García-Acosta JM, Delgado N, et al: Gender identity: the human right of depathologization. Int J Environ Res Public Health 16(6):97, 2019 30889934

Cavanaugh T, Hopwood R, Lambert C: Informed consent in the medical care of transgender and gender-nonconforming patients. AMA J Ethics 18(11):1147–1155, 2016 27883307

Coleman E, Radix AE, Bouman WP, et al: Standards of Care for the Health of Transgender and Gender Diverse People, Version 8. Int J Transgend Health 23(Suppl 1):S1–S259, 2022

Fenway Health: Personnel Manual. Boston, MA, Fenway Health, 2021

Grasso C, Goldhammer H, Thompson J, Keuroghlian AS: Optimizing gender-affirming medical care through anatomical inventories, clinical decision support, and population health management in electronic health record systems. J Am Med Inform Assoc 28(11):2531–2535, 2021 34151934

Kearns S, Kroll T, O'Shea D, Neff K: Experiences of transgender and non-binary youth accessing gender-affirming care: a systematic review and meta-ethnography. PLoS One 16(9):e0257194, 2021 34506559

Koh J: The history of the concept of gender identity disorder. (Japanese). Psychiatr Neurol Jpn 114(6):673–680, 2012

Kronk CA, Everhart AR, Ashley F, et al: Transgender data collection in the electronic health record: current concepts and issues. J Am Med Inform Assoc 29(2):271–284, 2022 34486655

National LGBTQIA+ Health Education Center: Addressing Unconscious and Implicit Bias. Boston, MA, The Fenway Institute, 2021. Available at: https://www.lgbtqiahealtheducation.org/courses/addressing-unconcious-and-implicit-bias-2021/. Accessed August 15, 2023.

Newsom KD, Carter GA, Hille JJ: Assessing whether medical students consistently ask patients about sexual orientation and gender identity as a function of year in training. LGBT Health 9(2):142–147, 2022 35104423

Puckett JA, Cleary P, Rossman K, et al: Barriers to gender-affirming care for transgender and gender nonconforming individuals. Sex Res Soc Policy 15(1):48–59, 2018 29527241

Puckett JA, Maroney MR, Wadsworth LP, et al: Coping with discrimination: the insidious effects of gender minority stigma on depression and anxiety in transgender individuals. J Clin Psychol 76(1):176–194, 2020 31517999

Suen LW, Lunn MR, Sevelius JM, et al: Do ask, tell, and show: contextual factors affecting sexual orientation and gender identity disclosure for sexual and gender minority people. LGBT Health 9(2):73–80, 2022 35073205

Suess Schwend A: Trans health care from a depathologization and human rights perspective. Public Health Rev 41(1):3, 2020 32099728

World Professional Association for Transgender Health: Standards of Care for the Health of Transsexual, Transgender, and Gender-Nonconforming People, Version 7. Philadelphia, PA, Taylor and Francis, 2012

Yuan N, Chung T, Ray EC, et al: Requirement of mental health referral letters for staged and revision genital gender-affirming surgeries: an unsanctioned barrier to care. Andrology 9(6):1765–1772, 2021 33960709

CHAPTER 25

Legal and Policy Considerations for Gender-Affirming Mental Health Care

Mason Dunn, J.D.
Alexander Chen, J.D.
Seran Gee, J.D.

GENERAL POLICY BACKGROUND: GENDER IDENTITY AND NONDISCRIMINATION

There are many legal considerations for transgender, non-binary, and/or gender-expansive (TNG) people living with mental health diagnoses. It should be noted that areas of gender identity and disability law are regularly expanding and changing; this text is up-to-date as of September 2022. For individualized guidance, TNG people and their clinicians should consult with an attorney in their state or jurisdiction to determine the most current status of law or policy.

For TNG people, one of the most commonly discussed areas of law pertains to nondiscrimination protections and rights. Given the reality of mistreatment, neglect, and abuse that TNG people face when accessing health care, it is clear why nondiscrimination laws are such a major focus (Romanelli and Lindsey 2020). The importance of nondiscrimination protestations further increases when considering the intersecting stigmas faced by TNG communities: mental health, disability, race, socioeconomic status, age, and other marginalizing factors (Hasenbush et al. 2019). For many years, gender identity nondiscrimination protections, including protections in health care, were addressed piecemeal at the state level. However, the Obama administration's rules pertaining to the Patient Protection and Affordable Care Act (ACA) (2010), affirmed and reinstated by the Biden administration, along with the *Bostock v. Clayton County, Georgia* decision (2020), unified many aspects of health care nondiscrimination protections at the federal level.

First, regarding the ACA, the Obama administration issued a 2016 rule (Nondiscrimination in Health Programs and Activities 2016) interpreting sex discrimination under Section 1557 (Patient Protection and Affordable Care Act 2010) of that act to include gender identity and sex stereotyping, and providing several explicit protections for TNG communities. Under this 2016 rule (Table 25–1), health insurance providers are banned from excluding gender affirmation care in coverage; likewise, clinicians are required to respect a patient's gender identity or gender expression. Although this rule has seen challenges at the federal level (including outright removal by the Trump administration in 2020), at the time of this writing, a number of courts have affirmed a TNG-inclusive interpretation of Section 1557 of the ACA.

In June 2020, the Supreme Court ruled (by a vote of 6–3) that Title VII of the Civil Rights Act of 1964 protects Two-Spirit, lesbian, gay, bisexual, transgender, queer, intersex, asexual, and more (2SLGBTQIA+) people from workplace discrimination, in the *Bostock v. Clayton County, Georgia* (2020) decision. The decision hinged on the interpretation of the word "sex" in Title VII to include sexual orientation and gender identity. Title VII deals only with employment, but most courts have considered the interpretation of protections on the basis of sex across federal laws through a consistent lens (Clark 2022). The court's interpretation in *Bostock* has and will continue to have resounding impacts on all federal protections, including Title IX and challenges to Section 1557.

AMERICANS WITH DISABILITIES ACT PROTECTIONS FOR TNG PEOPLE

In addition to the sex discrimination protections that apply to TNG people, people who experience gender dysphoria may satisfy the legal requirements for disability nondiscrimination protection and disability benefits due to their condition. Although some people are hesitant to associate gender identity with disability, the Americans With Disabilities Act (ADA) (1990) provides a legal definition for disability that is broader than the term's lay

---

TABLE 25–1. Section 1557 and 2016 rule

The 2016 rule defines gender identity as "one's internal sense of gender, which may be male, female, neither, or a combination of male and female," and is interpreted to "[encompass] 'gender expression' and 'transgender status'" (Nondiscrimination in Health Programs and Activities 2016).
Section 1557:
Applies to all health programs and facilities receiving federal financial assistance.
Requires providers treat TNG patients in a manner consistent with their gender identity, including access to facilities and use of affirming name and pronouns.
Prohibits most insurers from discriminating on the basis of sex (including gender identity) in health coverage. This includes
· blanket exclusions for gender-affirming care;
· limitation or outright denial of coverage for services for TNG people that would be covered for cisgender people; and
· denial of coverage for treatment that may be typically associated with one sex assigned at birth, when another sex is listed in medical records or identification.

---

meaning. Specifically, Section 12102(1) of the ADA defines disability as "a physical or mental impairment that substantially limits one or more major life activities of such individual; a record of such an impairment; or being regarded as having such an impairment."

It should be noted, however, that Section 12102(3)(A) provides that, for an individual to claim disability discrimination on the basis of "being regarded as having" a disability, the individual must further "establish...that [they have] been subjected to an action prohibited under this chapter because of an actual or perceived physical or mental impairment whether or not the impairment limits or is perceived to limit a major life activity" (ADA Amendments Act of 2008). In this way, the ADA uses a "social model" to define disability: the act defines disability in relation to society's failure to accommodate the full diversity of human abilities, rather than defining disability in terms of pathology (Barry et al. 2016).

Despite the ADA's inclusive definition of disability, certain stigmatized conditions and characteristics were explicitly excluded from the act's definition. Most pertinent to this chapter is Section 12211(b)(1) (ADA Amendments Act of 2008), which provides that the disability does not include "transvestism, transsexualism, pedophilia, exhibitionism, voyeurism, gender identity disorders not resulting from physical impairments, or other sexual behavior disorders" (*Blatt v. Cabela's Retail, Inc.* 2015). Contrary to that provision, fortunately, courts have recognized that individuals who experience gender dysphoria qualify as individuals with disabilities under the ADA (*Romer v. Evans* 1996). Additionally, it is noteworthy that the Department of Justice, under both the Obama and Trump administrations, conceded that such exclusion is not legally effective and declined to defend its constitutionality even when expressly invited to do so (Levi and Barry 2019).

Three legal theories have been invoked to find the exclusion ineffective. First, there is a long precedent of the Constitution forbidding Congress from legislating with "the bare desire to harm" an unpopular minority (*Romer v. Evans* 1996). The legislative record violates that prohibition in that the express purpose of the exclusion was to single out TNG people as undeserving of protections, without a principled, nondiscriminatory basis for doing so (Barry et al. 2016). Additionally, as the *Doe v. Massachusetts Department of Corrections* court (2018) observed, "[t]he pairing of gender identity disorders with conduct that is criminal or viewed by society as immoral or lewd [in the statute] raises a serious question as to the light in which the drafters of this exclusion viewed transgender persons."

Second, gender dysphoria may be considered to be a "gender identity disorder" (an outdated term that is considered offensive) that does "result...from physical impairments." Citing evidence of gender dysphoria having a basis in physical impairments, some courts have found that Section 12211(b)(1) (ADA Amendments Act of 2008), which excludes only "gender identity disorders not resulting from physical impairments," does not exclude gender dysphoria. For instance, the Superior Court of Massachusetts remarked, "in light of the remarkable growth in our understanding of the role of genetics in producing what were previously thought to be psychological disorders," the court could not "eliminate the possibility that all or some gender identity disorders result 'from physical impairments' in an individual's genome" (*Doe ex rel. Doe v. Yunits* 2001). This closely echoes the Department of Justice's position that "the burgeoning medical research underlying [gender dysphoria] points to a physical etiology" (*Blatt v. Cabela's Retail, Inc.* 2015).

Most significantly, in August 2022 the Fourth Circuit Court of Appeals became the first federal appellate court to take the affirmative step of finding people who experience gender dysphoria to be protected under the ADA and Rehabilitation Act (*Williams v. Kincaid* 2022). The Fourth Circuit ruled that as a matter of statutory interpretation (interpreting what a statute ought to be understood to mean), the exclusion does not apply simply because gender identity disorder as defined in the ADA is an "obsolete diagnosis" that has been superseded by the DSM-5 diagnosis of gender dysphoria (American Psychiatric Association 2013). Scholars have argued that the terms "transsexualism" and "gender identity disorder" differ from gender dysphoria because they are merely the medicalization of being TNG (Barry et al. 2016). In contrast, gender dysphoria does not refer to being TNG; rather, it is an experience of significant distress resulting from incongruence between one's gender and physical sexual characteristics (American Psychiatric Association 2013). Indeed, cisgender (i.e., non-transgender) individuals may experience gender dysphoria in some circumstances (e.g., a cisgender man who develops breast tissue during puberty and experiences clinically significant distress into adulthood as a result). Although this is still a developing area of the law, the *Williams* decision stands as an important advancement in the application of the ADA for TNG protections.

Regardless of which theory ultimately prevails, it is important to understand that people who experience gender dysphoria can be eligible for short-term and long-term disability benefits and cannot be discriminated against on the basis of their condition under federal law. Some individuals may hesitate to represent themselves as being disabled, but it is imperative that they be informed that they satisfy the legal definition and are thus entitled to protections and benefits. Further, it is important to recognize that the legal definition of disability is not a static status even for lifelong conditions. The ADA uses a social, rather than biomedical, definition of disability, so a person may cease to satisfy the definition after receiving satisfactory treatment or if societal shifts result in widespread accommodation availability (e.g., since eyeglasses became readily available, correctable vision impairments generally do not satisfy the ADA's definition of disability; Equal Employment Opportunity Commission 2014).

IDENTIFICATION DOCUMENTS

Identification documents (IDs; e.g., licenses, passports, school identification cards, credit or debit cards) are an essential tool and relied on in multiple facets of everyday life, from travel to employment to health care access. Obtaining these documents is a matter of human rights, and for TNG people, ensuring that IDs reflect and affirm gender identity is a matter of equity as well as health. Nonetheless, studies show alarming disparities in access to legal gender affirmation in the form of aligning IDs among TNG populations; the U.S. Transgender Survey of 2015 found that 45.1% of surveyed participants did not have documentation with their correct name or gender markers, and only 10% had fully correct and updated IDs (James et al. 2016). In that study, access to affirming IDs was inversely associated with psychological distress; those with fully congruent IDs had a lower prevalence of severe psychological distress and suicidal ideation (Scheim et al. 2020).

In addition to the mental health importance of gender-affirming IDs, clinicians should be aware of the process of updating ID documents to affirm gender identity, such as changing a name or gender marker. These processes can be confusing, cost-prohibitive, or even unachievable owing to institutional barriers. Clinicians should be aware of the policies, potential stressors, and requirements so that they may support patients in updating IDs.

For many TNG people seeking to update their IDs, the process can be confusing and potentially traumatic. To change one's first name, for instance, requires multiple sequential steps across numerous bureaucratic entities, many of which can take weeks or even months before one may proceed to the next step. These steps vary by state or country, can be costly, and may require individuals to confront transphobic and cisnormative institutions in person. For these reasons, some TNG people may avoid the process or only partially complete updating their IDs.

Many TNG and 2SLGBTQIA+ organizations at state and national levels have guides to assist in the process of name and gender marker updates for IDs. The process usually does not require legal representation, but a lawyer's assistance can ease some of the stress associated with navigating bureaucratic channels. To meet these needs, some nonprofit community organizations and law schools have created clinics and projects to provide legal assistance to TNG people seeking to update IDs (see Resources at the end of this chapter).

One of the many cisnormative factors to consider when updating IDs is the set of entrenched binary assumptions of gender, represented by the narrowed and oversimplified options of "M" or "F" gender markers. In recent years, some U.S. states have made strides in recognizing non-binary genders by providing an "X" option for gender markers on state IDs. At the time of writing, nine states allow an X gender marker on state IDs: yet once again, TNG people face a confusing mixture of frequently changing policies, as each state has different requirements for obtaining an X marker, and one's ability to update all documents to be in alignment with that X marker is not possible at this time. Further, X markers remain excluded from numerous essential services, such as federal financial aid applications, which further marginalizes non-binary individuals and disincentivizes selection of the X marker when it is available (Goetz and Arcomano 2022).

Clinicians should be prepared to provide support and assistance with navigating expectations for TNG patients working to update IDs. Given the stress and potential trauma involved in these processes, clinicians may be called on to help patients prepare or recuperate from challenging interactions. Given that many TNG people have a sense of urgency in updating IDs, it is important to understand that single steps can involve a wait of 4–6 weeks, delaying the entire process. Clinicians may need to provide support to manage the stress of waiting for documentation of name and gender markers.

Some states or countries may require letters from a treating clinician to change documentation of gender markers. Other state and federal documentation requires "self-attestation," without clinical documentation. For example, as of 2022, to change a gender marker on a U.S. passport, TNG people are no longer required to submit a letter from a clinician certifying that they have received "appropriate clinical treatment for gender transition." Passport applicants and holders now "can select male (M), female (F), or unspecified or another gender identity (X)" (U.S. Department of State 2022).

Many of the institutional policies relating to ID updates inherently pathologize gender affirmation. Requiring a treating clinician to write a letter of support assumes that changing a gender marker requires clinical evaluation and perpetuates the ongoing stigmatization and colonization of TNG bodies and experiences. Some states are eliminating this unnecessary clinical oversight and shifting to "self-attestation" for gender marker changes on IDs, although far too many state and federal policies continue to reinscribe pathologization of TNG identities. Clinicians may be limited in their ability to change or challenge these policies, but they should make space for patients to process the implications of institutionalized stigma.

STATE AND FEDERAL RESOURCES

NCTE ID Documents Center: https://transequality.org/documents
TLDEF Name Change Project: https://namechangeproject.wufoo.com/ forms/tldef-name-change-project-intake-form
NESL Identity Affirmation Project: https://nesl.edu/practical-experiences/ centers/center-for-law-and-social-responsibility/projects/identity-affirmation-project
GLAD/MTPC Transgender ID Project: https://www.glad.org/id/

REFERENCES

ADA Amendments Act of 2008, Public Law 110–325, 122 Stat. 3553, 2008
American Psychiatric Association: Diagnostic and Statistical Manual of Mental Disorders, 5th Edition. Arlington, VA, American Psychiatric Association, 2013
Americans With Disabilities Act of 1990, 42 U.S.C. § 12102(1) et seq., 1990
Barry K, Farrell B, Levi J, Vanguri N: A bare desire to harm: transgender people and the equal protection clause. Boston Coll L Rev 57(507), 2016
Blatt v Cabela's Retail, Inc., No. 5:14-cv-4822-JFL, 2015 WL 9872493 (E.D. Pa). Nov 16, 2015
Bostock v Clayton County, Georgia, 140 S. Ct. 1731, 590 U.S., 2020
Clark K: Interpretation of Bostock v. Clayton County regarding the nondiscrimination provisions of the Safe Streets Act, the Juvenile Justice and Delinquency Prevention Act, the Victims of Crime Act, and the Violence Against Women Act. United States Department of Justice, Civil Rights Division, 2022. Available at: https://www.justice.gov/crt/page/file/1481776/download. Accessed June 24, 2023.

Doe ex rel. Doe v Yunits, No. 00–1060A, 2001 WL 36648072 (Mass. Super.), 2001

Doe v Massachusetts Department of Corrections, 2018 WL 2994403, 2018

Equal Employment Opportunity Commission: Blindness and Vision Impairments in the Workplace and the ADA, 2014. Available at: https://www.eeoc.gov/laws/guidance/blindness-and-vision-impairments-workplace-and-ada. Accessed June 24, 2023.

Goetz TG, Arcomano AC: "X" marks the transgressive gender: a qualitative exploration of legal gender-affirmation. J Lesbian Mental Health 1–15, 2022

Hasenbush A, Flores A, Herman JL: Gender identity nondiscrimination laws in public accommodations: a review of evidence regarding safety and privacy in public restrooms, locker rooms, and changing rooms. Sexual Res Soc Pol 16(1):70–83, 2019

James S, Herman J, Rankin S, et al: The Report of the 2015 U.S. Transgender Survey. Washington, DC, National Center for Transgender Equality, 2016

Levi J, Barry K: Transgender tropes and constitutional review. Yale L Policy Rev 37(589), 2019

Nondiscrimination in Health Programs and Activities, 81 Fed. Reg. at 31,384, May 18, 2016

Patient Protection and Affordable Care Act of 2010, Pub. L. No. 111–148, 124 Stat. 119, 2010

Romanelli M, Lindsey MA: Patterns of healthcare discrimination among transgender help-seekers. Am J Prev Med 58(4):e123–e131, 2020 32001051

Romer v Evans, 517 U.S. 620, 627, 1996

Scheim AI, Perez-Brumer AG, Bauer GR: Gender-concordant identity documents and mental health among transgender adults in the USA: a cross-sectional study. Lancet Public Health 5(4):e196–e203, 2020 32192577

U.S. Department of State—Bureau of Consular Affairs: Selecting your gender marker. Travel.State.Gov, 2022. Available at: https://travel.state.gov/content/travel/en/passports/need-passport/selecting-your-gender-marker.html. Accessed November 11, 2022.

Williams v Kincaid 2022 WL 3364824 (4th Cir). August 16, 2022

CHAPTER 26

Transgender, Non-binary, and/or Gender-Expansive (TNG) Leaders

Dallas M. Ducar, M.S.N., A.P.R.N.

PSYCHIATRY AND MENTAL HEALTH CARE FOR 2SLGBTQIA+ COMMUNITIES: A LEGACY OF VIOLENCE

The history of psychiatry and mental health for Two-Spirit, lesbian, gay, bisexual, transgender, queer, intersex, asexual, and more (2SLGBTQIA+) individuals has been plagued with pathology and violence. Just 50 years ago, "Dr. H. Anonymous," or John Fryer (Robinson 2012), spoke out at the American Psychiatric Association (APA) annual meeting against the APA declaring homosexuality a mental illness; he did so in a mask and wig, with vocal distortion, to prevent personal attacks from his colleagues. His speech is often cited as a seminal event driving the subsequent removal of homosexuality from DSM (Byne 2014). More recently, the APA replaced the DSM diagnosis of *gender identity disorder* with *gender dysphoria*, which still requires TNG people to be diagnosed with a myopic categorization that erases the tremendous diversity of gender. Scholars have argued that the continued reliance on gender dysphoria as a diagnosis to access treatment has increased anti-TNG stigma (Nagoshi and Brzuzy 2010).

This marginalization of 2SLGBTQIA+ people was not isolated to the analyst's couch. To be out was to risk loss: family of origin, friendships, stable employment, health care, and free movement through the world. Mental health fields enacted stigma and overt harm, asserting nonnormative sexual orientation and gender identity as moral failings (Dickinson 2015). Such cisgenderist heterosexist stances perpetuated laws sanctifying anti-2SLGBTQIA+ discrimination and violence (McCreery 2020). This victimization continues today, particularly against Black TNG communities (Wirtz et al. 2020). The annual Transgender Day of Remembrance, in honor of Rita Hester who was murdered in 1998 in Allston, Massachusetts, is just one example of TNG communities working to remember these losses and push the needle of justice forward.

For cisgender individuals, hormone therapy and pubertal suppressants used to treat various conditions are generally accessible. To access the same medications, however, TNG people seeking gender-affirming hormone therapy (GAHT) are saddled with paperwork and insurance pre-authorizations; some clinicians still insist that patients "present as a certain gender" for a set time period. Cisgender straight people in power built systems that constrain our communities from authentic embodiment and intentionally left gaps in care. We need systems that are dedicated to advancing gender-affirming care; our institutions must be inclusive by design and sustain this movement. We need health care to become a space of liberation.

MENTAL HEALTH PROVIDERS HAVE A DUTY TO WORK TOWARD JUSTICE FOR TNG INDIVIDUALS

Mental health clinicians can do better. We play a crucial role in alleviating the burden of structural discrimination against transgender and gender-diverse communities (Hansen et al. 2018). Every clinician is in a position of power, and with that comes responsibility that can and must be used for good. This begins with starting to create an environment of trust in all clinical settings, one that begins as soon as the patient walks in the door and continues throughout the therapeutic relationship. This is incumbent on the clinician to create an environment of trust, collaboration, and allyship, while the system itself must be developed in a way to foster such interactions.

Those who experience discrimination are often the most vulnerable. It is not enough to provide services and create a safe space. We have a duty to fight injustice in every encounter, to ensure people are affirmed. A report from the Center for American Progress revealed that nearly half of transgender respondents, including 68% of transgender people of color, reported discrimination (Medina et al. 2021). Additionally, those who are discriminated against are less likely to attend to their own health needs and engage in clinical care in a timely manner (Reisner et al. 2014). Patient outcomes rely on trust first and foremost. A lack of trust increases morbidity and mortality. The right care does not just mean treatment or prevention, it also includes affirmation.

Fostering an environment of trust allows patients and clinicians to develop therapeutic alliances, which is crucial to supporting and advocating for TNG patients. This does not imply that mental health clinicians are poised to save TNG patients; rather, the patient-clinician relationship is an opportunity to remind the patient of their own power. Mental health clinicians must work with our communities in a collaborative, rather than authoritative, manner. William Madsen offers one approach: a relational stance of being an "appreciative ally." This aspect of collaborative helping positions clinicians in alliance with patients, such that patients experience us as "in their corner." Generally, this approach is grounded in a spirit of curiosity, connection, respect, and hope (Madsen 2009). Additional narrative approaches, such as externalization, deconstruction, and storytelling, can be crucial in working with TNG communities (Nylund and Temple 2017). Cultural humility and narrative humility may be helpful in this, by enhancing community participation in care and attending carefully and reflexively to a patient's story while also examining our own role in that story (DasGupta 2008; Tervalon and Murray-García 1998).

From a collaborative and allied approach, we can endeavor to remain curious about the patient's life without making assumptions. With a narrative therapeutic approach, we can establish a relational, rather than individualistic, perspective, allowing for curiosity, believing in possibilities, working in partnership, and empowering others (Madsen 2009). This narrative stance allows the patient to speak of experiences and intentions in their own voice, as the author of their own life (Combs and Freedman 2012). This proposed approach upends the Western historical marginalization of TNG communities and instead allows individual stories to be told and heard throughout society. The focus on working with others and seeing a person as the expert on their own story is crucial to working with TNG communities. This recognition does not remove the power imbalance, but it does help to promote a general collaborative approach, rather than imposing assumptions or normative interpretations.

LISTENING TO COMMUNITIES WHEN BUILDING GENDER-AFFIRMING CLINICAL ENVIRONMENTS

Addressing the needs of various TNG communities requires understanding the catchment area. We must listen to the people we serve. No community is a monolith, and all communities change over time. Recent surveys indicate that meeting needs for gender-affirming care requires the creation of more community agencies specializing in affirming care, as well as increasing clinical education (Temple 2013). Reisner et al. (2022) found that although TNG people often use gender-affirming mental health services, access barriers include lack of trained providers, mental health integration in primary care, and transportation; they also noted the lack of comprehensive definitions of gender-affirming care and of standard competencies for mental health clinicians providing gender-affirming care. In the absence of clear, shared terminology, assessments need to be specific and communities need to define gender-affirming care. Community-based participatory action research is one way to facilitate this: conducting research about the needs of TNG communities with their participation. Such work requires accountability, empowerment, collaboration with TNG researchers, and connecting outcomes to advocacy and social change (Singh et al. 2013).

Focus groups of TNG people in New England identified the need for increased clinician education (Loo et al. 2021). Participants valued attention to community feedback over years of experience, underscored the need to hire TNG clinicians when developing gender-affirming health care centers, and prioritized community outreach, engagement, health navigation services, and community resource mapping for building an affirming environment (Loo et al. 2021). Gender-affirming care includes primary care, sexual and reproductive health, gender-affirming hormone therapy (GAHT), and community support; all of this, including mental health care, is best provided in a wraparound model.

Gender-affirming practices may be embedded within primary care, fully integrated, or offered as a separate program entirely. Separate programs can be helpful when attempting to maintain patient safety and confidentiality and to focus entirely on caring for TNG patients. When providing primary care in the same location as gender-affirming medical care, a primary care clinician can also be trained to provide GAHT (White Hughto and Reisner 2016). Mental health treatment is required to address untreated or uncontrolled mental health difficulties (Coleman et al. 2012). Using an informed consent model, the primary care clinician can assess whether the patient is able to make an informed decision about their care (Morenz et al. 2020).

Mental health services should also be designed to provide care across the lifespan. About 25% of all 2SLGBTQIA+ children identify as non-binary (The Trevor Project 2021). With more children coming out younger, affirming conversations must also occur earlier—in pediatric care. Thus, it is essential for gender-affirming practices to integrate with other care environments or create networks with other clinicians. Families also may disclose mental health concerns first in primary care environments, and integrated systems with access to mental health providers are crucial to intervene with compassion and affirmation. We should also be skilled in taking care of older adults. TNG adults are more likely to experience subjective cognitive decline and depression, and an integrated system is helpful in identifying and treating these needs (Cicero et al. 2021) (see Chapter 13, "Working with TNG Youth and Their Families," and Chapter 14, "Mental Health Needs of TNG Older Adults").

THE PATIENT SHOULD BE IN THE DRIVER'S SEAT

As health care often enhances power differentials, it is crucial to center patient autonomy. All policies, procedures, and actions should include asking for consent: in how we chart, what words we use, how we touch the patient, how we refer to them, where we refer to them, and more. The entire clinical encounter and the surrounding health care information technology offer opportunities to engage patients in this collaborative decision-making.

Ask patients about sexual orientation, gender identity, and intersex status, and also inform them of where the data will be transmitted. This commitment to patient autonomy requires flexible systems that are responsive to patient needs and in turn can support people in being their most authentic selves.

To be gender-affirming, a space must provide basic safety and responsiveness to trauma (Hall and DeLaney 2021). At minimum, all staff should provide trauma-informed care to meet patient needs and prevent reenacting prior trauma (see Chapter 11, "Trauma-Informed Mental Health Care").

Mental health care, though just one facet of medical needs, is particularly important because it pertains uniquely to human experience: the existential narrative of finding oneself. Mental health services must be comprehensive and holistic. As gender-affirming mental health is variable in definition, it is important to tailor services to a patient's needs. Accordingly, at Transhealth, mental health services include psychiatry, psychotherapy, and nontherapeutic groups that foster support and build skills (Transhealth 2021). It is crucial that each of these services follows the basic principles of justice and autonomy, reducing the impact of discrimination and trauma and following informed consent models to collaborate with the patient in an alliance to foster an environment of empowerment.

TRANSHEALTH WAS DEVELOPED AS A COMMUNITY HEALTH CENTER, FOR US AND BY US

Transhealth was founded on May 4, 2021, offering comprehensive services: adult and pediatric primary care, GAHT, mental health care, and nonclinical services such as patient advocacy, to support TNG communities. We advance TNG health care through research, education, and advocacy. This first started by engaging a local TNG-identified funder who was committed to caring for the various needs of TNG communities. Whereas institutional buy-in is important for many environments that start as part of other organizations, especially academic medical centers, Transhealth's initial buy-in came from the TNG community. From start to finish, it was a project for and by our communities.

Accordingly, when hiring, we built a team that is deeply dedicated to this work, believes in the work, and invests themselves fully in the work. Our team collaboratively created every part of the organization, from workflows to hanging wall mounts. We hired individuals who belonged to the communities we served and were deeply rooted in the values of gender-affirming care. For interview guides, we created cases based on our values and mission.

We wanted to ensure that services were not implemented disparately; accordingly, we chose to provide wraparound services that allow all care—medical care, mental health care, resource navigation, social services, and community-based support—to be delivered in one space. We also operate using an informed consent model and a gender-affirming philosophy rather than specific published guidelines; our clinical focus is removing access barriers for every patient.

We believed it crucial to develop an organization that is TNG-led. Since our opening, we have strived to ensure that TNG individuals are distributed across formal and informal leadership. Active TNG participation in developing all clinical workflows is foundational to Transhealth; this has culminated in all staff being present in "startup mornings" one Thursday each month, for 4 hours, to collaborate on workflows together. Interprofessional care teams include primary care clinicians, case managers, social workers, and nurses. To improve access to care, we offer same-week internal mental health referrals provided by a comprehensive administrative staff. Additionally, based on TNG stakeholder input, we prioritized opening a community room, which offers robust program offerings both on-site and through external community services.

Transhealth has a CEO and COO, and the clinical component is led by a Primary Care Director and Mental Health Director who work in tandem with the Practice Manager. All clinicians practice at the top of their scope of practice and are eligible to serve as Clinical Directors. The Clinical Directorship is a rotating model, with term limits for 2 years, to encourage cross-disciplinary leadership.

Services are available to TNG individuals of any age and their families. All patients may opt in to an integrated visit, which includes both primary care and mental health care. Social determinants of health are addressed by community health workers, who follow patients in inpatient and outpatient settings, as well as in the community. Nurses and other staff members are provided time to pursue interdisciplinary education (i.e., professional development, continuing education), participate in community-building activities, engage in advocacy, and develop research projects. Ongoing and future work includes assessing clinical outcomes using patient-reported outcome measures that are relevant to the TNG people served by the clinic.

MENTAL HEALTH MODEL AT TRANSHEALTH

Trust is one of the most important values in our mental health team: this underlies the principles of autonomy and justice that underpin our care model. As outlined earlier, all care is provided following informed consent and trauma-informed models of care. We learned early on, as the needs assessment revealed, that there is a robust need for psychotherapeutic services for TNG communities. We sought to provide these services for all socioeconomic levels while still attempting to remain profitable, so that our mental health services could continue to expand. We also keep a 3:1 ratio of psychotherapists to prescribers and believe it is a core ethical requirement that all therapists receive supervision.

Psychotherapy services can function like a highway: if people are not able to transition out of psychotherapy in a timely manner, there is less access for others. We had to build both on-ramps to enable access and off-ramps to facilitate availability for new patients. To this end, we hired community health workers who are specifically trained to help guide patients from psychotherapy at Transhealth to community clinicians. We believe, due to this high demand, that there is an ethical requirement to justly allocate resources, and this means effective triage. Additionally, we worked with local and regional partners to try to expand access and specifically provide more care via telehealth, to increase access to psychotherapy across rural regions.

In learning from TNG communities, we wanted to target services to community needs. TNG patients may not desire what the medical-industrial complex considers evidence-based. In listening to our stakeholders, we needed to stray outside of evidence-based cognitive-behavioral therapy or dialectical behavioral therapy groups and provide nonclinical groups, including an art group for trauma survivors, makeup classes, weight-lifting classes, or social support classes. We sought meaningful coalitions with other local organizations, which required defining a "good partner" for Transhealth and imagining nontraditional mental health services, to foster empowerment, resilience, and gender euphoria. New projects include clothing closets, book exchanges, peer support, online groups, drama classes, meditation classes, and internet workstations. We developed robust resource lists and referral networks for patients to receive services that are not currently available at the center.

We also prioritize our values when designing other medical care. This means focusing on education, research, and advocacy, in addition to clinical expertise. As gender-affirming care lacks a standard certification, we tailor staff training to our stakeholders' needs and prioritize educating new clinicians across all disciplines in trauma-informed care. Aligned with this, we launched the Transhealth Gender-Affirming Care Access Program, through which any provider in the state can consult with our providers as needed. Accordingly, we decided to welcome clinical trainees already skilled in these areas. Ethically, we also chose to not pursue any research at Transhealth until establishment of a Transhealth Institutional Review Board, to ensure all research is "for us and by us." Finally, committed to advocating for our patients by working with local, regional, and national stakeholders, we collaborated with community health centers across the United States to expand mental health care access, build systems of accountability, increase reimbursement for mental health services, and provide avenues for patients to engage politically, such as voter registration and community organizing.

CHALLENGES IN CREATING INCLUSIVE AND AFFIRMING MENTAL HEALTH CARE

As described at the beginning of this chapter, psychiatry and mental health establishments have caused harm to 2SLGBTQIA+ communities. For this reason, many TNG individuals must navigate past traumas when building new models of clinical practice. Clinicians are also often forced to participate in ongoing systems that perpetuate stigma (Grinker 2018).

Dickinson (2015) offers one historical approach for clinicians: using subversive behaviors that defy health care tradition and hierarchy to practice in a way that is ethical and responsible. Doing so independently, however, can inflict secondary trauma and burnout; trauma-informed workplaces where clinicians may engage in this work as a community may offer respite. When we strive to create a truly inclusive mental health care environment and hire a team diverse in race, ethnicity, gender identity, gender expression, disability, religion, neurodivergence, and socioeconomic status, we also need to commit to a trauma-informed space for our colleagues. If we wish for our patients to show up authentically, we must create a space where our colleagues can do so as well. Of note, reimagining a mental health care environment may be limited by the U.S. health system; all practices need to advocate for broader changes to health care and fund time for team members to also participate in advocacy and community work.

Developing a gender-affirming mental health practice requires substantial administrative support. Building an organization from scratch can be daunting; we highly recommend having a founding team. Even if working within a larger health system, one needs a team with clinical and administrative skills (Morenz et al. 2020), and including experts within the organization can foster crucial buy-in. It is important to hire administrative staff skilled in strategy and long-term planning.

Effective planning and project management are crucial when developing a new practice. If building an independent clinical environment de novo, it is essential to develop a step-by-step outline of the type of organization you would like to become. This plan can be informed by legal, communications, and financial minds, and leadership should remain flexible and open to changing course when unexpected challenges arise. Keep in mind that a new practice often does not see increasing profits for at least two years. Legal consultation will be necessary to address name, description, type of corporation (or nonprofit organization), and any additional government regulations for a clinical practice. Credentialing new clinicians can take time; it is important to recruit early and start the credentialing process early, especially for new staff clinicians arriving from other jurisdictions, states, or countries. As branding and recruiting must start early in the planning process, it is important to bring in communications experts at the beginning. The organization's mission, vision, and values must be established early, so that all organizational goals align with the practice's mission. Establishing a charter during this time can also ensure a direct focus for the organization and educate new team members.

The singular organizational mission should be specific enough to guide all projects and sufficiently broad to provide flexibility to experiment with new models of care. Gender-affirming care is a highly dynamic field and requires ongoing dialogue with employees, patients, and communities. Laying a strong foundation for burnout prevention and fostering compassion is essential, especially when hiring marginalized individuals. At Transhealth, we implemented the Stress First Aid Model to foster peer support (Nash 2011), developed "startup mornings" that devote 4 hours to collaborating on new workflows, allocated time for team supervision, and consistently focused on our values to foster an engaged and loving work environment. We prioritized community engagement, including a weekly meeting on community projects, opportunities for all staff to engage with community partners, and therapeutic and nontherapeutic community classes open to all staff—as teachers or participants. Perhaps most important is sharing humor and fun: creating channels for jokes in our messaging systems, hosting monthly social hours, and sponsoring a Transhealth bowling team. At the end of the day, if you wish to hire members of communities who have been pushed to the margins, it is essential to develop a workplace that encourages participation, engagement, peer support, and humor.

Transhealth was created during the early COVID-19 pandemic, which required flexibility. During that time, Massachusetts expanded telehealth, and, with it, access to care for rural TNG people. Telehealth proved to be effective for varied clinical services, reducing geographic barriers to accessing culturally responsive care. No-show rates at Transhealth were below the national average, with a sevenfold increase in telehealth appointments over baseline. At first, we were unable to accept some insurance plans and adjusted to offer care at a reduced cost when necessary. We needed to establish quality clinical care first, before engaging in research or education, to gain the trust of the communities we serve. We continue to advocate for insurance and telehealth reform to reduce barriers to care for marginalized and underserved patients across state lines (Ducar 2021a, 2021b). TNG patients deserve integrated care.

NEXT STEPS IN CREATING AN AFFIRMING MENTAL HEALTH CARE ENVIRONMENT

Providing excellent care for our most minoritized communities is possible. Most gender-affirming care in the United States is provided in urban areas, and Transhealth has shown the need for and viability of such care in rural areas. When providing care in rural areas, access must be radically expanded, and this includes addressing social determinants of health. While mental health care clinicians are part of the system, they are not the whole story. TNG communities have often leaned on each other for support, and there must be a strong focus on community engagement, solidarity, and creating space for individuals from various backgrounds and experiences to engage in their own communal care.

Identity should never be medicalized. When creating a gender-affirming environment, we must assess our intersecting identities, reflect on our positionality, and consider how establishing this environment contributes to the greater liberation of TNG communities. Mental health care environments should be consistently dedicated to advocacy and work to reduce barriers to care, including those from the medical-industrial complex. The organization must consistently be ready to ask, "Who is empowered?" and act to empower TNG patients and team members.

Cisgender people in power have traditionally created systems that bar access to quality gender-affirming care. Instead, TNG communities should lead the way: reimagining the bounds of health care and fostering an activist health care environment that provides comprehensive care.

Leave the pathology, diagnosis, and DSM at the door and instead meet the person in front of you. Gender-affirming care offers a model for all of health care, one that is patient-centered and based on the human story. It is time for our communities to demonstrate how intentionality and community participation can radically transform health care delivery.

REFERENCES

Byne W: Forty years after the removal of homosexuality from the DSM: well on the way but not there yet. LGBT Health 1(2):67–69, 2014 26789613

Cicero E, Flatt JD, Wharton W: Transgender adults report greater cognitive and related functional challenges: findings from the 2015–2019 Behavioral Risk Factor Surveillance System. Presented at the Alzheimer's Association International Conference, Denver, CO, July 2021

Coleman E, Bockting W, Botzer M, et al: Standards of care for the health of transsexual, transgender, and gender-nonconforming people, version 7. Int J Transgend 13(4):165–232, 2012

Combs G, Freedman J: Narrative, poststructuralism, and social justice: current practices in narrative therapy. Couns Psychol 40(7):1033–1060, 2012

DasGupta S: Narrative humility. Lancet 371(9617):980–981, 2008 18363204

Dickinson T: 'Curing Queers': Mental Nurses and Their Patients, 1935–74. Manchester, UK, Manchester University Press, 2015

Ducar D: Expanding telehealth is vital to the trans community. The Hill, August 5, 2021a. Available at: https://thehill.com/opinion/healthcare/566488-expanding-telehealth-is-essential-to-the-trans-community. Accessed November 11, 2021.

Ducar D: How to expand health care coverage for trans and gender diverse populations. The Boston Globe, November 20, 2021b. Available at: https://www.bostonglobe.com/2021/11/20/opinion/how-expand-health-care-coverage-trans- gender-diverse-populations/?event=event12. Accessed December 23, 2021.

Grinker RR: Being trans is not a mental disorder. The New York Times, December 6, 2018. Available at: https://www.nytimes.com/2018/12/06/opinion/trans-gender-dysphoria-mental-disorder.html. Accessed November 9, 2021.

Hall SF, DeLaney MJ: A trauma-informed exploration of the mental health and community support experiences of transgender and gender-expansive adults. J Homosex 68(8):1278–1297, 2021 31799893

Hansen H, Riano NS, Meadows T, Mangurian C: Alleviating the mental health burden of structural discrimination and hate crimes: the role of psychiatrists. Am J Psychiatry 175(10):929–933, 2018 30269535

Loo S, Almazan AN, Vedilago V, et al: Understanding community member and health care professional perspectives on gender-affirming care: a qualitative study. PLoS One 16(8):e0255568, 2021 34398877

Madsen WC: Collaborative helping: a practice framework for family-centered services. Fam Process 48(1):103–116, 2009 19378648

McCreery P: Children in LGBT political discourses in the United States, in Oxford Research Encyclopedia of Politics. New York, Oxford University Press, 2020

Medina C, Santos T, Mahowald L, Gruberg S: Center for American Progress, 2021. Available at: https://www.americanprogress.org/article/protecting-advancing-health-care-transgender-adult-communities.

Morenz AM, Goldhammer H, Lambert CA, et al: A blueprint for planning and implementing a transgender health program. Ann Fam Med 18(1):73–79, 2020 31937536

Nagoshi JL, Brzuzy SI: Transgender theory: embodying research and practice. Affilia 25(4):431–443, 2010

Nash WP: US Marine Corps and Navy combat and operational stress continuum model: a tool for leaders. Combat Operational Behav Health 107:119, 2011

Nylund D, Temple A: Queer informed narrative therapy: radical approaches to counseling with transgender persons, in Social Justice and Counseling: Discourse in Practice. New York, Routledge/Taylor & Francis Group, 2017, pp 159–170

Reisner SL, White JM, Dunham EE, et al: Discrimination and Health in Massachusetts: A Statewide Survey of Transgender and Gender Nonconforming Adults. Boston, MA, Fenway Health, 2014

Reisner SL, Benyishay M, Stott B, et al: Gender-affirming mental health care access and utilization among rural transgender and gender diverse adults in five northeastern U.S. states. Transgend Health 7(3):219–229, 2022 36643056

Robinson VG: Forty years since John Fryer: that was then, this is now. J Gay Lesbian Ment Health 16(2):167–180, 2012

Singh AA, Richmond K, Burnes TR: Feminist participatory action research with transgender com, munities: fostering the practice of ethical and empowering research designs. Int J Transgend 14(3):93–104, 2013

Temple AL: Breaking the binary: addressing healthcare disparities within Sacramento's transgender community. Master's thesis, Sacramento, CA, Sacramento State, 2013. Available at: https://csu-csus.esploro.exlibrisgroup.com/esploro/outputs/graduate/Breaking-the-binary-addressing-healthcare-disparities/99257831368901671. Accessed July 18, 2023.

Tervalon M, Murray-García J: Cultural humility versus cultural competence: a critical distinction in defining physician training outcomes in multicultural education. J Health Care Poor Underserved 9(2):117–125, 1998 10073197

Transhealth: Our services. Transhealth, 2021.Available at: https://transhealth.org/our-services/. Accessed November 8, 2021.

The Trevor Project: 2021 National Survey on LGBTQ Youth Mental Health. West Hollywood, CA, The Trevor Project, 2021

White Hughto JM, Reisner SL: A systematic review of the effects of hormone therapy on psychological functioning and quality of life in transgender individuals. Transgend Health 1(1):21–31, 2016 27595141

Wirtz AL, Poteat TC, Malik M, Glass N: Gender-based violence against transgender people in the United States: a call for research and programming. Trauma Violence Abuse 21(2):227–241, 2020 29439615

INDEX

Page numbers printed in **boldface** type refer to figures and tables.